OBSTETRICS
BY TEN TEACHERS

EDITED BY
TLT LEWIS
CBE, MB BChir (Cantab) FRCS FRCOG
AND
GVP CHAMBERLAIN
MD FRCS FRCOG

FIFTEENTH EDITION

Edward Arnold
A division of Hodder & Stoughton
LONDON   MELBOURNE   AUCKLAND

© 1990 Hodder and Stoughton Ltd.

First published 1917 under the title *Midwifery*
by Edward Arnold (Publishers) Ltd.

Second edition	1920	Reprinted	1963
Reprinted	1921,1923	Eleventh edition	1966
Third edition	1925	(renamed *Obstetrics*)	
Reprinted	1927,1928	Reprinted	1970
Fourth edition	1931	Twelfth edition	1972
Fifth edition	1935	Reprinted	1975, 1976, 1978
Reprinted	1937	Thirteenth edition	1980
Sixth edition	1938	Reprinted	1982
Seventh edition	1942	First published in	
Reprinted	1944, 1946	paperback	1982
Eighth edition	1948	Reprinted	1982, 1984, 1985
Reprinted	1949, 1952	Fourteenth edition	1985
Ninth edition	1955	Reprinted	1986, 1989
Reprinted	1957	Fifteenth edition	1990
Tenth edition	1961	Reprinted	1991, 1992, 1993

British Library Cataloguing Publication Data

Obstetrics by ten teachers.—15th ed.
1. Obstetrics
I. Lewis, T.L.T. (Thomas Loftus Townshend)
II. Chamberlain, G.V.P.
618.2

ISBN 0–340–51650–X

Typeset in 10/11 pt Garamond by Wearside Tradespools,
Fulwell, Sunderland.
Printed and bound in Great Britain for Edward Arnold, a division of
Hodder and Stoughton Limited, Mill Road, Dunton Green,
Sevenoaks, Kent TN13 2YA by Butler & Tanner Ltd, Frome, Somerset

List of Contributors

including those contributing special chapters

Mary Anderson MB ChB FRCOG
Consultant Obstetrician and Gynaecologist, Lewisham Hospital, London

Michael Brudenell MB BS FRCS FRCOG
Obstetric and Gynaccological Surgeon, King's College Hospital, Denmark Hill, London

Geoffrey Chamberlain MD FRCS FRCOG
Professor of Obstetrics and Gynaecology, St George's Hospital Medical School, Cranmer Terrace, London

Tim Coltart PhD FRCS (Ed) FRCOG
Consultant Obstetrician and Gynaecologist, Guy's Hospital and Queen Charlotte's and Chelsea Hospital, Goldhawk Road, London

Robert Dinwiddie MB FRCP DCH
Consultant Paediatrician, The Hospital for Sick Children, Great Ormond Street, London

Denys Fairweather MD FRCOG
Professor, Department of Obstetrics and Gynaecology, University College London, Gower Street, London

Gedis Grudzinskas MD FRCOG FRACOG
Professor, Academic Unit of Obstetrics and Gynaecology, The London Hospital and St Bartholomew's Hospital, London

Frank Loeffler FRCS FRCOG
Consultant Obstetrician and Gynaecologist, St Mary's Hospital and Queen Charlotte's and Chelsea Hospital, Goldhawk Road, London

Gisela Oppenheim MB ChB FRCPsych DPM
Formerly Consultant Psychiatrist, Charing Cross Hospital and Queen Charlotte's Hospital for Women, Goldhawk Road, London

George Pinker KCVO MB BS FRCS(Ed) FRCOG
Consultant Obstetrician and Gynaecologist, St Mary's Hospital, Praed Street, London

Charles Rodeck FRCOG BSc MB BS FRCOG
Professor, Royal Postgraduate Medical School, Institute of Obstetrics and Gynaecology, Queen Charlotte's and Chelsea Hospital, Goldhawk Road, London

Marcus Setchell FRCS FRCOG
Consultant Obstetrician and Gynaecologist, St Bartholemew's Hospital and Homerton Hospital, London

Ronald Taylor FRCOG
Professor, Department of Obstetrics and Gynaecology, United Medical and Dental Schools of Guy's and St Thomas's Hospitals, Lambeth Palace Road, London

Ruth Warwick MRCP MRCPath
Consultant Haematologist, Department of Haematology, Queen Charlotte's and Chelsea Hospital, Goldhawk Road, London

Preface

In this book we have attempted to give a comprehensive description of modern obstetric practice. While we aim to provide the undergraduate student and those working for the DRCOG with all that it is necessary to know on the subject, we think that the text will serve as a basis to which more specialized knowledge can be added for those who are postgraduate and hoping to specialize.

We have given a full description of the newer methods of obstetric management with emphasis on modern imaging techniques and the assessment of fetal wellbeing.

We regret that the death of Sir Stanley Clayton removed an editor who had such an influence on the book over many years. We are grateful to Mr Hartgill, Mr Holmes and Mr Roberts who have given way to Mr Coltart, Professor Grudzinskas, Mr Loeffler and Professor Rodeck. Because of the increasing amount of litigation taking place in medicine generally, and in obstetrics in particular, a chapter on the medico-legal aspects of obstetrics by Dr M Anderson is included; Dr R Warwick has written a chapter on coagulation disorders; Dr G Oppenheim one on psychiatric disorders and Dr R Dinwiddie has revised extensively the paediatric section.

We thank the staff of our publishers for their unfailing guidance and courtesy.

TLTL
GVPC   1990

Contents

1

ANATOMY AND PHYSIOLOGY

OVULATION AND EARLY DEVELOPMENT OF THE OVUM

An oöcyte is released from the ovary during most normal menstrual cycles.

The cycle is described in two phases: the first half is known as the *follicular* or *proliferative phase*, during which the ovarian follicle enlarges and becomes distended with fluid. On about the 14th day of the cycle the follicle discharges an oöcyte into the peritoneal cavity, from where it is taken up by the uterine (fallopian) tube. The second half of the cycle is known as the *luteal* or *secretory phase*. In this phase the cells of the empty follicle become swollen with yellow lipid, and the follicle is now called the *corpus luteum*.

During the follicular phase the cells lining the follicle secrete oestrogens which cause proliferation of the glands and stroma of the endometrium. During the luteal phase the cells of the corpus luteum secrete both oestrogens and progesterone, and the combined action of these hormones causes further proliferation of the endometrium and also secretion of sugars, amino acids, mucus and enzymes by the endometrial glands. The endometrium reaches its maximum development in the late luteal phase, forming a decidua into which the oöcyte, if it is fertilized, can embed.

The complex hormonal control and details of the anatomical changes in the ovary and endometrium during the menstrual cycle are described in *Gynaecology by Ten Teachers*.

OVULATION

As early as the fourth week of life in the human embryo, germ cells migrate from the wall of the yolk sac to an area of mesenchyme on the posterior wall of the coelom. These invading cells form the primordial germ cells, which give rise to numerous primary oöcytes. These are large round cells, with relatively large, chromatin-rich nuclei. The primary oöcytes become surrounded by a single layer of smaller flattened cells to form primordial follicles.

At birth each ovary contains up to one million follicles, although many are lost before the menarche. In each menstrual cycle between 10 and 20 follicles start to mature, but one dominant follicle (the *primry oöcyte*) outstrips the others, and reaches full development, although multiple pregnancy may be due to ripening and fertilization of more than one oöcyte in the cycle.

THE OVARIAN FOLLICLE

During maturation of the follicle the flat cells that surround the primordial ovum multiply, become rounded and arranged in several layers (the *granulosa cells*). Their growth is eccentric, so that the oöcyte comes to lie at one side of the mass of granulosa cells, and eventually clear fluid appears among these cells, so that a follicle is formed with the oöcyte placed to one side (*see* Fig. 1.1). The clump of granulosa cells that is directly related to the oöcyte forms a hillock (the *cumulus*) that projects into the cavity of the follicle, and at this stage the oöcyte is surrounded by a clear membrane, the *zona pellucida*, within which it can rotate. The granulosa cells that are immediately related to the zona pellucida become arranged in a radial fashion and form the *corona radiata*. The oöcyte itself enlarges slightly during maturation of the follicle, chiefly by increase in the volume of the cytoplasm, and reaches a diameter of about 0.15 mm.

The cells of the ovarian stroma which surround the granulosa cells also proliferate, becoming swollen by the accumulation of lipid. These cells form the *theca interna* and play an important part in the formation of the corpus luteum at a later stage. The ovarian stromal cells outside the theca interna become somewhat compressed by the growth of the follicle and form the *theca externa* (Fig. 1.1).

As the follicle increases in size it approaches the surface of the ovary, where it is seen as a transparent vesicle which varies in size, and which may reach a diameter of 18 mm. The follicle eventually projects from the surface of the ovary, and at about the midpoint of the cycle the cell layers dehisce and the oöcyte, still surrounded by the corona radiata, is discharged into the peritoneal cavity. This takes 2 or 3 minutes.

CORPUS LUTEUM

After ovulation the walls of the follicle collapse and are thrown into folds; there is usually a little haemorrhage into the now empty cavity. The granulosa cells become swollen by the accumulation of yellow lipid, and are now *granulosa-lutein cells*. Similar changes also occur in the theca interna, the cells of which are now termed *theca-lutein cells*. If the oöcyte that was discharged from the follicle is not fertilized then degenerative changes (luteolysis) begin in the corpus luteum at about the 22nd day of the cycle, but if the oöcyte *is* fertilized some of its cells produce *human chorionic gonadotrophin (hCG)*, a hormone which causes the corpus luteum to persist and enlarge further, maintaining its production of oestrogen and progesterone for about 12 weeks, until this function is taken over by the placenta.

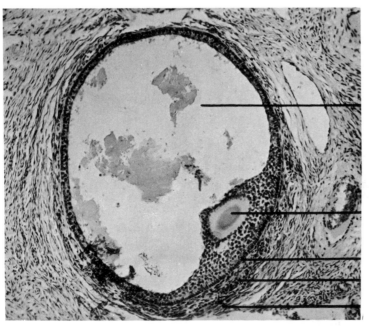

Liquor folliculi

Oöcyte

Granulosa cells

Theca interna

Theca externa

Fig. 1.1   Ripe ovarian follicle

FORMATION OF DECIDUA

The changes in the endometrium during the menstrual cycle occur in preparation for the possible reception of the fertilized ovum. If the ovum is fertilized and embeds in the endometrium all these changes are accentuated and the endometrium is described as the *decidua of pregnancy*. If fertilization and embedding do not occur the endometrium undergoes necrosis, except for the basal layer, from which its regeneration in the next cycle occurs.

During the *follicular*, or *proliferative phase* of the menstrual cycle, under the influence of oestrogen produced by the follicle, the endometrium becomes more vascular, the cells of the glandular epithelium and stroma proliferate and the endometrium becomes thicker, with long straight glands.

In the *luteal*, or *secretory phase*, when the corpus luteum produces both oestrogen and progesterone, the gland cells become tall and columnar and pour out their secretions of glycogen and mucin into the lumina of the glands. The glands become convoluted (Fig. 1.2) and the stromal cells swell. These changes do not affect the deepest parts of the endometrial glands; the stromal changes are most marked in the superficial layer and result in a great contrast between the basal layer of endometrium

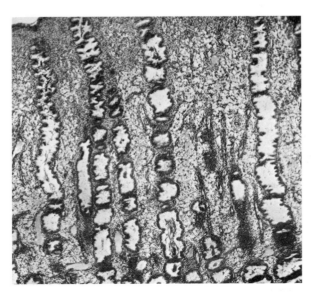

Fig. 1.2 Photomicrograph of endometrium at the end of the secretory or progestational phase of the menstrual cycle

with straight glands, the spongy intermediate layer with distended convoluted glands and the superficial compact layer. The arterioles have a spiral arrangement, and there is a great increase in vascularity.

MATURATION OF THE OVUM

The nuclei of human body cells each contain 46 chromosomes; this number is maintained throughout successive divisions of the cells. The chromosomes are responsible for the transmission of all the inheritable qualities. The reproductive cells (the oöcyte and the spermatozoon) differ from the ordinary body cells in that they each contain only 23 chromosomes. When fertilization occurs the oöcyte and spermatozoon unite and the total of 46 chromosomes is re-established. The male and female cell each contribute half of the total, so that some inherited qualities are derived from the father and some from the mother. The number of chromosomes in the germ cells is reduced during their maturation by a special type of cell division called *meiosis*.

In ordinary division of body cells (*mitosis*) each chromosome replicates and the two halves of each chromosome separate and pass into two daughter cells.

In the meiotic division of germ cells the chromosomes first become arranged in pairs, then they replicate and one member of each pair passes to one of four daughter cells, so halving the number of chromosomes in the mature germ cells.

The ovum undergoes the first maturation division when it is still in the ovary. The primary oöcyte divides by meiosis into two cells of unequal size – a large secondary oöcyte and a small polar body; the latter comes to lie in the perivitelline space within the zona pellucida. After this meiotic (reducing) division the secondary oöcyte contains only 23 chromosomes. The subsequent division of the secondary oöcyte, which takes place in the uterine tube, is a mitotic division. At this division a second polar body is extruded, but the final mature ovum still contains only 23 chromosomes.

A similar meiotic division takes place in the spermatozoon, when the primary spermatocyte divides into two equal secondary spermatocytes, which each contain 23 chromosomes. By a further mitotic division each of these divides to form two spermatids, so that the original primary spermatocyte gives rise to four spermatozoa, each with 23 chromosomes.

The adult cells of a normal female contain two X chromosomes, and after meiotic division each oöcyte will contain one X chromosome. The adult cells of a normal male contain one X and one Y chromosome; when meiotic division occurs these separate so that each secondary spermatocyte contains either an X or a Y chromosome, and eventually there will be two types of spermatozoa, those with an X chromosome (gynaecogenic) and those with a Y chromosome (androgenic). During fetilization, if conjugation of an X sperm and an X oöcyte occurs, the final combination will be XX, and will give rise to female genetic structure; but if conjugation of a Y sperm and an X oöcyte occurs the final combination will be XY, and will give rise to male genetic structure. There are recognizable sexual differences in the nuclei of adult cells, particularly seen as a small club-shaped projection of chromatin in the nuclei of polymorphonuclear leucocytes, and as a peripherally placed coiled mass of chromatin (Barr body) in other cells, in the female. This Barr body is the inactive X chromosome of the cell.

TRANSIT AND FERTILIZATION OF THE OVUM

The mechanism by which the ovum reaches the lumen of the fallopian tube has been much discussed. The ciliated cells of the fimbriae at the abdominal ostium of the tube set up a flow of fluid which can carry small particles from the recto-vaginal pouch into the tube. The fimbriated end of the tube is brought into close contact with the ovary at the time of ovulation; the mechanism of this is uncertain. Once the ovum has reached the cavity of the tube it is carried towards the uterine cavity by ciliary action. The tubes show peristaltic movements, but these are less important than the action of the cilia in moving the ovum down the tube.

Successful fertilization depends on coitus occurring at the correct time in the cycle and semen of an adequate quality being deposited in the region of the cervix.

Semen is a suspension of spermatozoa in seminal plasma, which is a combined secretion of the epididymis, seminal vesicle and prostate gland. It contains, among other substances, fructose (chiefly from the vesicle and an essential nutrient for spermatozoa) proteins, fibrinolytic and proteolytic enzymes (chiefly from the prostate), and prostaglandins. Immediately after ejaculation the semen coagulates, and then after about 15 minutes reliquefies; these changes are caused by the prostatic enzymes. Prostaglandins may cause tubal and uterine contractions.

Spermatozoa contain hyaluronidase, which is readily released into the seminal plasma. This assists the sperm to penetrate the cervical mucus and the corona radiata around the ovum. At the time of ejaculation the sperms are not so motile, they only become so after the semen has undergone liquefaction.

Fertilization of the ovum normally takes place in the ampullary portion of the fallopian tube, and spermatozoa reach the tube between 30 minutes and 3 hours after coitus. The transit of the spermatozoa results partly from their own motility, and partly from uterine and tubal peristalsis, the stimulus for which may be seminal prostaglandins.

Sperm are attracted to the ovum by chemotaxis, and after coitus many spermatozoa can be found in the tubes. Several may penetrate the zona pellucida, but as soon as one sperm makes its way into the ovarian cytoplasm the ovum separates from the zona pellucida and becomes impervious to further penetration. The head of the spermatozoon represents the nucleus of the male cell, and it fuses with the nucleus of the oöcyte to form the segmentation nucleus, whose complement of 46 chromosomes is again complete. The fertilized ovum is carried down the tube by ciliary and peristaltic action, and reaches the uterine cavity 5 to 6 days after ovulation.

EARLY DEVELOPMENT AND EMBEDDING OF THE BLASTOCYST

After the formation of the segmentation nucleus the zygote starts to divide, and soon a solid clump of cells called the *morula* is formed. A cavity appears among the cells of the morula so that it becomes vesicular, and it is then termed the *blastocyst*. This stage of development is reached while the zygote is still in the fallopian tube.

The outermost cells of the blastocyst form the *trophoblast*, which has the power of eroding and digesting the surface epithelium of the decidua. The fertilized ovum sinks into the thickness of the decidua, lying in a cavity in the stroma between adjacent endometrial glands. The glands are dis-

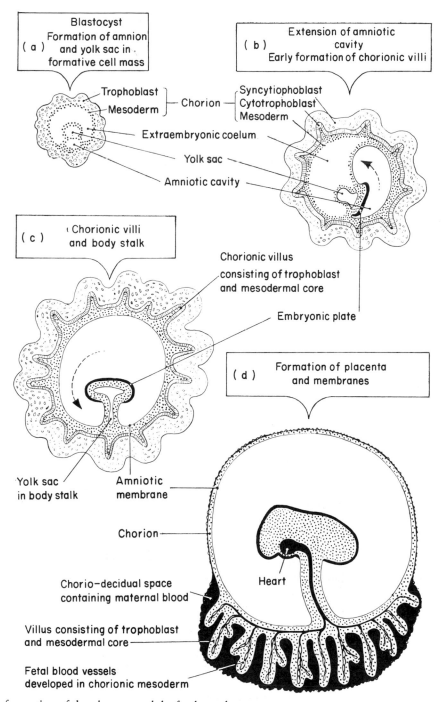

Fig. 1.3 The formation of the placenta and the fetal membranes

torted and pushed aside by the enlargement of the growing zygote. The aperture through which the zygote entered the decidua is sealed over with a plug of fibrin. Maternal blood vessels are invaded and eroded by the trophoblast, and extravasation of maternal blood occurs around the zygote.

The structure of the blastocyst is indicated in Figure 1.3(a). The inner cell mass, from which the embryo will develop, is seen projecting into the blastocyst, and two small cavities appear in the cells of the inner cell mass, from which the amniotic cavity and the yolk sac develop. The diagrams indicate the progressive extension of the amniotic cavity, which comes to surround and envelop the embryo, and ultimately the amniotic membrane covers the body stalk up to the point at which it becomes continuous with the embryonic ectoderm at the umbilicus.

Very soon, while it is eroding into the maternal decidua, the trophoblast becomes arranged in projecting masses, at first in a labyrinthine formation, but later arranged as villi which grow and branch. Maternal blood vessels are opened by the cytolytic action of the trophoblast, so that maternal blood lies in the intervillous spaces, and the embryo starts to secure its nutrition from this.

The trophoblast becomes differentiated into two layers. There is a thick outer layer of *syncytiotrophoblast*, in which the nuclei are scattered in a mass of cytoplasm that has no evident division into separate cells (Fig. 1.4). The inner layer of cytotrophoblast (*Langhans' layer*) is thinner, and consists of a single layer of rounded cells.

The blastocyst is lined with extraembryonic mesoderm, and it will be seen from the diagrams (Fig. 1.4) that this is continuous with the

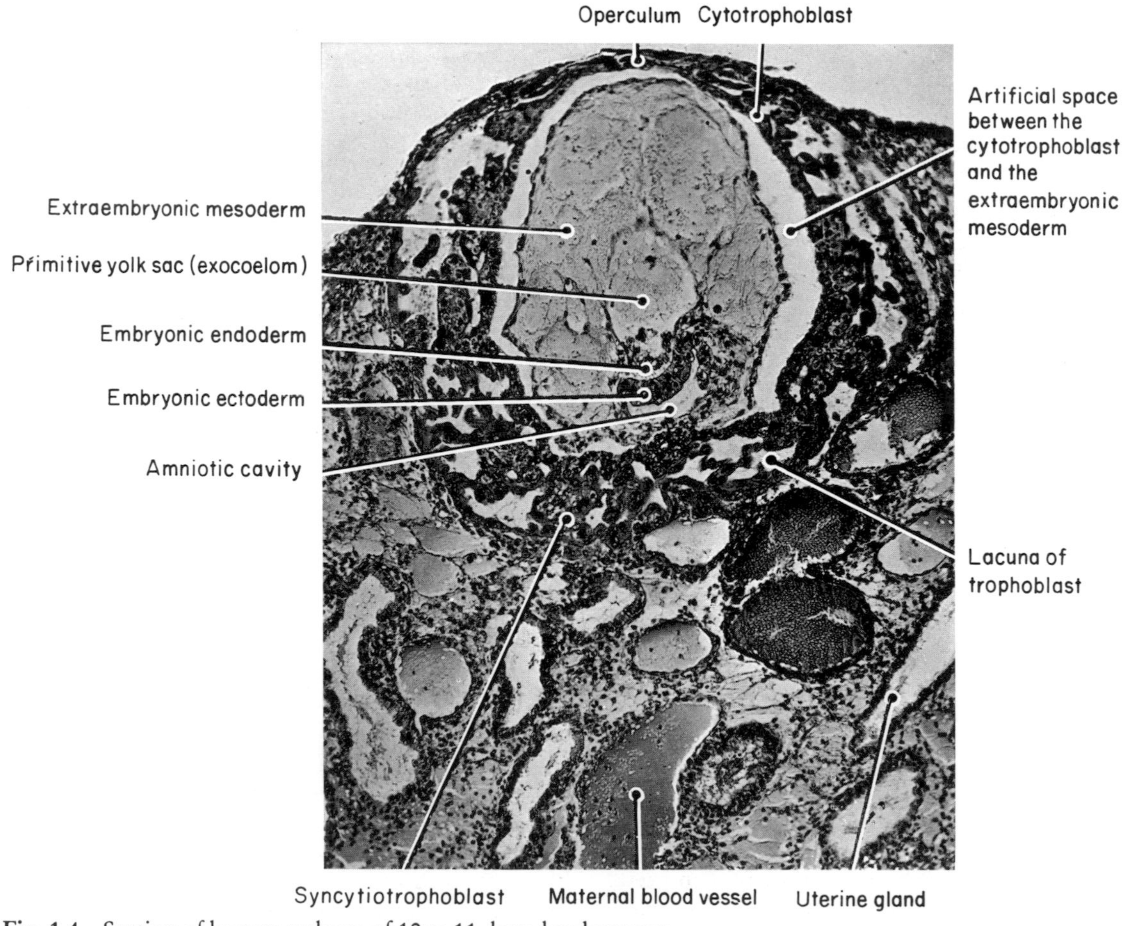

Fig. 1.4   Section of human embryo of 10 to 11 days development

mesoderm of the embryo itself. The extraembryonic mesoderm is continuous with the central tissue of the villi, so that each villus has an outer covering of trophoblast and a central mesodermal core. Lacunae appear in the mesoderm and gradually become joined to form a pattern of primitive blood vessels, extending through both the body of the embryo and the extraembryonic mesoderm. By this arrangement the placental circulation is ultimately formed; the fetal heart not only pumps blood through the tissues of the fetus itself, but also through the tissues of the placenta.

The combined layer of trophoblast and underlying mesoderm is termed the chorion. Within it is the amniotic membrane that bounds the amniotic cavity.

The zygote embeds in the stratum compactum of the decidua, the most frequent site of implantation being the upper and posterior part of the uterine cavity; it produces a slight projection into the uterine lumen. According to its relations to the embryo three parts of the decidua are distinguished (Fig. 1.5):

Decidua basalis

This is the portion of the decidua which lies between the embryo and the muscular wall of the uterus. It bounds the deeper half of the implantation cavity and later on forms the site of attachment of the definitive placenta. A number of thin-walled sinuses pass through it, bringing blood to the intervillous spaces. It also serves as a barrier against the invasion of the muscle by the syncytiotrophoblast, and normally the chorionic tissue does not penetrate through the decidua into the muscle.

Decidua capsularis

This is the portion of the decidua which intervenes between the embryo and the uterine cavity and which bounds the superficial half of the implantation cavity. As the ovum grows it bulges into the cavity, and by the 12th week the growing embryo fills the cavity, so that the decidua capsularis becomes fused with the decidua vera.

Decidua vera

This is the portion of the decidua that is not related to the site of implantation and which lines the rest of the cavity of the uterus.

Two other terms need definition. The *decidual space* is the space bounded by the decidua vera and the decidua capsularis. It is obliterated by the 12th week of pregnancy. The *choriodecidual space* is the space between the chorionic villi and the decidua basalis. It contains maternal blood.

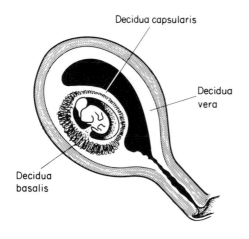

Fig. 1.5 Uterus containing an embryo of about 9 weeks

Labels in figure: Decidua capsularis, Decidua vera, Decidua basalis

THE PLACENTA, CORD AND MEMBRANES

In the primitive mammalian placenta the fetal chorion is merely applied to the surface of the maternal decidua, so that exchange of nutrients and excretory products between maternal and fetal blood takes place through several layers (epitheliochorial placenta).

In the human placenta the trophoblast erodes into the decidua, so that the endothelium of the maternal blood vessels is destroyed and maternal blood is in direct contact with the chorion, without the intervention of any decidual tissue (haemochorial placenta).

At first the syncytiotrophoblast forms an open reticulated network, whose lacunae are filled with maternal blood, and so, in part, the trophoblast replaces the maternal endothelium. The trophoblast soon becomes arranged in trabeculae, which are covered by syncytiotrophoblast and have a core of cytotrophoblast. When the embryonic mesoderm appears it extends into each of these trabeculae and finally the vascularization of the mesoderm completes the formation of chorionic villi by about the 16th day after fertilization.

At some points the trophoblast comes into direct contact with the decidual plate, thus anchoring the main villi to the maternal tissues at the junctional zone. Here, lying between the invading trophoblast and the decidua, a wavy layer of fibrin – the fibrinous layer of Nitabuch – can be seen. The number of anchoring villi is small but, by budding from both them and the chorion, true chorionic villi are formed. These differ from the anchoring villi in that their outer ends protrude free into the intervillous space. The capillaries in the terminal parts of the villi are very convoluted, but adjacent villi are not joined, i.e. the villi do not form a reticulum (Fig. 1.6).

The trophoblast extends for a variable distance into the maternal spiral arterioles where they enter the intervillous space, partly replacing the maternal vascular endothelium. The vessels in the trophoblast are converted into funnel-shaped deltas, so that the peripheral resistance to maternal blood flow is reduced and the flow to the placental bed is increased. Conversely, if this extension of trophoblast does *not* occur, there is a reduction in placental bed blood flow. This may lead to intrauterine growth retardation, pre-eclampsia or hypoxia in labour.

Structure of chorionic villus

A villus has a core of mesoderm and a covering of trophoblast; there are numerous fetal blood vessels in the mesoderm core. In the main villous stems the arteries and veins have connective tissue walls, but in the terminal villi only capillaries are present. The arteries are branches of the umbilical arteries. They end as capillaries in the terminal villi, from where oxygenated blood is collected into venous radicals and passed back into the veins of the main villous stems, and from there to the umbilical vein of the cord (Fig. 1.7).

From the time of their formation in the third week until the end of the first trimester the villi are covered by a single layer of cytotrophoblast and an outer layer of syncytiotrophoblast which is in immediate contact with the blood in the intervil-

Chorionic villi   Syncytiotrophoblast covering villus

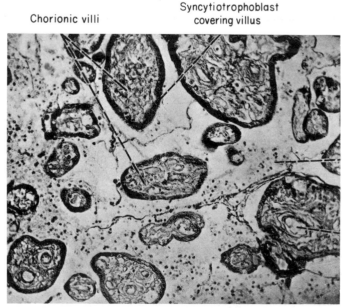

Maternal blood in intervillous spaces

Fetal blood vessel

Fig. 1.6   Microscopical section of placenta at term. ×170

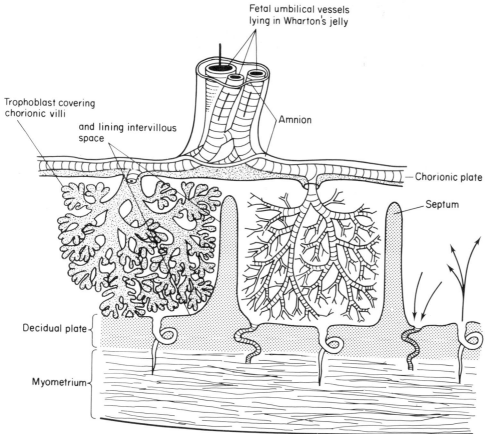

Fig. 1.7 The structure of the placenta. For clarity only the fetal arterioles are shown. The real villi are much more finely branched

lous space. After the 20th week the cytotrophoblast begins to disappear until finally only a thin layer of syncytium remains.

Further development of the placenta

The chorionic villi are formed in immense numbers and constitute the bulk of the placental area. They form an arrangement over a great surface, so that thin-walled vessels carrying fetal blood are only separated from the maternal blood by thin layers of villous connective tissue and syncitiotrophoblast.

At first villi are formed all over the surface of the gestation sac, so that an ovum of four weeks' growth appears as a translucent, thin-walled sac covered by a spherical halo of soft villi (Fig. 1.8). As growth proceeds the decidua capsularis becomes thinner, and between the 12th and 16th weeks

the villi on the capsular surface of the embryo degenerate rapidly, leaving this side of the chorion smooth (*chorion laeve*). In compensation, the villi on the surface opposed to the decidua basalis undergo a great deal of hypertrophy (*chorion frondosum*) and become matted into a solid disc, which is the fully developed placenta. This is formed by the 12th week, though proportionately it then comprises a much larger part of the ovular surface than it does at term.

Increase in size of the placenta

From the end of the fourth week, when the villi have penetrated towards the decidua basalis, there is no further invasion. Further growth in thickness of the placenta is now due to growth of the chorionic villi with an accompanying expansion of the intervillous sinuses. Until the end of the 16th

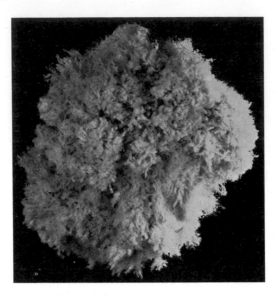

Fig. 1.8 Embryo showing chorionic villi

week, the placenta grows both in thickness and circumference. Subsequently it continues to increase in size circumferentially until near term. The growth is proportionate with that of the fetus and of that part of the wall of the uterus to which the placenta is attached.

The placenta at term

The placenta at term is circular in shape, forming a spongy disc 20 cm in diamter, and about 3 cm thick. Its weight is usually about 500 g but there is a direct relationship with the fetal weight.

The placenta has a fetal and a maternal surface. The fetal surface is covered by smooth amnion underneath the chorion. The blood vessels are visible beneath this as they radiate from the insertion of the umbilical cord.

The maternal surface is rough and spongy, and presents a number of polygonal areas known as *cotyledons*, each being somewhat convex and separated from those adjoining it by a shallow groove. Each cotyledon is formed by, and corresponds to, a main villous stem and its system of branch villi. The number of cotyledons, between 15 and 20, depends on the number of end arteries into which the umbilical artery divides. A cotyledon is made up of between ten and 20 lobules, each lobule corresponding to the opening of a maternal utero-

placental vessel. The colour is a dull red, with a thin, greyish, somewhat shaggy layer on the surface, which is the remnant of that part of the decidua basalis which has come away with the placenta. Numerous small greyish spots are frequently seen on the maternal surface. These are due to the deposition of calcium in degenerate areas and are the result of normal senescence. They are more numerous in placentae after term, often amounting to 30 per cent of the surface. These deposits do not occur in the villi nor do they interfere with the maternal circulation in the intervillous spaces; they are of no apparent significance.

The chorion spreads away from the edge of the placenta to form the outer layer of the two, membranes which enclose the fetus and liquor amnii. Though the line of demarcation between the placental edge and the chorion is sharp they are essentially one structure, for the placenta is a specialized part of the chorion.

The umbilical cord usually reaches the fetal surface of the placenta at about the middle of its disc, although sometimes it is at its edge (*battledore placenta*). It brings with it two umbilical arteries and one umbilical vein.

The area supplied by each umbilical artery varies. However, shortly after they have reached the placenta, there is always a communication between the two which serves to equalize the pressure in the two systems. Except for this communication, the main trunks into which the arteries divide are terminal, and each ends in a tuft of capillary vessels which drains into the corresponding tributary of the umbilical vein.

The substance of the placenta is made up almost entirely of a multitude of chorionic villi, most of which protrude in an arborescent manner into the intervillous blood spaces. The placenta can be described as a space containing maternal blood, which is bounded on the maternal side by a decidual plate, and on the fetal side by a chorionic plate from which the chorionic villi branch into the maternal blood (Fig. 1.7).

The intervillous space can be thought of as a lake of maternal blood which has left the maternal vessels to flow slowly round in a space bounded by fetal trophoblast. To supply and drain this space arteries and large sinuses perforate the decidual plate. It was formerly maintained that the blood flows to the edge of the placenta to be collected in a marginal sinus before leaving the intervillous space, but vessels serving the arterial inflow and venous drainage are now known to be scattered over the entire decidual plate.

The lobules of each coyledon consist of a group of villi which are based on one large fetal artery which branches and rebranches to supply the villi. The maternal blood enters the intervillous space via about 200 arterioles which perforate the decidual (basal) plate. Each maternal arteriole spurts a jet of blood into the centre of a corresponding fetal lobule. The blood percolates through the branching villi of the lobule and then returns to the basal plate where it flows out through the decidual veins.

Placental bed

The placental bed is covered with decidua which the spiral arteries pierce to deliver blood to the maternal lake which bathes the villi. The ends of the arteries are narrow at first, but from about the sixth week after conception trophoblastic cells invade their walls and the arterial ends open out like river deltas. By 16 weeks, in the normal woman, this process of invasion is complete and each of the 200-odd spiral arteries ends in a funnel-like delta. This results in a much lower pressure at the distal end of the blood vessel, allowing greater flow. The trophoblast invasion

may be absent in those who subsequently develop intrauterine growth retardation and pre-eclampsia.

FUNCTIONS OF THE PLACENTA

The placenta is essentially a fetal organ; it is the only means of transfer of anabolites and catabolites and, as such, is the main interface between the fetus and the outside world. The placenta:

- enables the fetus to take oxygen and nutrients from the maternal blood
- serves as the excretory organ where carbon dioxide and other waste products pass from the fetal to the maternal blood
- forms a barrier against the transfer of infection to the fetus, although some organisms, for example the rubella and HIV viruses are able to cross it
- secretes large amounts of chorionic gonadotrophin, oestrogen and progesterone in large amounts, but also secretes other hormones which play an essential part in the maintenance of the decidua and the growth of the uterus and breasts.

Placental transport

The transport of oxygen to the fetus is discussed on page 17.

In general the trophoblast and underlying endothelium of the fetal vessels behave as a semipermeable membrane, allowing the free passage of water and soluble substances of relatively low molecular weight according to the laws of osmotic equilibrium, but there are also mechanisms of active transport, which allow more rapid diffusion of solutes, as well as the transfer of larger protein molecules.

Substances with a molecular weight of less than 1000 are, in general, able to pass the placental barrier, and most anaesthetic agents and drugs fall into this class. The concentrations of water, sodium chloride, magnesium, urea and uric acid are equal in maternal and fetal blood. A few substances, including amino acids, nucleic acid, calcium and inorganic phosphorus, have a higher concentration in fetal than maternal blood and the trophoblast has some power of selective transfer of these substances, most of which are necessary for the building of fetal tissues. Glucose is found in higher concentration in maternal than in fetal blood, not because it does not cross the placenta freely, but probably because of its continual rapid utilization by the fetus.

Much of the fat in fetal tissues is synthesized from carbohydrate, especially in late pregnancy. Synthesis of fatty acids, triglycerides, cholesterol and lipids mostly takes place in fetal tissue, although there is also a contribution by direct transfer of maternal lipids.

The serum iron concentration in the fetus is higher than that in the mother, but the mechanism of transfer is uncertain.

Oestrogens, androgens and thyroxine cross the placenta but insulin, parathyroid hormone and posterior pituitary hormones do not. The vagina of the newborn female child shows evidence of the oestrogenic action of maternal oestrogens *in utero*.

The syncytium has a high degree of selective activity, permitting passage of some IgG gamma-globulins, but not IgA or IgM globulins.

Despite the separation of the nucleated red cells in the vessels in the villi from the maternal red cells in the intervillous space, fetal red cells and fragments of villi may escape into the maternal circulation. The entry of red cells from a fetus whose blood group differs from that of its mother accounts for the development of haemolytic disease in certain circumstances. *See* Chapter 9, page 319.

Placental permeability increases as pregnancy progresses, probably because the trophoblast becomes thinner, and also because the villi become finer and more branched.

The functional efficiency of the placenta

Placental transfer will depend upon the maternal blood flow through the intervillous space, the effective surface area of the chorionic villi, and the fetal blood flow through them.

The maternal blood flow through the placental bed is about 1000 ml per minute at term. The pressure in the intervillous space, which is of the order of 15 mmHg, will be affected by uterine contractions in late pregnancy, as well as in labour. As the uterus contracts the veins in the myometrium are occluded first, so that the venous outflow ceases. The inflow of blood will continue until the uterine pressure equals the pressure of the arterial inflow. These pressures are not usually present until labour. With a strong contraction the inflow also ceases, and the blood in the intervillous space

is temporarily stagnant but the space does not empty because the veins are closed.

The capacity of the intervillous space is about 140 ml. The blood in it is exchanged several times per minute. The area of the surface of the chorionic villi which is exposed to this 140 ml of blood has been estimated to be about 11 square metres. The blood therefore forms a very thin film over the surface of the villi. This large area, resulting from the fine branching of the villi, does not take into account the microvilli on the trophoblast, which can be seen with the electron microscope.

The volume of the fetal capillaries has been estimated to be about 60 ml and the fetal blood flow to be about 300 ml per minute, giving a total replacement of the fetal blood in the placenta of about five times per minute. The pressure in the fetal capillaries in the villi is of the order of 30 mmHg.

Placental hormones

Oestrogens, progesterone, chorionic gonadotrophin, lactogen, thyroid-stimulating hormone, a hormone resembling adrenocorticotrophin, and possibly relaxin (a hormone which causes relaxation of pelvic ligaments in some species) are secreted into the maternal blood by the placenta.

During pregnancy there is a progressive increase in the blood oestrogen and urinary oestrogen concentrations; these reach their peak just before the onset of labour. The oestrogen found during pregnancy is chiefly oestriol glucuronate. The placenta converts precursors, which are formed in the fetal adrenal gland and liver, to oestriol sulphate. This passes into the maternal blood before being conjugated with glucuronic acid in the maternal liver, and is finally excreted by the maternal kidney (*see* pp. 26 and 132).

Until the end of the eighth week the corpus luteum continues to secrete progesterone. With the gradual cessation of function of the corpus luteum, the placenta becomes responsible for the secretion of progesterone which, like oestrogen, reaches a peak just before labour. The concentration of progesterone in maternal plasma is about 24 ng/ml at the eighth week, and is derived from the corpus luteum, and 180 ng/ml at term, when it is derived from the placenta.

Chorionic gonadotrophin can be detected in the maternal plasma by radioimmunoassay as early as

6 days after fertilization of the ovum, and is found in the urine soon after that. It reaches its peak concentration in the blood and urine at 10–11 weeks gestation. The concentration then falls to a lower level at which it remains steady. The presence of chorionic gonadotrophin in the urine forms the basis of the routine tests for pregnancy. It eventually disappears from the urine after delivery if the fetus dies but may persist for a time if placental tissue is retained.

THE CHORIONIC MEMBRANES

After the definitive placenta is formed the rest of the chorion atrophies and persists only as a thin, friable membrane intervening between the amnion and the decidua. On its outer surface vestiges of decidual cells and of the trophoblastic layer that formerly covered it can be distinguished microscopically, but the bulk of it is a fragile connective tissue, loosely attached to the amnion.

THE AMNION

The first appearance of the amnion is a hollow space in the embryonic ectoderm. It is lined by cubical cells. These quickly become more columnar at the part which eventually forms the embryonic plate and the embryo. At first more or less spherical, the amniotic cavity soon becomes flattened down upon the embryo and closely applied to it. As the head and tail appear and the body walls fold round to enclose the embryonic coelom, the amnion attached at their margins is also carried round, so that embryo is pushed up and projects into the amniotic cavity. When the body cavity of the embryo is quite closed up, the amnion is attached all round the place at which the ventral stalk emerges (*see* Figs. 1.5(b) and 1.5(c) on p. 15).

At this period the embryo is relatively very small, and has the amnion closely applied to it, while the cavity of the blastocyst is relatively very large. Now a great change begins. The amniotic cavity enlarges out of proportion to the embryo, and becomes distended with fluid, while the embryo is gradually carried more and more into the amniotic cavity by elongation of the ventral stalk, which becomes the umbilical cord.

The enlargement of the amniotic cavity which brings about the complete investment of the umbilical cord likewise brings the amnion into close contact with the fetal surface of the placenta. This surface is, therefore, completely covered by the amnion. The amnion is loosely attached to the placenta and chorion, and can be separated up to the insertion of the cord.

The amnion is lined by a single layer of cubical or flattened epithelial cells which is attached to a layer of connective tissue. The epithelium contains granules, fat droplets and vacuoles. The connective tissue on the outer side of the amniotic membrane is closely applied to the similar connective tissue on the inner side of the chorion; the two merely stick together, and are not organically united. They can easily be separated from one another at all periods of pregnancy. That portion of the amnion which covers the umbilical cord, however, is very closely incorporated with the connective tissue of the cord and cannot be stripped off.

AMNIOTIC FLUID

The amniotic fluid is usually slightly turbid from the admixture of solid particles derived from the fetal skin and the amniotic epithelium. It may also be stained a green or brown colour if any meconium has been passed into it. The solid matter is composed of lanugo hairs, epithelial cells and sebaceous material from the fetal skin, and cast-off amniotic epithelial cells.

The volume of the amniotic fluid at term is about 800 ml, with a wide range from 400 to 1500 ml in normal cases. At 10 weeks the average volume is 30 ml, at 20 weeks 300 ml and at 30 weeks 600 ml. The rate of increase is therefore about 30 ml per week, but the rate falls off near term. This is evident on clinical examination. On palpation at 30 weeks there seems to be a lot of liquor relative to the size of the fetus; nearer term there is relatively less liquor, and when the expected date of delivery is passed the uterus seems to be full of baby.

At term the liquor has a specific gravity of 1010. It contains 99 per cent water and its osmolality is less than that of maternal or fetal plasma. The liquor has organic, inorganic and cellular constituents. Concentrations of some of the important contents near term are as follows:

sodium 130 mmol/L
urea 3–4 mmol/L
protein 3 g/L

lecithin 30–100 mg/L

α-fetoprotein 0.5–5 mg/L.

In addition traces of steroid and non-steroid hormones and of enzymes are present. It is mildly bacteriostatic.

The liquor is of both maternal and fetal origin, and the relative importance of the different mechanisms of production alters as pregnancy progresses.

In very early pregnancy there is secretion from the amnion.

Later, diffusion through the fetal skin accounts for much of the liquor, and there is increasing diffusion through the fetal membranes, including the part of the amnion that covers the fetal vessels in the cord and on the surface of the placenta. By the 20th week the skin loses its permeability, and from this time onwards the fetal kidneys play an increasing role in the production of liquor.

By term about 500 ml per day is secreted as fetal urine and tracheal fluid accounts for as much as 200 ml. Studies with radioisotopes have shown that near term 500 ml of water are exchanged hourly between the maternal plasma and the amniotic fluid. Disposal of the fluid is partly by absorption through the amnion into maternal plasma and partly by fetal swallowing and absorption in the intestine to enter the fetal plasma.

In cases of renal agenesis there is oligohydramnios (a deficiency of liquor amnii) and in conditions of defective swallowing such as anencephaly and oesophageal atresia there is polyhydramnios (an excess of liquor amnii).

Functions of the liquor amnii

The liquor guards the fetus against mechanical shocks, equalizes the pressure exerted by uterine contractions and allows, at least in the early months, plenty of room for fetal movement. Since the temperature of the fluid is maintained by the mother, the fetus is not subjected to loss of heat. Fetal metabolism is devoted entirely to growth and differentiation, and not dissipated in making good heat loss. Some of the fluid is swallowed, but it can hardly be regarded as a source of nutrition for the fetus since the content of protein and salts is so small.

During labour, the liquor contained in the bag of forewaters forms a fluid wedge which, with the uterine contractions, dilates the internal os uteri and cervical canal. When the membranes rupture during labour the liquor flushes the lower genital tract with fluid that is aseptic and bactericidal.

Investigation of the amniotic fluid

Samples of liquor can be obtained during pregnancy for various diagnostic purposes by abdominal amniocentesis. Not only can a variety of chemical estimations be made for normal and pathological constituents, but fetal amniotic cells can be obtained for tissue culture and chromosomal study. Details are given on page 273.

THE UMBILICAL CORD

The umbilical cord forms the major connection between the fetus and the placenta. It is derived from the ventral stalk and receives a close covering of amniotic epithelium. The constituents of the umbilical cord are:

the covering epithelium, which is a single layer of amnion

Wharton's jelly, which is composed of cells with elongated anastomosing processes in a gelatinous fluid, and is part of the extraembryonic mesoderm

blood vessels. At first these are four in number; two arteries and two veins. The embryonic umbilical veins fuse before the third month leaving a single vessel. The two umbilical arteries are derived from the internal iliac (hypogastric) arteries of the fetus, and carry reduced blood from the fetus to the placenta. The umbilical vein carries oxygenated blood from the placenta to the fetus

the umbilical vesicle and its duct, the shrivelled remnant of the yolk sac, may be found as a very small yellow body near the attachment of the cord to the placenta

the allantois, which occasionally occurs as a blindly-ending tube just reaching into the cord, is continuous inside the fetus with the urachus and bladder.

The cord is approximately 50 cm in length, but its length varies greatly, and may be as long as 180 cm, or as short as 7.5 cm. It is about 1 cm thick, but is not uniform, presenting nodes and swellings which are sometimes caused by dilatation of the umbilical vein, but more often by local increase in Wharton's jelly. At the earliest stage the cord is straight, but as early as the 12th week it shows a spiral twist.

In addition to the nodes mentioned above (sometimes called false knots) on rare occasions the cord has one or more true knots, due to the fetus passing through a loop in the cord. If such a true knot becomes drawn very tight the fetus will perish from obstruction to its circulation. The cord is often coiled round the fetal body, limbs or neck, but this seldom gives rise to any serious trouble. Further reference will be made to anomalies of the cord on page 74.

THE FETUS

SIZE OF THE FETUS

The diameter of the embryonic sac at 5 weeks is 8 mm and it increases by about 1 mm per day up to 12 weeks. Obviously the size of the sac must be sufficient to enclose the flexed fetus.

The length of the fetus is a more reliable index of its age than its weight. In the early weeks the measurement of the fetus is commonly taken from the vertex of the head to the coccyx (crown–rump length), but from the 20th week onwards the measurement is taken from the vertex to the heels. For antenatal care the biparietal diameter of the fetal head is a more useful measurement, and this can be determined accurately with ultrasound. Table 1.1 and Fig. 1.9 shows the approximate measurements (p. 20):

A rough guide to the vertex–heel length of the fetus (in cm) after the 20th week is given by multiplying the number of lunar months by five.

Other characteristics of the growing fetus are useful in determining the age.

At 8 weeks the 2.3 cm fetus lies in the enlarging amniotic cavity, but the amnion is not yet in contact with the chorion and the extraembryonic coelom is not yet obliterated. The ventral stalk and yolk sac have united to form the umbilical cord which is invested by amnion, and the primitive small intestine is contained in the dilated proximal part of the cord. The facial form has been completed by the formation of the nose and its separation from the mouth. The ears are completely formed externally, and the eyelids have appeared around the eyeball. The limbs are enlarging and show their jointed appearance, and the fingers and toes are formed. The flexion of the trunk has diminished, so that the vertex of the head rather than the back of the neck now forms the upper end of the embryo.

At 12 weeks the placenta is discoid. The amnion entirely fills the chorionic sac. The umbilical cord, still short and thick, shows a spiral twist. The primitive intestine is completely withdrawn into the body cavity. Nails have appeared on the fingers and toes, and the external sexual organs are differentiated. The crown–rump length is 6 cm and the weight about 14 g.

At 28 weeks the fetus weighs about 1100 g. The subcutaneous fat is becoming more evident, and the skin wrinkles begin to disappear. The testicles are in the inguinal canals. The eyelids have opened. At this period the fetus is said to be viable, and the law assumes that it can survive after birth. However, with modern intensive neonatal care many infants survive earlier delivery, so that the present legal convention needs revision.

After this the weight of the fetus increases with

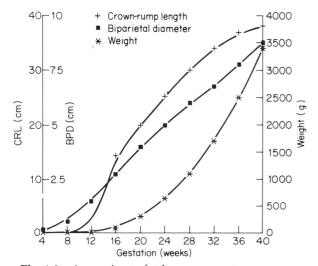

Fig. 1.9 Approximate fetal measurements

comparative rapidity. The fetus becomes completely covered with *vernix caseosa*, a greasy substance composed of the secretion of sebaceous glands mixed with desquamated epithelial cells. The scalp hair increases in length. The short colourless hairs known as lanugo, which have previously appeared on the body and head, tend to disappear. The red colour of the skin changes to flesh colour owing to the thickness of subcutaneous fat. Just before the 36th week one testicle has usually descended into the scrotum. The nails reach the ends of the fingers but not of the toes.

At 40 weeks the fetus measures 50 cm from vertex to heels and, as a rule, weighs between 2700 and 3600 g. The signs that the fetus has reached term are not always certain, but the length and weight are important. The nails usually project beyond the ends of the fingers and have reached the ends of the toes. The skin is pink and the lanugo has almost disappeared, except over the shoulders. The whole of the intestine contains meconium. The umbilicus is almost at the centre of the body. Both testicles have descended into the scrotum. As a rule only one epiphysis has started to ossify, that at the lower end of the femur, but the centres of ossification of the upper epiphysis of the tibia and of the humerus may have appeared.

Babies weighing more than 4500 g at birth are rare. If a baby weighs less than 2500 g at term it is probably growth-retarded (dysmature) and on this account may have a diminished chance of survival. It is different with twins; both may weigh less than 2500 g, and they tend to be born before term, and yet both are likely to survive. The heaviest children are likely to be born when the mother's age is between 25 and 35 years. Very young mothers commonly have small babies. The weights of the children tend to increase in successive pregnancies, provided that the mother's age is under 35. On average male babies are heavier than female ones at birth.

FETAL CIRCULATION

The fetal circulation differs from that of the adult in several respects. Oxygen and nutrients are carried back from the placenta in the single large umbilical vein. Although there is free diffusion of oxygen across the thin barrier between the maternal and fetal circulations in the placenta, the oxygen saturation in the umbilical venous blood is already reduced from the 95 per cent level in maternal arterial blood to about 80 per cent because the active metabolism of the placenta has already used some of the oxygen. On entering the body of the fetus the vein communicates with the portal vein, so that some blood passes through the liver to the hepatic vein and inferior vena cava, but most of the oxygenated blood passes more directly through the ductus venosus to the vena cava (Fig. 1.10). In the inferior vena cava it mixes with the stream of desaturated blood returning from the lower limbs and abdominal organs, so that the oxygen saturation is reduced to less than 70 per cent by the time the blood enters the right atrium. By a remarkable anatomical arrangement most of the blood entering the right atrium from the inferior vena cava is directed through the foramen ovale into the left atrium, and from thence it passes into the left ventricle and out into the ascending aorta. By this arrangement the coronary arteries and the brain receive the most highly oxygenated blood.

Blood returning from the head and upper limbs through the superior vena cava streams towards the tricuspid valve to enter the right ventricle, taking with it a portion of the blood which has entered through the inferior vena cava. The unexpanded fetal lungs offer such high resistance to blood flow that the greater part of the right ventricular output passes from the main pulmonary artery through the widely patent ductus arteriosus into the aorta, to be distributed to the lower part of the body of the fetus, and along the paired umbilical arteries to the placenta. The blood in the descending aorta has a saturation of about 60 per cent, which is lower than that in the ascending aorta because of the admixture of blood which has come from the ductus arteriosus.

In the fetus only 5 to 10 per cent of the total cardiac output goes directly to the lungs and returns to the left atrium via the pulmonary veins. Although the left ventricle is pumping the most highly oxygenated blood to the brain and coronary arteries, the right ventricle is contributing more to the total cardiac output, and its wall is as thick as that of the left ventricle.

The greater part of the blood descending in the aorta leaves the body by the hypogastric (umbilical) arteries to be oxygenated in the placenta.

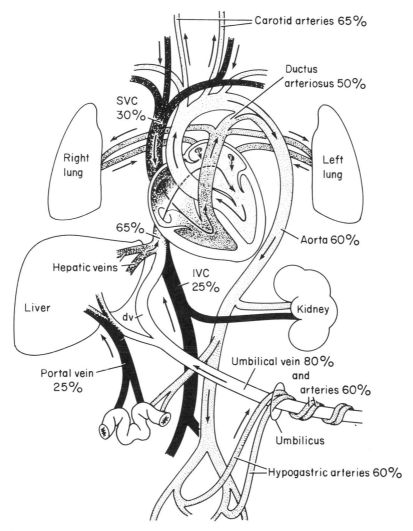

Fig. 1.10 Fetal circulation. SVC, superior vena cava; IVC, inferior vena cava; dv, ductus venosus. The percentage figure represents the oxygen saturation of the blood

CHANGES IN THE CIRCULATION AT BIRTH

See page 240.

OXYGEN SUPPLY TO THE FETUS

As the fetus grows it requires ever increasing amounts of oxygen. This is achieved by:

an increase in placental transfer of oxygen due to reduction in the diffusion distance

an increase in the haemoglobin content of fetal blood

fetal haemoglobin (HbF), which is made in the liver and spleen rather than the bone marrow, and has a different structure from adult haemoglobin (HbA).

Instead of two alpha- and two beta-globin chains as in HbA, HbF has two alpha and two gamma chains. The oxygen dissociation curve of HbF is shifted to the left so that it is more saturated than HbA at the low Po_2 levels present *in utero*.

The fetal red cell count rises progressively from 1.5 million per mm^3 at 10 weeks to 5.5 million at term. The cells are macrocytic, and the haemoglobin content at term is about 18 g per 100 ml. The maternal blood at term often contains less than 12 g per 100 ml.

The effect of these differences between maternal and fetal blood is that 100 ml of maternal blood can carry 16 ml of oxygen if it is fully saturated, but the same volume of fetal blood can carry 21 ml. In other words, the fetal blood can easily take up oxygen from the maternal blood. Maternal arterial blood is nearly fully saturated and carries about 15.7 ml of oxygen per 100 ml, whereas fetal blood in the descending aorta is only about 60 per cent saturated, but carries 13 ml of oxygen per 100 ml.

NUTRITION OF THE FETUS

Although the fetus is completely dependent on the maternal blood and the placenta for its nutritional requirements, it is a separate physiological entity, and it will take what it needs from the mother, even at the cost of reducing her reserves of some substances, for example calcium and iron. For nearly every substance the rate of fetal intake increases progressively, and is greatest in the late weeks of pregnancy.

EFFECT OF TERATOGENS ON THE FETUS

A variety of agents will interfere with the development of the embryo, for example rubella virus (p. 113), drugs (p. 46) and radiation. The effect of a teratogen depends on the stage of development reached at the time of exposure. In early pregnancy abortion may occur, and major malformation may arise if the agent acts at the time of organogenesis. Minor malformations and functional defects are likely to be produced at a later stage of pregnancy.

ANATOMY OF THE NORMAL FEMALE PELVIS AND THE FETAL SKULL

Knowledge of the shape and dimensions of the normal female pelvis and of the fetal skull is essential for proper understanding of the mechanism of labour and its abnormalities.

THE PELVIS

Although some sexual differences may be recognizable at birth the female pelvic characteristics are chiefly developed between that time and puberty. Radiological surveys have shown that variations in the shape of the pelvis are very common. What is described as the normal female pelvis, the rounded *gynaecoid pelvis*, occurs in only 40 per cent of white women. Other women have pelves with male characteristics (*android pelvis*), in some there is a slight increase in the anteroposterior diameter of the pelvis (*anthropoid pelvis*) while in the remainder the pelvis is slightly flattened (*platypelloid pelvis*) (*see* also p. 202). Only the typical gynaecoid pelvis will be described here.

The part of the pelvis above the brim is described as the false pelvis and that below the brim as the true pelvis. The obstetrician is only concerned with the latter. The true pelvis may be described in terms of the brim, the cavity and the outlet.

The pelvic brim

The pelvic brim (Fig. 1.11) lies in one plane bounded in front by the symphysis pubis, on each side by the upper margin of the pubic bone, the illiopectineal line and the ala of the sacrum and posteriorly by the promontory of the sacrum. The brim is oval in shape, with the transverse diameter slightly greater than the anteroposterior (Fig. 1.12).

The pelvic cavity

This is sometimes described in terms of an imaginary plane bounded in front by the middle of the symphysis pubis, on each side by the pubic bone, the obturator fascia and the inner aspect of the ischial bone and posteriorly by the junction of the second and third pieces of the sacrum. The ischial spines lie slightly below this plane. In the

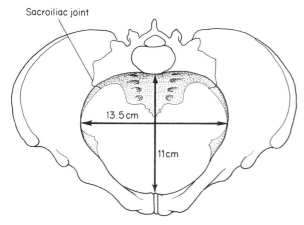

Fig. 1.11 The pelvic brim

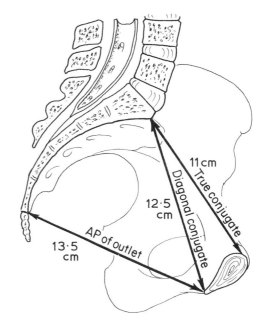

Fig. 1.12 Sagittal section of pelvis. The true and diagonal conjugate diameters are shown as is the anteroposterior diameter of the outlet

gynaecoid pelvis the cavity is circular and roomy because the sacrum is inclined backwards, is well curved and the sacrosciatic notches are wide.

The pelvic outlet

The pelvic outlet (Fig. 1.13) is roughly diamond-shaped and is bounded in front by the lower margin of the symphysis pubis, on each side by the descending ramus of the pubic bone, the ischial tuberosity and the sacrotuberous ligament and posteriorly by the last piece of the sacrum (*not* the coccyx, which is mobile). Unlike the brim, the outlet does not have boundaries which lie in a single plane, but an imaginary plane of the outlet is described, passing from the lower margin of the symphysis pubis to the last piece of the sacrum. It will be noted that the ischial tuberosities lie well below this plane. In a gynaecoid pelvis the sub-pubic arch is wide and the tuberosities are far apart. The shape of the outlet is oval with the long axis in the anteroposterior diameter.

During pregnancy the ligaments of the sacroiliac joints and the symphysis pubis become softened and there is slightly increased mobility at these joints. The sacrococcygeal joint allows the coccyx to move freely backwards during delivery.

The pelvic axis

The axis of the pelvis is an imaginary curved line which shows the path which the centre of the fetal head follows during its passage through the pelvis. It is obtained by taking several anteroposterior

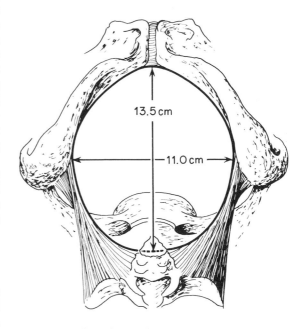

Fig. 1.13 The pelvic outlet

diameters of the pelvis and joining their centres (Fig. 1.14).

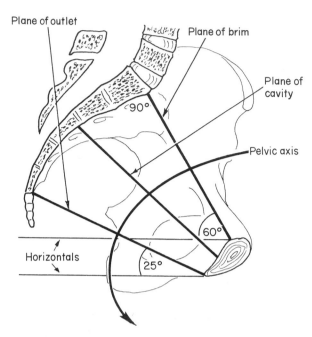

Fig. 1.14 The planes and axis of the pelvis

Pelvic inclination

The pelvic inclination is the angle that any pelvic plane makes with the horizontal. In the erect position the brim is normally inclined at 60 degrees. In negroid women this angle may approach 90 degrees, referred to as steep inclination of the brim, and because of this the head may be slow to engage during labour.

The pelvic outlet is inclined at about 25 degrees to the horizontal.

The inclination of the sacrum is measured differently. It is the angle between the front of the first piece of the sacrum and the plane of the pelvic brim. It may affect the available space in the upper part of the pelvic cavity. (Fig. 1.14).

AVERAGE DIMENSIONS OF THE NORMAL PELVIS

It must be clearly understood that the pelvic diameters vary just as much as women's heights vary, and that the diameters will also be affected by the pelvic shape. What matters during delivery is not the absolute size of the pelvis but the size relative to that of the fetal head. However, in a woman of average height with a normal pelvis the following measurements are to be expected.

Diameters of the brim

The anteroposterior diameter of the brim (or true conjugate) is measured from the back of the upper part of the symphysis pubis to the promontory of the sacrum and is 11 cm. The transverse diameter of the brim measures 13.5 cm (*see* Fig. 1.11).

Diameters of the pelvic cavity

The plane of the cavity has already been defined. The anteroposterior and transverse diameters both measure 12 cm.

Diameters of the pelvic outlet

The outlet does not lie in a simple plane like the brim. The anteroposterior diameter of the outlet is measured from the lower part of the symphysis pubis to the lower end of the sacrum (*not* the coccyx) and is 13.5 cm. The transverse diameter is measured between the inner surfaces of the ischial tuberosities and is 11 cm (*see* Fig. 1.13).

The average normal measurements are summarized in Table 1.1.

Table 1.1 Average dimensions of the normal pelvis

	Anteriorposterior (cm)	Transverse (cm)
Brim	11	13.5
Cavity	12	12
Outlet	13.5	11

The brim is a transverse oval, the cavity is round and the outlet is an anteroposterior oval.

CLINICAL EXAMINATION OF THE PELVIS

A pelvic examination is sometimes made early in pregnancy to confirm to diagnosis of pregnancy and its duration, to exclude abnormalities of the pelvic organs and to assess the capacity of the pelvis. If the patient has miscarried, or has threatened to miscarry previously, it is wise to postpone any internal examination until later. In any case, a further pelvic examination is usually performed at about the 36th week, when a better assessment of pelvic capacity can be made, since at this time the pelvic floor is more relaxed; the size of the fetal head can also be related to that of the pelvic brim at this time.

Vaginal assessment of the pelvis

The brim

The sacral promontory cannot be reached with an examining finger in a normal pelvis unless the patient is anaesthetized. If it can be felt it is likely that the true conjugate is considerably reduced, and in such a case it may be possible to estimate the diagonal conjugate with the exploring finger. This is the distance between the promontory and the lower margin of the symphysis pubis. The true conjugate may be derived by subtracting 1.5 cm from the diagonal conjugate (*see* Fig. 1.12, p. 19).

The pelvic cavity

On vaginal examination a general idea of the capacity of the pelvic cavity can be gained. The anterior surface of the sacrum is palpated from above downwards, noting whether it is straight or concave. The position of the ischial spines may be assessed by palpation of the sacrospinous ligaments, which should be of a length that will accommodate three finger-breadths. The spines are sometimes unduly prominent, but it is the distance between them rather than their prominence that matters.

The pelvic outlet

The intertuberous diameter can be determined by external palpation, but vaginal examination gives the best assessment of the width of the subpubic arch and of the position of the sacrum.

The pelvic floor

Although this is not part of the bony pelvis it is mentioned here because it forms part of the birth canal and plays an important part in the mechanism of labour. The two levator ani muscles, with their fascia, form a musculofascial gutter during the second stage of labour, with the opening of the vagina looking forward between the sides of the gutter (Fig. 1.15). The pelvic floor directs the most salient portion of the presenting part forwards under the subpubic arch.

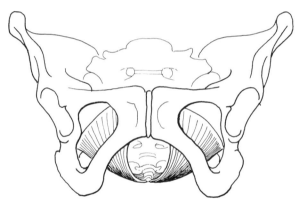

Fig. 1.15   The levator sling

THE FETAL SKULL

The fetal skull may be divided into the vault, face and base. By the time of birth the bones of the face and base are all firmly united, but the bones of the vault are not so well ossified, being joined only by unossified membranes at the sutures. During labour the bones of the vault can undergo *moulding*, by which the shape of the skull can be altered by overriding the cranial bones with reduction of some of its diameters.

The bones which form the vault are the parietal bones, and parts of the occipital, frontal and temporal bones (Fig. 1.16). At birth the frontal

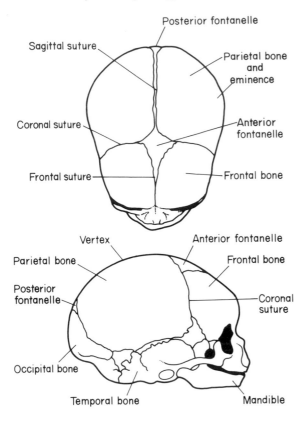

Fig. 1.16   The fetal skull. Superior and lateral views

bone is divided into two parts. Three sutures are of obstetric importance:

  the sagittal suture lies between the superior borders of the parietal bones
  the frontal suture, which is a forward continuation of the sagittal suture, lies between the two parts of the frontal bone
  the coronal suture lies between the anterior borders of the parietal bones and the posterior borders of the frontal bones.

Fontanelles

The points of junction of the various sutures are termed *fontanelles*; the anterior and posterior fontanelles are important in obstetrics.

The anterior fontanelle lies where the sagittal, frontal and coronal sutures meet.

The posterior fontanelle lies at the posterior end of the sagittal suture, between the two parietal bones and the occipital bone.

The position of these two fontanelles, when felt on vaginal examination, indicates in which direction the occiput is pointing and the degree of flexion or extension of the head.

The anterior fontanelle (or bregma) is much the larger of the two, is roughly kite-shaped, has four sutures running into it, is always patent at birth and takes about 20 months to close.

The posterior fontanelle is triangular in shape, has three sutures running into it, in most cases cannot be felt as a space during labour and closes soon afterwards.

The area of the fetal skull bounded by the two parietal eminences and the anterior and posterior fontanelles is termed the *vertex*. It is the part of the head which presents in normal labour.

DIAMETERS OF THE FETAL SKULL

The diameters of the fetal skull which are important in the mechanism of labour may be divided into vertical, longitudinal, and transverse.

Vertical and longitudinal diameters

The fetal head is ovoid in shape. In normal labour the head is well flexed so that the least diameters of the ovoid, namely the *suboccipitobregmatic* and *biparietal (transverse) diameters* are those which

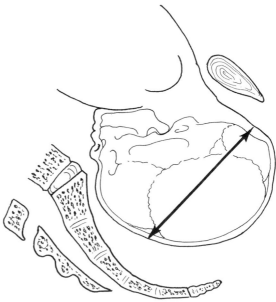

Fig. 1.17   The suboccipitobregmatic diameter of 9.5 cm, engaged in the pelvis when the head is fully flexed

engage. The suboccipitobregmatic diameter is measured from the suboccipital region to the centre of the anterior fontanelle (bregma) and in the normal head at term is 9.5 cm (Fig. 1.17).

If the head is less well flexed the *suboccipitofrontal diameter* is involved. This is taken from the suboccipital region to the prominence of the forehead and measures 10 cm. This is the diameter of the head which passes through the vulval orifice at the moment of delivery of the head (*see* Fig. 4.7, p. 160).

With further extension of the head the *occipitofrontal diameter* engages. This is measured from the root of the nose (glabella) to the posterior fontanelle and is 11.5 cm. This diameter meets the pelvis with a persistent occipitoposterior position (Fig. 1.18).

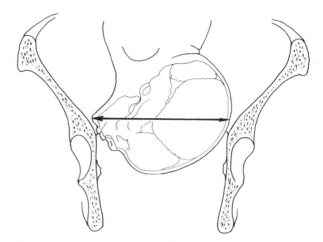

Fig. 1.19 The mentovertical diameter of 13 cm meeting the pelvis in a brow presentation

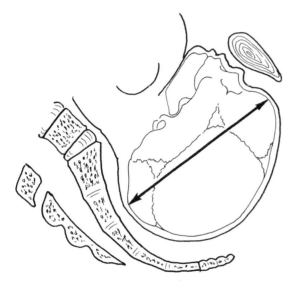

Fig. 1.18 The occipitofrontal diameter of 11.5 cm, engaged in the pelvis in an occipitoposterior position

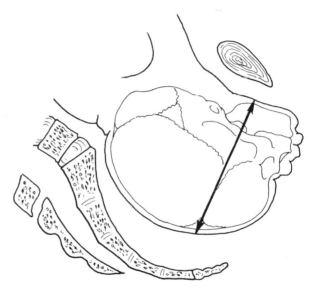

Fig. 1.20 The submentobregmatic diameter of 9.5 cm, engaged in the pelvis in a face presentation with the head completely extended

The greatest longitudinal diameter is the *mentovertical*, which is taken from the chin to the furthest point of the vertex and measures 13 cm. This is the diameter which is thrown across the pelvis in a brow presentation (Fig. 1.19) and is too large to pass through a normal pelvis.

Beyond this point further extension of the head so that the face presents results in a smaller vertical diameter, i.e. the other end of the ovoid presents. The *submentobregmatic diameter* is taken from below the chin to the anterior fontanelle and measures 9.5 cm (Fig. 1.20).

Transverse diameter

The biparietal diameter, measured from one parietal eminence to the other, is 9.5 cm (Fig. 1.21).

PROCESSES OF THE DURA MATER

The great folds of the dura mater, the falx cerebri and the tentorium cerebelli, act in some degree as internal ligaments, resisting too great deformation

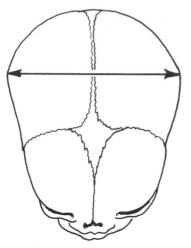

Fig. 1.21   Biparietal diameter, 9.5 cm

of the fetal head both in the longitudinal and the transverse directions. If moulding is excessive, or if the fetal head is subjected to severe and sudden stresses, these parts of the dura mater are liable to be torn; some of the great venous sinuses are then in danger of rupture. These are the inferior longitudinal sinus, running in the free edge of the falx cerebri and receiving the great cerebral veins of Galen from the brain, and the straight sinus running between the falx cerebri and the tentorium cerebelli.

DIAMETERS OF THE FETAL TRUNK

The *bisacromial diameter* is taken between the parts furthest apart on the shoulders and is 12 cm. The *bitrochanteric diameter* measures 10 cm.

MATERNAL PHYSIOLOGY

Although the anatomical and physiological changes that occur during pregnancy chiefly involve the genital tract and the breasts, many other interrelated changes occur in other systems of the body. The most important alterations in maternal physiology during pregnancy may be summarized thus:

Endocrine and paracrine changes

Placental hormones and proteins influence ovarian and pituitary function, maintain the decidua, initiate the growth of the myometrium, increase the vascularity of the whole genital tract and cause proliferation of the glandular tissue of the breasts (Fig. 1.22). These substances have secondary effects, including the retention of water in the body, relaxation of smooth muscle, and possibly relaxation of pelvic ligaments.

Changes due to uterine enlargement

The increased blood flow through the uterus causes substantial changes in the maternal circulation, and the enlarged uterus alters the general posture and affects the mechanism of respiration.

Metabolic changes

The fetal requirements of oxygen and food substances, the growth of the uterus and preparation for lactation affect the mother's metabolism and dietary needs.

Details of some of these changes are as follows:

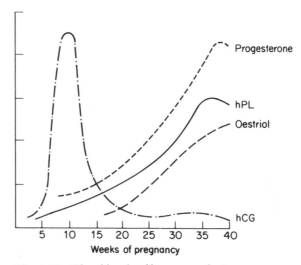

Fig. 1.22   Blood levels of hormones during pregnancy

ENDOCRINE AND PARACRINE SYSTEM

Trophoblastic hormones and proteins

The trophoblast produces large amounts of human chorionic gonadotrophin (hCG), particularly in the first trimester of pregnancy (*see* Fig. 1.22). During pregnancy large quantities of hCG are present in the blood and urine, and high concentrations of this substance prolong the lifespan of the corpus luteum, which in turn continues to produce oestrogen and progesterone and so to maintain the uterine decidua until the output of oestrogen and progesterone from the placenta rises. The decidua (gestational endometrium) in turn increases the rate of synthesis of prostaglandins and secretory proteins.

The cardinal symptom of pregnancy, amenorrhoea, is dependent upon continuing production of progesterone and oestradiol by the corpus luteum to sustain the decidua (Fig. 1.23). The luteotrophic action of rising concentrations of hCG extends the life of the corpus luteum and gonadal steroid production for at least eight to 10 weeks, until the developing placenta is sufficiently mature to assume the synthesis of progesterone and oestriol. Thereafter, involution of the corpus luteum of pregnancy occurs.

It is interesting to note that the principal function of the ovary in early pregnancy is to produce these two hormones and little else, as evidenced by successful pregnancy following ovum donation in women with ovarian agenesis or premature menopause who seem only to require synthetic progesterone and oestrogen for the first trimester. In addition, the extensive structural changes in the endometrium as it becomes decidua are reflected by at least a quantitative alteration in the synthesis of secretory proteins by the various cell types of the endometrium. The most striking change is seen in the rate of production of the major secretory protein of the glandular epithelium, progestogen-dependent endometrial protein, and also of the stromal cell types which produce insulin-like growth factor binding protein. Current research may reveal that serum levels of these proteins will provide the first non-invasive tests of endometrial and decidual function.

Embryonic development can also be reflected in the maternal bloodstream by changes in serum concentrations of alpha-fetoprotein (AFP) which in pregnancy is derived from endodermal tissues.

AFP and other substances of embryonic origin are present in the highest concentrations in amniotic fluid, and in lesser amounts in maternal peripheral blood (Fig. 1.24). These and other endocrine events are largely responsible for initiating the metabolic and physiological adaptations which prepare for pregnancy and parturition.

The common symptoms of pregnancy – morning sickness, breast changes and urinary frequency

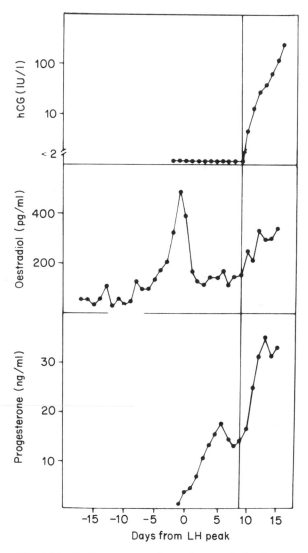

Fig. 1.23 Daily concentrations of oestradiol and progesterone throughout a spontaneous conception cycle indicating the changes in steroid hormones in relation to hCG

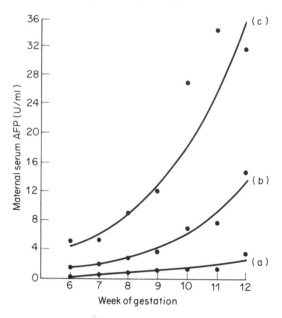

Fig. 1.24 Maternal serum AFP: (a) 5th centile; (b) Median; (c) 95th centile

– which happen early in the first trimester (*see* pp. 33–34) are most likely to be caused by the hormonal changes, and as the second trimester is entered, abdominal swelling or distention due to the growing uterus is evident.

Large amounts of oestrogens and progesterone are found in the blood and urine during pregnancy, at first secreted by the corpus luteum, then by the placenta after the 12th week. The oestrogen which appears in the largest quantity in maternal urine during pregnancy is oestriol. This is formed in the placenta from precursors which come from the fetal suprarenal cortex and liver.

The blood progesterone level rises during pregnancy, and therefore the urinary excretion of the metabolite pregnanediol increases. Even if the corpus luteum is removed in early pregnancy the hormone levels continue to rise as the placenta produces large quantities of these hormones. Oestrogen and progesterone maintain the decidua of pregnancy, cause the growth and hyperaemia of the uterus and lower genital tract, and the hyperaemia and development of the breasts. Oestrogen stimulates synthesis of prolactin via the pituitary gland, but together with progesterone it inhibits the lactogenic effect of human placental lactogen (hPL) and prolactin.

Other maternal endocrine changes

During pregnancy the anterior lobe of the pituitary gland undergoes hypertrophy, with an increase of both acidophil and basophil cells due to the influence of increased oestrogen. No anatomical changes are evident in the posterior lobe of the pituitary gland.

The thyroid gland is slightly enlarged during pregnancy, and the basal metabolic rate is increased (*see* p. 29 and 121).

There is an increased concentration of adrenal hormones in both the blood and the urine. The observation that rheumatoid arthritis often undergoes a remission during pregnancy may be explained by the increased secretion of glucocorticoids. There is also some increase in the excretion of mineralocorticoids (aldosterone).

THE UTERUS

During pregnancy the uterus is adapted to contain the growing fetus and placenta, and it also undergoes changes in preparation for its task of expelling the fetus during labour. The changes include development of the decidua, hypertrophy of the muscle coat, increased vascularity, formation of the lower segment and softening of the cervix.

At term the uterus is about 35 cm long and 23 cm in diameter. It weighs 1 kg, in contrast to the non-pregnant uterus which weighs 65 g. The pregnant uterus is usually slightly rotated on its long axis, so that the anterior surface faces a little to the right, and the fundus may also be inclined to one or other side, most often the right. The enlargement of the uterus is greatest at the fundus, so that the points of entry of the fallopian tubes appear to lie well below the top of the uterus.

The enormous growth of the myometrium during pregnancy is caused by two factors – hormonal stimulation and distension. During early pregnancy the embryo does not fill the uterine cavity, and distension has no influence at this stage. An identical uterine enlargement occurs in cases of ectopic pregnancy when the embryo is outside the uterus. The growth is brought about by the action of oestrogen and progesterone. Later on, as the fetus and placenta become larger, the distension of the uterus provides a further stimulus to growth.

In early pregnancy active mitosis can be seen in the connective tissue and muscle cells, and the enlargement of the uterus is largely due to an increase in the number of cells. Later in pregnancy the enlargement is chiefly due to hypertrophy of the individual cells, and cell division is less active. At term each muscle cell is about ten times as long as it was before pregnancy. The blood supply to the uterus is greatly increased and, especially under the placental site, the veins become converted to large sinuses, thicker than a pencil.

At term the wall of the uterus appears thin in relation to the enormous enlargement of the cavity, but in fact it is still about 1 cm thick. In late pregnancy there are three layers in the muscular wall of the uterus:

- a thin outer layer of fibres that arches over the fundus and is continuous laterally with the muscle of the round ligaments
- a thick intermediate layer, consisting of a meshwork of interlacing fibres, which surrounds the blood vessels. The contraction of this layer will stop the blood flow in the vessels, and it is the strong contraction of this layer which prevents dangerous haemorrhage from the large placental sinuses in the third stage of labour
- a thin inner layer arranged in a circular fashion, especially around the internal os and around the tubal openings.

During pregnancy the uterus contracts from time to time (Braxton Hicks contractions), and contractions can be stimulated by abdominal palpation. These contractions are not so strong or regular as those of labour, and are painless.

The ovarian and uterine arteries and veins are greatly enlarged.

THE CERVIX

Although the cervix hypertrophies to some extent during pregnancy, it does not do so to the same extent as the body of the uterus. The cervix becomes softer because of increased vascularity and a great increase in the gland spaces. The glands are distended with mucus, and the pattern of the glands becomes far more complex, so that the cervix seems to contain a honeycomb filled with mucus, this is sometimes described as a mucus plug. On inspection the cervix has a purple tinge from venous congestion.

Since effacement does not usually take place until the onset of labour, the cervix remains elongated until the end of pregnancy, although in

multiparae the external os tends to be patulous. An intact and effective internal os is of importance in retaining the embryo safely within the uterine cavity; with an incompetent cervix there is a considerable risk of abortion, or of premature rupture of the membranes.

Because of the great activity of the columnar epithelium of the cervix, and the increased secretion of mucus, it is common for the stratified epithelium on the vaginal surface of the cervix to be replaced by an outward extension of columnar epithelium – referred to as cervical ectropion. Such an appearance is not to be regarded as abnormal during pregnancy, and it will usually disappear in the puerperium.

The Vagina and Vulva

The increased vascularity already described in the cervix affects the vaginal walls a little later, and they eventually show the purple coloration right down to the vulva. The vaginal walls become softened and relaxed, and the same change occurs in the perineal body.

The watery transudation that normally occurs through the vaginal wall is increased during pregnancy. The hypertrophied cervical glands secrete more mucus, and this is added to the vaginal transudate and desquamated vaginal cells, so that the total discharge from the vagina is increased. The vaginal secretion is acid in reaction (pH 4.5 to 5) and is some protection against ascending infection.

Under the influence of placental hormones the vaginal epithelium is very active, and in a smear desquamated cells often have their lateral edges rolled over, so that they appear boat-shaped (navicular cells), these cells are usually clumped together. This normal epithelial activity should not be mistaken for carcinoma *in situ*.

As pregnancy advances the vulva shares in the increased vascularity and shows some swelling in consequence. Varicose veins may appear.

THE BREASTS

During pregnancy the secretion of oestrogen in large amounts causes thickening of the skin of the nipple and active growth and branching of the underlying ducts. The added action of progesterone causes proliferation of the glandular epithelium of the alveoli. Neither of these hormones causes the active secretion of milk, which only begins after delivery when the level of oestrogen falls and that of prolactin, from the anterior lobe of the pituitary gland, rises (*see* p. 247).

Slight changes in the breasts occur in the menstrual cycle, under the influence of oestrogen and progesterone, and the breasts may become tense and uncomfortable for a few days before the onset of the period. If pregnancy occurs these changes are more marked. The earliest change is a swelling of the breasts, especially at the periphery. The lobules of the gland can be felt easily and are harder than normal, these changes producing a knotty feeling in the breast. At the same time the breasts become a little tender, and the patient often describes a 'prickly' sensation in them. The increased blood supply is shown by a very obvious network of veins under the skin. As a result of congestion, followed by actual growth of the glandular tissue, the breasts become more prominent. Plethysmographic studies have shown that each breast may increase in volume by about 200 ml, an increase of about one-third.

By about the 12th week of pregnancy the glands begin to secrete an almost clear fluid, which will appear in droplets if the breast is squeezed towards the nipple. Towards the end of pregnancy the secretion becomes more copious and is yellow in colour and creamy in consistence. It is then known as *colostrum*, and consists of water, fat, albumin, salts and colostrum corpuscles. The latter are cells shed whole from the gland acini, and filled with fat droplets. When the milk secretion is eventually established colostrum corpuscles are not found in it, because the fat is discharged from the secreting cells into the lumina of the acini, and the cells themselves are not detached.

Changes also occur in the nipple, which becomes larger and more readily erectile. The areolar skin is active and slightly raised above the surrounding skin. The areola becomes pigmented to a greater or lesser degree, the change being most marked in women with darker hair and skin. Once the pigmentation has occurred it persists as a permanent change. The sebaceous glands on the areola are very active in pregnancy, and can be seen as a ring of about 12 to 20 small tubercles (Montgomery's tubercles).

At about the 20th week of pregnancy, in dark-skinned women, further pigmentation may occur on the skin beyond the margin of the areola. This is termed the secondary areola, and is not a uniform pigmentation, but takes the form of patchy streaks. The secondary areola disappears after pregnancy.

The stretching of the skin over the breasts may produce striae like those which occur on the abdomen.

Sometimes outlying lobules of mammary tissue are found in the axillae; they enlarge during pregnancy and may form comparatively large swellings. Such breast tissue has inadequate drainage to the main duct system, and so may become tense and painful when lactation begins.

THE ABDOMINAL WALL

The muscles of the abdominal wall become stretched to accommodate the enlarging uterus, and although, in perfect health, subsequent recovery is complete, in not a few multiparae some loss of tone of these muscles persists. In late pregnancy the umbilicus may be flattened out, or even protrude.

Stretching of the abdominal skin may cause the formation of *striae gravidarum*. These are due to rupture of the elastic fibres of the skin, and they appear as curved lines, roughly concentric with the umbilicus, which may also be seen on the loins or thighs, and sometimes on the breasts. At first the striae are pink or red, but after delivery they become silvery-white, and are then called *striae albicantes*. Not all women develop striae; perhaps one-third do not. It is unusual to see striae in other conditions in which the abdominal wall is stretched, such as large ovarian cysts or ascites. The fact that they are frequently seen in Cushing's syndrome, when there is high level of glucocorticoids in the blood, as there is in pregnancy, has led to the suggestion that the striae are partly due to the action of these hormones.

Pigmentation of the line from the pubes to the umbilicus (the linea nigra) may be seen, especially in dark-skinned women, and may persist in part after the pregnancy.

THE PELVIC JOINTS

The pelvic hyperaemia causes some softening and slight relaxation of the ligaments of the sacroiliac joints, and of the ligaments and fibrocartilage of the symphysis pubis, and the mobility at these joints is slightly increased in pregnancy. In some animals a specific hormone, relaxin, derived from the ovary or in some species from the placenta, causes relaxation of the pelvic joints, but it is uncertain whether such a hormone plays any part in human physiology.

The changes so far described have mostly been those directly related to the genital tract and the breasts. Numerous other changes occur in the rest of the body, and nearly every system is involved in some change. Yet pregnancy is a physiological and not a pathological process, and many women both feel and appear to be in better general health during pregnancy than at other times. Given good previous nutrition and sound emotional adjustment, the physiological changes of pregnancy are not to be regarded as a strain on the mother's health, but merely as a temporary adaptation to a normal function.

MATERNAL METABOLISM DURING PREGNANCY

Weight gain

The body weight increases during pregnancy. The total gain varies between 7 and 17 kg in normal cases, with an average of 12.5 kg. After the 12th week the average normal gain is about 0.35–0.45 kg per week.

A fetus weighing 3.4 kg, a placenta of 0.65 kg, amniotic fluid weighing 0.8 kg, a uterus of 1 kg, and an increase in the weight of the breasts of 0.8 kg would account for a total gain of 6.65 kg. The average additional gain of 6 kg represents the weight gained by the rest of the maternal tissues, and this is partly due to fluid retention (1.5 kg), and partly due to increase in the body fat and protein.

During pregnancy, apart from the water contained in the fetus, placenta and liquor amnii, there is a considerable retention of water in the maternal tissues, chiefly in the extracellular compartment, including the blood plasma. The following figures illustrate the typical increase in body water found in maternal tissues at term:

increase in intracellular water	550 ml
increase in extracellular water	
intravascular (plasma)	900 ml
extravascular	1850 ml
	3300 ml

Corresponding quantities of sodium are retained and at present it is believed that this retention of salt and water is due to the high concentrations of sex steroids during pregnancy, although the part played by mineralocorticoids has not yet been fully determined.

Metabolic changes

The basal metabolic rate during pregnancy is increased by between 10 and 25 per cent, but if allowance is made for the metabolism of the fetus and its supporting tissues the basal metabolic rate of the maternal tissues is probably unaltered. Free thyroxine levels in the blood are normal or slightly reduced.

During pregnancy the total need for calories is increased by 80 000 kcal, this is to maintain the fetus and additional maternal tissues. Apart from fluid retention in cases of hypertension, abnormal weight gain during pregnancy and the puerperium is often due to simple overeating, chiefly by an excessive intake of carbohydrate.

During pregnancy the renal threshold for the excretion of sugar from the blood is often lowered, so that glucose may appear in the urine although the blood sugar level is normal. This condition is of no importance but it must be distinguished from true or gestational diabetes, by a glucose tolerance test if necessary. Glycosuria is probably the result of increased glomerular filtration, which allows so much glucose to enter the tubules that they are unable to absorb it all. Lactose may appear in the urine during lactation, but is not found during pregnancy.

A high protein intake, amounting to a total extra requirement of 900 g, is needed to supply the growing fetus, placenta, uterus and breasts. In spite of an increased excretion of amino acids during pregnancy, sufficient nitrogen is retained for the maternal and fetal needs.

There are also changes in lipid metabolism during pregnancy; the total lipid requirement during pregnancy being 3.5 kg. Plasma levels of triglycerides, cholesterol and free fatty acids rise, and there is a greater tendency to ketosis.

The maternal diet must not only supply the protein, carbohydrate and fat required, but also the essential minerals and vitamins. An ordinary diet provides adequate amounts of most of these substances, but in the case of iron and calcium there is some risk of a deficit, particularly during the last trimester when the fetal uptake is greatest.

The fetal body at term contains about 30 g of calcium, but even with this large demand a mother taking a first class diet will maintain her calcium reserve during pregnancy. However, with a less favourable diet there may be a deficiency in late pregnancy which leads to decalcification of the maternal bones and dentine. Recalcification quickly occurs after lactation has been completed if the diet contains adequate calcium.

In the case of iron only about 1.2 mg is usually assimilated daily, an amount insufficient to meet the fetal needs, especially in late pregnancy. In addition the mother forms additional red cells during pregnancy. The blood volume is increased, and although the amount of haemoglobin per millilitre may be reduced, the increase in blood volume outweighs this, so that the total amount of haemoglobin in the maternal body is increased. Even in health, and with a normal diet, the maternal iron reserves in the liver, spleen and marrow may therefore be reduced during pregnancy. Not all the iron so used is lost; apart from the iron in the fetal tissues and blood, and the maternal blood lost at delivery, the iron built up into additional maternal red cells during pregnancy is later returned to her reserves. Further details of iron metabolism are given on page 102.

CHANGES IN THE BLOOD DURING PREGNANCY

The total blood volume is increased during pregnancy by about 30 per cent. The uterine wall and the maternal blood spaces in the placenta contain a large volume of blood, perhaps 800 ml. The increase in blood volume is an adaptation to supply the needs of the new vascular bed. Although the total number and volume of red cells increase by about 20 per cent, the plasma volume increases by about 50 per cent, with the result that the blood becomes more dilute and the red cell count and the haemoglobin concentration fall. A red cell count of 4 million per mm^3 and a haemoglobin concentration of 11 g per 100 ml are usually accepted as normal during pregnancy. Although such levels are commonly observed in completely healthy women in pregnancy, if supplemental iron is given in a form that is well absorbed then in many of these women the red cell count and haemoglobin concentration remain higher. The question which is still by no means decided is whether this gives any additional benefit. However, many women

have poor iron reserves and inadequate diets, and for them iron supplements are essential.

A very high leucocytosis is often observed during labour and the early puerperium, but not during normal pregnancy, when the count does not exceed 11 000 per cubic millimetre. The platelet count is normal. The erythrocyte sedimentation rate is much increased during normal pregnancy. Readings of up to 100 mm per hour are not unusual without any detectable abnormality.

CHANGES IN THE CIRCULATION DURING PREGNANCY

The cardiac output rises from 4.5 L/min to 6 L/min during the first ten weeks of pregnancy, remaining at the higher level until after delivery. The systolic blood pressure is unaltered during normal pregnancy but the diastolic pressure is reduced in the first and second trimester, returning to non-pregnant levels by term. The pulse rate rises by between eight and sixteen beats per minute so that the greatly increased cardiac output must be achieved by the expulsion of 70–80 ml more blood from the heart at each beat. This extra cardiac work is well within the reserve of the normal heart. The heart is displaced upwards in late pregnancy and the apex is rotated outwards, so that the apex beat is displaced outwards and the electrical axis is altered. There may be slight left axis deviation in an electrocardiograph, but there is little evidence of muscular hypertrophy.

The large blood flow through the uterus may be regarded as an arteriovenous shunt across the main circulation, and the increase in cardiac output and in the blood volume may be related to this. In addition there is increased renal blood flow and some dilatation of peripheral vessels. The hands and feet are often noticeably warm during pregnancy, and the skin capillaries are dilated.

The enlarged uterus interferes with the venous return from the legs, so that there is stasis in the large veins and slight oedema of the ankles may occur, even in normal pregnancy. Because of this interference with venous return, some women complain of faintness when lying on their backs (supine hypotension); haemorrhoids or varicose veins may appear for the first time or become worse during pregnancy.

Changes in the respiratory system during pregnancy

Pulmonary ventilation is increased by about 40 per cent, as a result of increased tidal volume. Oxygen requirements only increase by 20 per cent and the overbreathing leads to a fall in P_{CO_2}. The low P_{CO_2} gives rise to a sensation of dyspnoea, which may be accentuated by elevation of the diaphragm. When the fetal head engages in the pelvis in late pregnancy the breathlessness diminishes.

Changes in the alimentary tract during pregnancy

The most striking change in the digestive function in pregnancy is nausea or morning sickness, which occurs to a greater or lesser degree in about a third of pregnancies. It begins at the 6th week and stops spontaneously before the 14th. Although it is generally limited to the early morning it may occur at other times of the day. Usually the symptoms are slight; excessive or prolonged vomiting is certainly pathological. The cause is uncertain. *See* also page 45 for further discussion and description of the treatment.

Appetite and thirst increase during pregnancy, but minor digestive upsets are common, probably due to the relaxant effect of progesterone on smooth muscle. Sometimes gastric or intestinal distension occurs, and especially in early pregnancy this causes a feeling of abdominal enlargement. Heartburn is a common complaint, and is caused by relaxation of the cardiac sphincter of the stomach. In a few of the more severe cases this symptom is caused by a hiatus hernia. The emptying time of the stomach is prolonged during pregnancy, and even more so during labour (a fact of considerable importance in relation to the risk of vomiting during anaesthesia). The gastric acidity is often reduced, and peptic ulcers almost invariably become quiescent during pregnancy.

Constipation is not uncommon, and this, together with the pelvic hyperaemia and pressure of the enlarged uterus, may lead to the formation or increase in size of haemorrhoids.

Changes in the urinary tract during pregnancy

There is progressive increase in the glomerular filtration rate and renal plasma flow, starting in early pregnancy and reaching 50 per cent at term. A progressive fall in plasma creatinine levels from 73 μmol/L to 47 μmol/L at term occurs, and there is a similar fall in plasma urea from 3.5 to 3.1 mmol/L. Values considered normal in a non-pregnant woman may therefore indicate impaired renal function during pregnancy. The cumulative water retention in pregnancy is 7.5 L, together with 950 mmol sodium. This is due largely to increased aldosterone, renin and angiotensin I and II.

Frequency of micturition occurs during the first 12 weeks, when the enlarging uterus is still in the pelvic cavity and presses on the bladder. It may also occur in the last month of pregnancy when the presenting part of the fetus is engaging in the pelvis.

From about the 16th week of pregnancy onwards there is considerable and progressive dilatation of the renal pelvis and of the ureters down as far as the level of the pelvic brim. Direct measurement of the intraureteric pressure shows that it is lowered rather than raised, and the dilatation is chiefly caused by loss of muscle tone, although pressure from the uterus, displaced to the right by the descending colon, may explain the greater degree of change which is usually seen on the right side. The reduction in tone, which is thought to be caused by progesterone, is important in relation to pyelonephritis during pregnancy. The dilatation disappears during the puerperium, so long as there is no infection of the tract.

Changes in the skin during pregnancy

The striae gravidarum and linea nigra of the abdomen, and the primary and secondary areolae of the breast have already been mentioned. Pigmentation also occurs on the face, mainly as irregularly shaped brown patches on the forehead or cheeks, known as the chloasma or mask of pregnancy. These patches completely disappear after pregnancy. The cause of these changes is unknown, but may be related to oestrogen, progesterone, adrenal hormones or an increase in melanocyte-stimulating hormone.

Palmar erythema and spider naevi often occur in normal pregnancy. They are caused by increased oestrogen levels and disappear after pregnancy.

Emotional changes during pregnancy

See Chapter 3, page 122.

Changes in immune reactivity

The fetus contains antigens derived from the father and is therefore an allograft which is foreign to the mother. The reasons why the mother's immune system does not reject the fetus are not fully understood. One suggestion is that the mother produces blocking antibodies which inhibit the cell-mediated rejection process. The immunological changes in pregnancy seem to be relatively minor. They include a 30 per cent increase in neutrophils, a decrease in helper T-cells, a slight reduction in IgG, an increase in IgD and a slight depression in cell-mediated immunity. These and other unknown factors may limit, rather than abolish, the immunological response and a restrained rejection process may be necessary to prevent excessive growth of the placenta. Many diseases which are thought to have an autoimmune basis tend to remit in pregnancy.

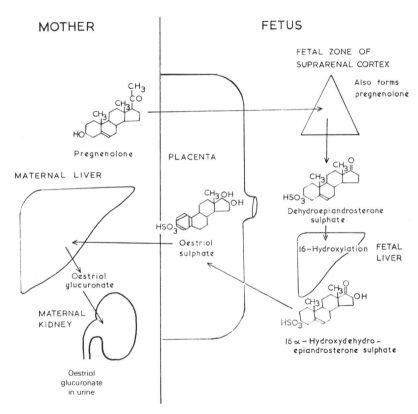

Fig. 1.25 Formation of oestriol during pregnancy

2

NORMAL PREGNANCY

THE DURATION OF PREGNANCY

In cases in which pregnancy has followed a single coitus the average duration of pregnancy from the date of intercourse is 266 days. If the calculation is made from the first day of the last menstrual period the average duration is 280 days because ovulation most frequently occurs on the 14th day of a 28 day menstrual cycle. However, there is considerable variation in the duration of normal pregnancy, even in cases in which the menstrual cycles were previously regular and of normal length, and also in cases in which the date of a single coitus is known. The method of estimating the most likely day of delivery is discussed on page 38.

SYMPTOMS OF PREGNANCY

AMENORRHOEA

Amenorrhoea is the earliest symptom of pregnancy. In a healthy woman whose menstrual periods were previously regular, if there is a sudden cessation of the periods the presumption must always be that she is pregnant unless some other cause of the amenorrhoea can be found. Amenorrhoea has not the same significance in the case of a woman whose periods were previously irregular, nor may it have any significance in a woman of menopausal age. Pregnancy has been known to occur in a young girl before a menstrual period has been observed, and it may arise during a period of amenorrhoea, for example during lactation or following discontinuation of oral contraception.

Conversely, difficulty may arise if there is bleeding during early pregnancy. Such bleeding may come from the cavity of the uterus before the decidua capsularis fuses with the decidua vera, but it is not be regarded as menstrual bleeding. Women with slight bleeding in the early weeks of pregnancy may prove to be completely normal, but such bleeding may be the first indication that the embryo is dead or dying.

MORNING SICKNESS

This may start as early as the first missed period. *See* pages 31 and 45.

BREAST SYMPTOMS

In the early weeks of pregnancy some tenderness and fullness of the breasts may be noticed.

FREQUENCY OF MICTURITION

During the first 12 weeks, when the uterus is still a pelvic organ, there is often some frequency of micturition, because the enlarging uterus presses on the bladder slightly, particularly in the daytime when the woman is standing.

ABDOMINAL ENLARGEMENT

Many women notice some abdominal fullness in early pregnancy at a time when the uterus is not much enlarged. This can only be the result of slight intestinal distension. Later on the uterine enlargement becomes evident, and sometimes it is this that first brings the patient to the doctor, especially in a case in which the menstrual periods were previously irregular. On the other hand, a woman sometimes thinks that she is pregnant because of abdominal swelling from some other cause, such as fat or an ovarian cyst.

QUICKENING

A primigravida usually first feels fetal movements between the 18th and 20th weeks of pregnancy, but multiparae may recognize the movements about two weeks earlier. At first the movements are slight, and may be confused with wind in the intestine. This very subjective symptom is not of much value in the diagnosis of pregnancy, as a woman who believes that she is pregnant will commonly declare that she feels movements.

SIGNS OF PREGNANCY

It will be seen that it is not possible to make a certain diagnosis of pregnancy from any of the symptoms given above, although a combination of them may be highly suggestive. The clinical diagnosis of pregnancy, especially in the first half, depends on a combination of symptoms and signs, and in every case an examination to seek confirmatory physical signs is required. Only when the pregnancy has advanced far enough for the parts of the fetus to be recognized clearly, for fetal movements to be palpable, or the fetal heart sounds to be heard, can the physical signs be said to be absolute.

The ultrasound demonstration of the embryonic heart movements, which is now possible using a transvaginal probe, within six weeks of the last menstrual period (LMP), or four weeks after implantation is an absolute sign of pregnancy. Subsequently, fetal structures can be easily visualized with ultrasound either by abdominal or vaginal routes.

SIGNS DUE TO CHANGES IN THE UTERUS

Enlargement of the body of the uterus

A slight enlargement of the body of the uterus is the earliest alteration which can be detected, but it is difficult to be certain of this if the patient has had a previous pregnancy. On bimanual examination the body is felt to be globular, and as progressive enlargement occurs the diagnosis becomes more evident.

Softening of the uterus

Softening of the uterus due to its increased vascularity is a useful sign, since although there are many other causes for uterine enlargement they do not, as a rule, cause softening. The lowest part of the body of the uterus softens first and, because of this, on bimanual examination the globular fundus may feel distinct from the still unsoftened cervix until about the ninth week of pregnancy (Hegar's sign). Deliberate attempts to elicit this sign should not be made, as they may cause unnecessary discomfort and even vaginal bleeding.

Softening and blue discolouration of the cervix

These changes soon follow the softening of the uterus, and are usually complete by the 16th week. When they are marked they are reliable signs of pregnancy, but in a few cases the cervix remains firm throughout pregnancy.

Progressive enlargement of the uterus

By the 12th week the fundus of the uterus is palpable in the abdomen just above the symphysis pubis and progressive enlargement of the uterus follows (Fig. 2.1). The fundus reaches the level of the umbilicus at about the 22nd week, and is just below the xiphisternum at the 36th week. If the presenting part of the fetus then sinks into the pelvis the fundus descends slightly, so that at term it is again at the level it occupied at the 34th week. The level of the fundus may be higher than expected from the duration of the pregnancy in cases of multiple pregnancy, polyhydramnios or fibromyomata, and at a lower level than expected with an abnormal, growth-retarded or dead fetus. If the fundus is at an unexpected level an error in the dates is of course to be considered.

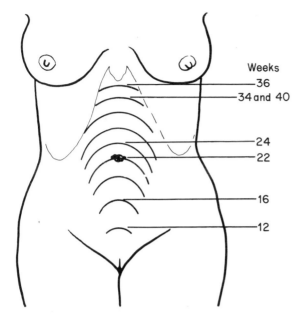

Fig. 2.1 Height of the fundus

Painless contractions

The pregnant uterus varies in consistency on palpation because it has intermittent painless contractions. If the patient is easy to examine these may be felt even when the uterus is still in the pelvis. When the uterus rises up into the abdomen the contractions are more easily felt, and are reliable evidence that any swelling under examination is in fact the uterus.

Uterine souffle

Because the blood flow through the vessels in the broad ligament is greatly increased during pregnancy, on auscultation with a stethoscope pressed firmly against the side of the uterus the uterine souffle may be heard at any time after the 20th week. It is a blowing murmur, synchronous with the maternal pulse. It is not diagnostic of pregnancy, as it may also be heard with some large uterine fibromyomata.

SIGNS DUE TO THE PRESENCE OF THE FETUS

Ballottement

From the 16th week until about the 30th week ballottement may occcasionally be observed. It depends upon the fact that at this stage of pregnancy the fetus is floating in a relatively large amount of liquor amnii.

Internal ballottement is felt on vaginal examination. A finger is placed in the anterior fornix with the patient lying on her back. If the fetus can be felt it is pushed upwards, when it will be felt to float away, and then fall back on the finger.

External ballottement is elicited on abdominal examination of a breech presentation, when the head may be felt to move between the two hands placed on either side of the fundus of the uterus.

Palpation of fetal parts

Abdominal palpation of fetal parts is usually possible from the 24th week onwards, and at a later stage the definite recognition of the head, back and limbs of the fetus is an absolute sign of pregnancy.

Fetal movements

During palpation fetal movements may be felt, and this is also an absolute sign. In a thin patient the movements can often be seen as well.

Fetal heart sounds

On auscultation of the abdomen with the fetal stethoscope the fetal heart sounds may be heard after the 24th week. The fetal heart rate varies between 120 and 160 beats per minute, and is therefore at roughly double the rate of the maternal pulse. The sounds are described as resembling the ticking of a watch under a pillow; there is a double sound to each beat, but more equal than the maternal heart beat, and at a different pitch.

Fetal heart movements can be detected from the sixth week with a real-time ultrasound scan, or from the 10th week with a simple Doppler-effect ultrasound machine. (*See* p. 37).

Funic souffle

The funic souffle is occasionally heard if the fetal stethoscope happens to lie directly over the umbilical cord. It is a soft, blowing murmur synchronous with the fetal heart sounds.

SIGNS DUE TO CHANGES IN THE BREASTS AND THE SKIN

These have already been described (*see* pp. 27, 28). The primary areola persists after the first pregnancy and this sign is therefore useless in the diagnosis of any subsequent pregnancy. Similarly, secretion can often be expressed from the breasts of any woman who has once been pregnant, even when she is not again pregnant.

DIAGNOSIS BY DETECTION OF HUMAN CHORIONIC GONADOTROPHIN

Pregnancy tests depend on the detection of large quantities of the gonadotrophic hormone produced by the trophoblast. This is found in the maternal circulation and is excreted in maternal urine after implantation. Human chorionic gonadotrophin (hCG) is a glycoprotein. The α subunit is also found in other hormones (e.g. LH, FSH) but the β subunit is specific for hCG.

TESTS PERFORMED ON MATERNAL URINE

The most certain results are obtained if the urine is concentrated, and for that reason it is best to test the first morning specimen.

Immunochemical tests

If the patient is pregnant her urine will contain hCG soon after the time of implantation. When anti-hCG is added to the urine it combines with the hCG and is neutralized. The mixture is now tested for anti-hCG with a suitable indicator and if none is found the test is positive for pregnancy.

If the patient is not pregnant, the urine does not contain hCG and the anti-hCG remains unfixed and will react with the indicator. A change in the indicator shows that the patient is *not* pregnant.

Anti-hCG is obtained from rabbits or sheep which have been immunized against hCG. Various indicators have been used, including hCG-coated latex particles or hCG-coated red blood cells. If the patient is not pregnant the latex particles are precipitated or the red cells are agglutinated.

The urinary output of hCG, which parallels the maternal blood levels during pregnancy, rises rapidly to reach a peak at about 12 weeks and then falls again to a much lower level (*see* Fig. 1.22). Tests for hCG are constructed to be negative until seven to 10 days after the missed period, and may even give negative results after the 16th week, but by then the diagnosis is easily made clinically or by ultrasound.

TESTS PERFORMED ON MATERNAL SERUM OR PLASMA

Immunoassays, such as radioimmunoassays and enzyme-linked immunoassays can be used to detect hCG or its β subunit at implantation, i.e. seven to 10 days after conception, even before the period has been missed. However, these tests require expensive reagents and laboratory equipment and are not used for clinical purposes. Assays for the detection of the β subunit are much less likely to give false-positive results due to cross-reaction with LH.

Radioimmunoassays are now being replaced by enzyme-linked immunosorbent assays (ELISA). These involve a double reaction, with the hCG sandwiched between the standard-phase antibody and the enzyme-labelled antibody. When urine containing hCG is run into a tube which has been coated with this double antibody binding occurs, and the enzyme-linked antibody becomes bound to the already captured hCG. The addition of an enzyme substrate, which is broken down by the bound enzyme, results in a blue colour – a positive end-point if pregnancy is present. In general ELISA tests are much more sensitive and just as specific as the agglutination tests, they can detect pregnancy at lower levels of hCG and so can predict gestation at eight to 10 days after fertilization (i.e. before the missed period).

High concentrations of hCG are seen in multiple pregnancy, and also in hydatidiform mole and choriocarcinoma when quantitative tests are routinely used. The detection of hCG is also of assistance in the diagnosis of ectopic pregnancy, a positive result in women with lower abdominal pain alerting the clinician to the possibility of this life-threatening condition, and a negative result virtually excluding it.

Very sensitive hCG tests such as these may give positive results for many weeks after a pregnancy has been delivered, failed or terminated, as small fragments of trophoblastic tissue continue to metabolize hCG in minute, but still detectable amounts.

False-positive results may occur rarely due to cross-reaction with LH when elevated levels are seen in the polycystic ovary syndrome, or together with elevated FSH in the climacteric or postmenopausally.

ULTRASOUND DIAGNOSIS OF PREGNANCY

With a real-time ultrasound scan (*see* p. 55) the gestation sac can often be diagnosed as early as five weeks from the first day of the last menstrual period, and a week later echoes representing the embryo within the sac can be obtained and cardiac pulsation may be recognised, particularly if a transvaginal transducer is used. Simple and easily portable machines (e.g. Sonicaid, Doptone) are available which employ a different principle. Ultrasonic waves are emitted by the head of the machine, which is placed against the skin of the abdomen. If the waves strike a moving surface, such as flowing blood, the reflected waves have an altered wave length, according to the Doppler principle. The alteration is detected by the apparatus, and in the case of the fetal heart the rhythmic changes in wave length are converted into audible signals, which are surprisingly similar to the fetal heart sounds. Blood flowing in any large maternal vessel will give the same effect, but the characteristic rate of the fetal heart makes the source of the signals clear. With these machines the fetal heart beat can be recognized at the 10th week.

DIFFERENTIAL DIAGNOSIS OF PREGNANCY

The pregnant uterus has to be distinguished from other abdominopelvic swellings, of which the commonest are fibromyomata, ovarian cysts and a distended bladder. Pregnancy may also be associated with these.

Uterine fibromyomata

When these tumours are deeply placed in the uterus they may enlarge it symmetrically, and they are sometimes soft enough to simulate the consistency of the pregnant uterus. However they do not cause amenorrhoea and pregnancy tests are negative.

Ovarian cysts

In many cases, on bimanual palpation, the unenlarged uterus can be felt separately from the ovarian cyst. Ovarian neoplasms will not cause amenorrhoea except in the unlikely event of their being bilateral and totally destroying both ovaries. A thrill or fluctuation is common with ovarian cysts, but is only felt in the pregnant uterus in cases of hydramnios. There is no clinical evidence of the presence of a fetus, and the pregnancy test is negative. Ultrasound examination will show the cyst wall, an empty uterus and absence of fetal parts.

Distended bladder

The bladder may become distended and then be mistaken for the uterus if there is retention of urine from incarceration of a retroverted gravid uterus (*see* p. 63). The direction of the cervix and the passage of a catheter disclose the diagnosis.

Pregnancy associated with fibromyomata

It can sometimes be difficult to diagnose pregnancy in a uterus with multiple fibromyomata. Pregnancy tests and ultrasound examination will be of value in early pregnancy. Later on small tumours can easily be mistaken for fetal parts. A fibromyoma in the uterine wall is immobile, unlike a fetal limb which alters its position from time to time. When the uterus contracts fetal parts become more difficult to feel, whereas a fibromyoma may become more evident. A fibromyoma in the pelvis may even be mistaken for the fetal head.

Pregnancy associated with an ovarian cyst

Two swellings are usually evident, the pregnant uterus and the cyst, but in some cases they are in such close juxtaposition that it is not easy to distinguish them. The combined swelling will then be larger than expected for the duration of pregnancy. Ultrasound scan will reveal the fetus within the uterus with the cyst as a separate cavity.

PSEUDOCYESIS

Pseudocyesis is a psychological disorder in which the patient has a false but fixed idea that she is pregnant. The term does not include the uncommon instances of wilful and conscious deception; the patient honestly believes that she is pregnant. Pregnancy fantasies may occur with other delusions in psychoses, but most patients with pseudocyesis do not have serious mental illness.

It is frequently, but not always, seen near or after the menopause, and not invariably in patients without children. There may be amenorrhoea, and the patient may declare that she has morning sickness and breast enlargement, and that she can feel fetal movements. The abdomen may appear distended, either by air collected in the stomach by aerophagy, by intestinal distension, by persistent contraction of the diaphragm with exaggerated lumbar lordosis or sometimes just by fat. The shape of the swelling is not that of the pregnant uterus, fetal parts cannot be felt and the fetal heart cannot be heard. If the patient is fat a pregnancy test or ultrasound scan may be required. The difficulty is to convince the patient that she is not pregnant.

ESTIMATION OF THE EXPECTED DATE OF DELIVERY AND ASSESSMENT OF MATURITY

Since there is no exact means of knowing the time at which conception occurred, it is usual and convenient to calculate the date on which delivery is to be expected from the first day of the last menstrual period, with the assumption that ovulation took place about 14 days after that. A simple practical method is to count forward nine calendar months (or backwards three months) from the first day of the last period, and to add seven days. This gives an average of 280 days, with a little variation as the lengths of the calendar months are not uniform. If the previous menstrual cycles were irregular or prolonged no reliance can be put on this method. Even if the previous cycles were regular, in as many as 40 per cent of cases labour begins more than seven days before or after the calculated date (*see* Fig. 2.2).

An attempt has often to be made to estimate the probable date of delivery or the maturity of the gestation when the date of the last menstrual period has been forgotten, when conception occurred during a phase of amenorrhoea, for example during lactation, or when conception took place soon after discontinuation of oral contraception. When decisions have to be made towards the end of pregnancy about the optimum moment for

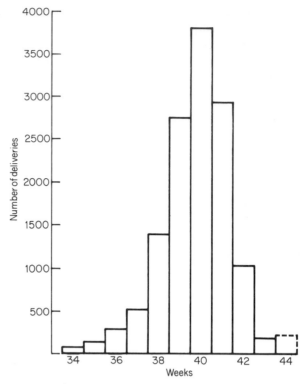

Fig. 2.2   Numbers of patients delivered each week in a sample of 13 634 single pregnancies (with certain dates of last menstrual period)

delivery an accurate record of observations made in early pregnancy may be found to be extremely useful; these early observations sometimes prove to be more reliable than those made later on.

Clinical observations

The date at which the patient first felt fetal movements gives a rough indication of maturity. Primigravidae usually feel fetal movements between 18 and 20 weeks, and multiparae may recognize the movements a little sooner, but a patient who cannot remember the date of ner last period is seldom able to give an accurate report of the date of quickening.

Bimanual examination by an experienced clinician performed between six and 12 weeks gives a fairly accurate assessment of uterine size. Subsequent repeated measurements of the height of the uterine fundus give only approximate estimates, with an error of perhaps ±4 weeks, and measure-

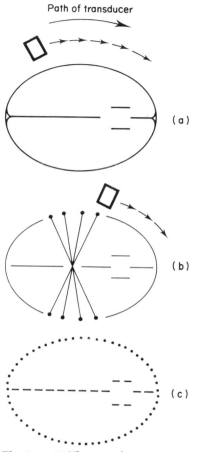

Path of transducer

(a)

(b)

(c)

Fig. 2.3 (a) The transducer moves over the head; (b) Series of retarded images; (c) Coalescing images make up a two dimensional image of the fetal head

ments of the abdominal girth are also an imprecise guide.

Ultrasound scan

Ultrasound measurements of the fetus provide a quick, safe and accurate method of dating a pregnancy, especially in the first 20 weeks. The crown–rump length is measured in the first trimester, thereafter the biparietal diameter, the abdominal circumference and the femur length are the most useful observations to record. The measurements are compared with standard curves showing normal increments of growth, and there is a straight-line relationship between the size of the fetal head and the duration of pregnancy before the 24th week; subsequently there is more variation.

Hormone assays

A novel application for assays of placental hormones and proteins is the assessment of gestational age at four to six weeks of pregnancy. A single determination of blood hCG, human placental lactogen (hPL) or schwangershaftsprotein 1 (SP1) can be applied to a formula that relates the logarithm of the hormone or protein result to the day of gestation. Since the error range is of the same order as accurate menstrual data and ultrasound scan, this may be useful in women with uncertain dates who decline to have an ultrasound scan at this time.

ANTENATAL CARE

Antenatal care and investigation is an important part of preventive medicine. Its object is to maintain the mother in health of body and mind, to anticipate difficulties and complications of labour, to ensure the birth of a healthy infant, and to help the mother rear the child.

If it is well conducted it does more than detect and treat abnormalities. It should establish contact and promote understanding between the woman and those who will look after her in pregnancy and labour. Some hospital clinics have justly been criticized as impersonal and overcrowded. Long waiting times, uncongenial decor and furnishing,

lack of privacy, poor facilities for children and inadequate time for the woman to talk to the doctor or midwife are faults which can often be rectified by better organization.

PREPREGNANCY COUNSELLING

It may be said that antenatal care should start before pregnancy. In a perfect world every woman might endeavour to secure that her health was in its best possible state before embarking on pregnancy. This idea should be more widely spread by all agencies responsible for health education.

The main structure of the organs of the embryo is laid down in the first eight weeks of pregnancy, and it is during this time that major congenital abnormalities arise. Much effort is devoted to the care of the pregnant woman and her fetus from about the 12th week onwards, but there is little medical support for the early embryo. Dietary, smoking and drinking habits may well call for advice from the doctor or midwife, and women of poor physique and those with social problems may need help.

Facilities will hardly permit every woman to seek medical advice before every possible conception, either from her general practitioner or from a hospital clinic, but prepregnancy counselling is of especial value for women with problems and anxieties. Such counselling may be the first medical examination that a young woman has had since leaving school, and health problems may be found which would otherwise only have been discovered at an antenatal booking clinic.

A prepregnancy counselling clinic might give advice to women with any of the following conditions:

women who have had an unsuccessful pregnancy from abortion or preterm labour, obstetric complications, intercurrent disease or fetal genetic abnormalities

women with some continuing disease who are anxious to know whether pregnancy would exacerbate this, or whether the child might be harmed. The list of possible conditions is unlimited, but includes heart disease, hypertension and renal disease, diabetes, haemoglobinopathies, epilepsy, thromboembolism, mental disease and treated malignant disease. Some women may be taking drugs for the control of their disease, and possible effects on the fetus might call for variation in the drugs or their dosage

women with a family history of disease. Such conditions as diabetes, epilepsy, haemophilia, sickle-cell disease, muscular dystrophy and Huntington's chorea, although some of them are rare, will call for advice about the possibility of inheritance. Genetic problems may require special investigation, including chromosomal studies by experts.

ANTENATAL CARE

The number of times a woman needs to be seen during her pregnancy will vary. The first visit, when she comes to make arrangements, should be as early in pregnancy as possible. Thereafter she should be seen every four weeks until the 30th week, fortnightly until the 36th week, and then weekly until the onset of labour. If complications arise more frequent visits will be necessary. However, a woman who has had at least one normal pregnancy may not need so many visits.

Today hospital delivery is advocated for the majority of women, but not all antenatal care has to be in hospital clinics. Shared care between the hospital and the woman's general practitioner or midwife is preferable in many normal cases, as this may save the patient travelling, promote better doctor–patient relationships, and allow individual care by reducing the numbers of patients attending hospital clinics. Women having shared care should attend the hospital to see the obstetrician for a booking visit. Thereafter, if all is well, the hospital visits are usually at 30 and 36 weeks, and weekly from term until the onset of labour, all other visits being to the general practitioner or midwife.

BOOKING VISIT

At the first visit the following procedure is followed:

General medical history

It is important to know whether the woman has had any significant illness, including cardiac disease, renal disease, diabetes, rubella, or a blood transfusion. Tactful enquiry should be made about possible exposure to HIV infection, whether or not she has taken drugs, her level of alcohol intake and how many cigarettes she smokes, as well as a brief survey of her general social and environmental circumstances. Previous surgical treatment, particularly gynaecological operations, may be relevant.

Family history

Any disease with a hereditary tendency, including diabetes and hypertension, is recorded. A family history of twins may be significant.

Past obstetric history

If the woman has been pregnant before, she is questioned about previous pregnancies and labours. For example, a history of repeated abortion or premature labour might suggest cervical incompetence, and intrauterine fetal death might suggest the possibility of hypertension, diabetes or rhesus incompatibility. A history of raised blood pressure might suggest pregnancy-induced hypertension, with the possibility of recurrence.

The history of previous labours is a guide to what may be expected in the coming labour. For example, if the woman has had a long labour ending in instrumental delivery, resulting perhaps in the birth of a dead or injured child, it is possible that she has pelvic contraction. A history of postpartum haemorrhage would be a warning of possible recurrence. It is essential to know the birthweights of any previous children. The cause of any stillbirth or neonatal death should be ascertained whenever possible, sometimes by writing to the doctor who was then in charge of the patient.

It is important to know whether the children were breast-fed, and of any feeding difficulties which may possibly be overcome by special advice.

History of the present pregnancy

This should then be taken. The date of the first day of the last menstrual period must be carefully recorded, with a note of the woman's normal cycle and of any irregularities. If she was using oral contraception this may be relevant, as may a history of subfertility.

The doctor will then proceed to examine the patient:

General examination

The woman is weighed, and her height and development are noted, including any abnormal gait or deformity. The breasts are examined to exclude a tumour, and to check the structure of the nipples for breast-feeding. The blood pressure is recorded, and the heart and lungs examined. The teeth should be inspected for the presence of gum infection and caries, and dental care encouraged. The legs should be examined for the presence of varicose veins, oedema and any other abnormality.

Abdominal examination

An examination of the abdomen is made, including auscultation of the fetal heart sounds if the pregnancy has reached 24 weeks. Before this time fetal blood flow may be detected with the portable ultrasound apparatus. Details of the method of abdominal examination are given on page 49.

Vaginal examination

In most clinics a vaginal examination is made at the woman's first visit. By this time the position of the uterus (anteverted or retroverted) and its size in relation to the menstrual history are determined, and any extrauterine abnormalities such as an ovarian cyst or a fibromyoma may be discovered. A cervical smear is taken for cytological examination. Some idea of the general shape of the pelvis may be gained, but efforts to estimate pelvic capacity are usually better postponed until the 36th week, when the tissues are more relaxed. For details *see* page 206.

Investigation

A chest X-ray is no longer performed as routine but it may be wise in women coming from countries where tuberculosis is still common. A midstream specimen of urine is examined for bacteria and tested for glucose and protein.

Blood is taken for determination of ABO and rhesus blood groups, and is screened for the presence of abnormal antibodies. Haemoglobin concentration is estimated, and for women of Afro-Caribbean, Asian and Mediterranean origin haemoglobin electrophoresis is performed to screen for haemoglobinopathy. Serological tests for syphilis are carried out, as well as rubella antibody screening, and if the woman is not rubella-immune a note is made to offer vaccination in the puerperium. In many clinics the serum is examined for α-fetoprotein at 16–18 weeks, a high level indicating a possible neural tube defect or other congenital abnormalities, and a low level predicting an increased risk of Down's syndrome. The presence in the blood of hepatitis B antigen should also be detected, so that precautions can be taken to avoid infection of attendants during venepuncture or delivery, and arrangements made to vaccinate the neonate. HIV antibody screening should be done in at risk women. A random blood sugar estimation is often performed.

Ultrasound examination

In many clinics a routine ultrasound scan is performed at the 16th week to confirm the gestational age and to exclude any gross fetal abnormality. A full anomaly scan may be done between the 18th and 20th week.

SUBSEQUENT VISITS

At every subsequent visit the blood pressure is recorded and the urine is tested. A careful check is kept on the woman's weight. Provided that it is within normal limits at the outset, the increase should not exceed 12 kg during the pregnancy. There is little, if any, increase during the first 12 weeks. From the 16th to the 28th week the average gain is about 6 kg, and thereafter weight is gained at about 2 kg every four weeks. Excessive weight gain should raise suspicion that the woman is developing hypertensive disease, or that she has an excessive intake of carbohydrate which needs to be checked.

The haemoglobin concentration is estimated again at the 30th and 36th weeks, and many clinics repeat the blood sugar estimation.

At every visit the height of the fundus is recorded, and from the 32nd week onwards the presentation of the fetus. After the 36th week it is important to determine whether the widest diameter of the fetal head has entered the brim of the pelvis, or if it has not done so, whether it can be made to engage. Any suspicion that fetal growth is impaired calls for full investigation of the case, usually by ultrasound measurement of the fetus.

What has been described is routine antenatal care. Any abnormality will demand further investigation and treatment, with more frequent visits to the clinic or admission to hospital for observation. Some special tests are described in the next section.

ANTENATAL MONITORING OF THE FETUS

Measurements of fetal growth

The most reliable indication of fetal well-being is normal growth. Assessment of fetal size by abdominal palpation is not to be undervalued, especially if the observations are made by one observer and carefully recorded. The fundus–symphysis pubis height is often measured, in centimetres, with a tape measure. Repeated ultrasound examination of the biparietal diameter of the fetal head and ultrasound measurement of the abdominal circumference of the fetus are more precise measurements which may be applied to any case in which there is clinical suspicion of retarded growth, or reason to fear it, for example in cases of hypertension.

Investigation of circulatory and other fetal responses

Apart from asking the mother to keep records of the fetal movements ('kick counts') antenatal recording of the fetal heart rate over a period of 20 minutes or so may be made with a cardiotocograph.

A normal fetus has periods of inactivity during which the heart rate shows little variation, and episodes of active movement, during which the heart rate shows increased beat-to-beat variation and accelerations. Uterine contractions of pregnancy may cause temporary slowing of the rate. A fetus that shows none of the normal variations in heart rate, or one that shows prolonged slowing of the heart rate with a uterine contraction, may be at risk of hypoxia. Blood flow in the placental, umbilical and fetal vessels may be assessed with modern Doppler blood flow machines.

Assay of hormones and enzymes to assess fetoplacental function

The placenta produces several hormones and enzymes and various measurements of these substances in maternal blood or urine have been used as placental function tests. Biophysical tests have largely superseded these, but human placental lactogen (hPL) and oestriol assays are still sometimes performed, either as a screening test or serially after the 30th week. The formation of oestriol by the fetus and placenta is described on page 12.

Investigations to exclude fetal abnormalities

Ultrasound screening will demonstrate the fetal sac and the fetus from very early in pregnancy but abnormalities of the fetus are only likely to be shown after the 16th week. In late pregnancy radiological examination is occasionally used if fetal abnormality or fetal death is suspected.

Liquor amnii may be obtained by abdominal paracentesis so that fetal cells found in it can be grown in tissue culture for chromosomal analysis, for example in cases of Down's syndrome (*see* p. 273). In some other inherited diseases biochemical study of the liquor is also helpful.

Chorionic biopsy is a new technique under trial, which allows earlier examination of fetal cells for chromosomal study. A cannula attached to a syringe is passed through the cervical canal or transabdominally into the uterine cavity and a sample of villi is obtained by aspiration.

In cases of open neural tube defects α-fetoprotein may be found in excess in maternal serum, and amniocentesis is then performed so that estimation of α-fetoprotein in the liquor can be done for confirmation (unless an ultrasound scan has confirmed the lesion).

Estimations of rhesus antibody titres in maternal blood and bilirubin concentrations in liquor amnii are frequently used in the management of cases of haemolytic disease (*see* p. 319).

Fetoscopy, performed by passing a fine cannula and fibreoptic system into the uterus through the abdominal wall, will allow inspection of the fetus, and aspiration of a blood sample for electrophoresis and other tests.

The technique of cordocentesis allows aspiration of blood from the umbilical cord under ultrasound visualization (*see* p. 272).

ADVICE TO THE PATIENT DURING PREGNANCY

During pregnancy the woman should be advised to attend the education classes which are now generally available at antenatal clinics. Usually, each woman is given a booklet, which she can read at leisure, with explanations of events in pregnancy and labour, advice about the care of her health and information about services available. With the advent of so many special investigations such as blood tests and ultrasound many clinics also have leaflets to explain these. The woman will also need information about financial grants and social services.

It is important to allay any anxiety about labour. A simple explanation of the stages of labour should be given to the woman so that she will know what

to expect. This is a convenient time to discuss analgesia and to demonstrate the use of gas and oxygen or trilene apparatus. It is helpful if the labour ward staff can meet the woman so that when she arrives in labour she does not find herself among complete strangers. If the woman's partner is to be present during labour he should also be given preparatory instruction.

DIET

A number of investigations on the effect of diet on the outcome of pregnancy have been made. It has been shown that a poor quality diet predisposes to premature labour and increased perinatal mortality, but claims that hypertension can be prevented by modification of the diet during pregnancy have not been substantiated.

There is no need for a large increase in calorie value of the diet; 2400 calories is recommended, but the distribution of its constituents requires consideration. Protein should be increased, and at least two-thirds of the protein should be of animal origin, i.e. meat, milk, eggs, cheese and fish. If these are taken the intake of fats will be adequate. Carbohydrates can be reduced slightly to compensate for the increased calorie value of the protein, and more severely restricted if weight reduction is necessary.

In the latter half of pregnancy there is need for a considerable increase in the intake of calcium, phosphorus and iron, and probably of other trace elements, to supply the needs of the growing fetus and to prepare for lactation. Milk, cheese, eggs, meat and fresh green vegetables are foods rich in mineral salts, and a well-balanced diet will contain sufficient minerals, except perhaps for calcium and iron.

Calcium

The amount of calcium required daily by an adult is 0.5 g; during pregnancy the amount is increased to 1.5 g. Calcium is contained in milk, cheese, some vegetables and bread. It is difficult to be sure that all the calcium taken is absorbed; for example, the phytic acid of bread flour produces an insoluble salt of calcium.

Iron

Many women have poor iron reserves at the beginning of pregnancy, so it is necessary to check the haemoglobin level throughout pregnancy. The daily absorption of iron from an ordinary diet is about 1.2 mg, while the requirement during pregnancy averages 3.5 mg (*see* p. 102). An iron supplement is therefore often given. The preparation commonly used is ferrous sulphate 200 mg three times daily. This may cause gastric irritation in some patients and constipation in others; ferrous fumarate 300 mg daily, or a slow-release preparation, may be used in these patients. During pregnancy anaemia from deficiency of folic acid may occur, and in many clinics combined pills are used, containing iron with a daily dose of 0.5 mg of folic acid.

REST AND EXERCISE

Although violent exercise is imprudent during pregnancy, the woman should be encouraged to continue all ordinary activities. Adequate sleep must be secured, with a sufficient number of hours in bed. Sleeplessness is occasionally troublesome towards the end of pregnancy. It may be treated, if it is severe enough, with sedatives such as promezathine hydrochloride 10 mg, benzodiazepines such as temazepam (Normison) 20 mg or flurazepam (Dalmane) 15 mg.

REGULATION OF THE BOWELS

Constipation is a troublesome complication in many pregnant women. With a diet containing plenty of fruit, vegetables and bran a daily action of the bowel can usually be ensured; otherwise mild aperients such as senna and lactulose may be prescribed.

COITUS

Women can be reassured that coitus is not harmful during pregnancy except when there is a threat to miscarry or a previous history of abortion. It should be avoided if there has been antepartum haemorrhage.

PREPARATION FOR LACTATION

The best preparation for lactation is to ensure that the expectant mother is aware of the normal course of events following delivery and is mentally prepared for breast-feeding.

Attention must be given during antenatal ex-amination to the nipples. A poorly developed, retracted or inverted nipple cannot be drawn into the infant's mouth, and may be traumatized because the baby cannot fix onto the nipple properly. The nipples should be examined to see whether they are retracted or inverted, and to ascertain whether they will protract. The external appearance of the nipple is not a certain guide and the base of the nipple should be gently pinched to make it protrude. If the nipples are retracted the mother should wear glass nipple shells during the day, and at night during the latter part of pregnancy, and this will in some cases correct the abnormality.

There should be no attempt to harden the nipples with spirit; only ordinary washing is necessary. Dry skin on the nipples may be treated with an occasional application of lanoline. Expression of the breasts during the last few weeks of pregnancy has been advocated as a way in which congestion may be prevented, but this requires special instruction to the mothers, and not all of them find it easy.

The breasts should be supported by a well-fitting brassiere which does not press upon the nipples.

ANTENATAL EXERCISES

In many clinics women are given instruction in antenatal exercises. These are directed more to posture and general physique than to the muscles especially concerned with childbirth. Many women benefit from instruction in muscular relaxation, so that they can relax voluntarily during the uterine contractions of the first stage of labour. Relaxation may also be achieved by deep breathing during pains. This is the basis of the method of so-called psychoprophylaxis. Other classes give instruction in yoga or 'active birth'.

DISORDERS OF PREGNANCY

The more serious disorders of pregnancy, such as abortion, antepartum haemorrhage, hypertensive conditions and polyhydramnios are described separately in later chapters. The complications mentioned here of less consequence.

VOMITING OF PREGNANCY (MORNING SICKNESS)

From about the sixth to the 12th week of pregnancy nausea or vomiting in the early morning is so common that it is accepted as a symptom of normal pregnancy. It usually occurs soon after waking, and is often retching rather than vomiting. It nearly always stops before the 14th week and does not disturb the patient's health or her pregnancy.

Since morning sickness sometimes occurs when the woman does not know that she is pregnant it seems to be caused by something other than a psychological reaction to pregnancy, and the increased incidence of vomiting in cases of twins and hydatidiform mole has led to the theory that it is the result of higher levels of chorionic gonadotrophin, or of sensitivity to it. The vomiting occurs at the time of peak output of this hormone in normal pregnancy, but studies comparing hormone levels and sensitivities in cases of excessive vomiting with those of normal controls have not consistently supported this theory.

If the vomiting is persistent and disturbs the patient's health it is termed *hyperemesis gravidarum*. In these severe cases the only biochemical abnormalities which have been found are those which are secondary to vomiting, starvation and dehydration, namely ketosis, electrolyte imbalance and vitamin deficiency. In the years before the management of electrolyte imbalance was understood hyperemesis was a significant cause of maternal mortality, and in fatal cases severe weight loss, tachycardia and hypotension, oliguria, neurological disorders from vitamin B deficiency and jaundice from hepatic necrosis were seen. In the last 20 years the incidence of hyperemesis in the United Kingdom has greatly diminished, and maternal deaths or cases requiring termination of pregnancy are now virtually unknown.

In some of the persistent cases there may be psychological factors. Mere removal to hospital without any other treatment often leads to dramatic and immediate improvement. Hyperemesis is almost unknown in so-called underdeveloped countries.

Management

In any case of severe or persistent vomiting it is essential to exclude any other possible cause for it such as pyelonephritis, intestinal obstruction, infective hepatitis or cerebral tumour.

Ordinary morning sickness can be simply treated by reassurance and sometimes by giving one of the antiemetics which have been proven to be non-teratogenic such as meclozine 25 mg, cyclizine 50 mg or promezathine 25 mg, up to three times daily.

If the vomiting is severe the patient is admitted to hospital. If it continues her dehydration, ketosis and electrolyte imbalance require treatment by intravenous fluids and antiemetics, and sometimes with vitamin supplements. The treatment is regulated by twice daily studies of the blood chemistry and cessation of vomiting, normal urinary output and weight gain are indications of recovery. Oral feeding is begun as soon as possible, starting with fluids and progressing to semi-solids and eventually to a full diet. The possible need for psychotherapy must be considered.

PTYALISM

An apparent increase in the amount of saliva occasionally occurs during early pregnancy. In extreme cases the patient spits out her saliva instead of swallowing it and lives in an aura of wet handkerchiefs. Treatment is unsatisfactory. Psychological factors should be borne in mind.

VARICOSE VEINS

Varicose veins of the legs may cause considerable discomfort during pregnancy, and may be associated with oedema and thrombosis. Fortunately pulmonary embolism from such thrombi is extremely rare. Support by elastic stockings may give some relief. Surgical treatment is not advised during pregnancy because the condition often improves considerably after delivery. The residual lesion should be assessed about three months after delivery before deciding on surgical treatment.

Vulval varices

Vulval varices may be uncomfortable during pregnancy, and are an occasional cause of a vulval haematoma during labour.

HAEMORRHOIDS

Haemorrhoids may first appear or be made worse during pregnancy. Surgical treatment is not advised during pregnancy except to evacuate a painful perianal haematoma under local anaesthesia. Aperients should be prescribed. The anal region should be carefully washed and dried after defaecation and analgesic ointment applied.

PRURITUS VULVAE AND VAGINAL DISCHARGE

An excess of vaginal discharge from any cause may lead to vulval pruritus. The commonest cause during pregnancy is infection with *Candida albicans* which may be associated with the lowered renal threshold for sugar which occurs in many pregnant women. In all cases of pruritus the urine should be tested for glucose, and if there is any reason to suspect the possibility of diabetes a glucose tolerance test will be required. In candidiasis there may be vulvitis with redness of the skin, or vaginitis with masses, or plaques, of white cheesy material lightly adherent to the epithelium. Microscopical examination of a little of the discharge in a drop of normal saline will show mycelial threads, and *Candida* will be grown on culture. A variety of fungicides may be used for treatment, including nystatin pessaries 100 000 units to be inserted for 14 successive nights with nystatin cream to the vulva, or clotrimazole (Canesten) pessaries and cream for three nights.

Vaginitis during pregnancy may also be caused by *Trichomonas vaginalis*, which causes a profuse offensive, purulent discharge, in which the organisms can be found on microscopical examination. Metronidazole tablets 200 mg three times daily by mouth for seven days may be used during pregnancy. No adverse effect on the fetus has ever been shown with this drug, but it may be wiser to rely on local treatment before the 12th week.

CRAMPS IN THE LEGS

Transient nocturnal painful spasms of the small muscles of the feet or of the muscles of the legs sometimes occur during pregnancy. Such cramps have been attributed to calcium deficiency, but there is no satisfactory evidence to support this. It is more likely that they are due to temporary circulatory insufficiency. The cramp tends to improve spontaneously in late pregnancy, but can be troublesome during labour.

ACROPARAESTHESIA

This is not uncommon during pregnancy. There is a sensation of pins and needles in the hands with some sensory loss, and sometimes weakness of the small muscles. The patient finds it difficult to use her hands for fine work. Acroparaesthesia has been attributed to oedema in the carpal tunnel involving the median nerve, and this will explain the cases in which the signs have the appropriate distribution, but in many cases the ulnar border of the hand, and sometimes even the forearm, is involved, and in these cases pressure on the lowest part of the brachial plexus near the first rib must be considered.

Some, but not all, patients obtain relief from diuretics such as chlorothiazide. Splinting the wrists at night is sometimes helpful. Recovery after delivery is the rule.

HARMFUL EFFECTS OF DRUGS ON THE FETUS

After the discovery that the drug thalidomide, when given to pregnant women, could cause gross fetal deformities, all drugs used during pregnancy have come under close scrutiny.

Thalidomide was used as a sedative and antiemetic but was withdrawn in 1962 after it was found to cause gross limb deformities (phocomelia) and other fetal abnormalities if given to the mother between the 30th and 70th days of pregnancy. Yet care is necessary before attributing any solitary case of deformity to a particular drug. In every 1000 viable births there will be about five perinatal deaths from congenital malformation and more than 10 other infants with malformations of clinical significance. The great majority of these malformations occur as a result of genetic disturbance or pathological events entirely unrelated to any drugs which the mothers may have taken during pregnancy. Properly controlled statistical study is always necessary in studying such relationships.

There are few drugs which do not pass the placental barrier, and possible effects on the fetus must always be considered when drugs are prescribed during pregnancy. It is an important principle of teratology that it is not so much the nature of any harmful agent as the time in embryonic development at which it acts that chiefly determines the abnormality produced. In general, the earlier in pregnancy that a teratogenic agent acts the more severe will be the malformation. Furthermore, there is a short critical period during which each developing structure is particularly vulnerable. In addition there seem to be many maternal factors which affect the outcome, such as the standard of nutrition and hormone levels. It should be a general principle to avoid the administration of any drug during the early weeks of pregnancy unless it is clearly necessary for the treatment of a maternal condition.

In Great Britain there is an expert Committee on the Safety of Drugs which insists that adequate tests are carried out on pregnant animals before a drug is used for women. There is a scheme for the voluntary notification by doctors to the General Register Office through regional medical officers of all malformations present at birth, whether the baby is born alive or is stillborn. A central register is kept, and it is hoped that any national or regional incidence of malformations will be noticed and investigated.

A brief account of possible teratogenic and other adverse effects of drugs during pregnancy follows.

SEDATIVES AND ANALGESICS

Morphine and pethidine

Morphine or pethidine, given within two or three hours of delivery, will depress the fetal respiratory centre. This effect can be antagonized by an injection of naloxone.

Heroin

If the mother is a heroin addict the baby may show withdrawal symptoms after delivery, with restlessness and failure to feed, and consequent loss of weight.

Aspirin

Non-steroidal anti-inflamatory drugs such as aspirin and indomethacin may inhibit prostaglandin synthesis and produce premature closure of the fetal ductus arteriosis. They may postpone the onset of labour.

Diazepam

Diazepam (Valium) administered in large doses before delivery will depress the fetal medullary centres and cause loss of the normal base-line variation of the heart rate, and there is hypotonia after delivery.

Phenytoin

Phenytoin (Epanutin) given to control epilepsy is a folic acid antagonist, and if it is used during pregnancy additional folic acid must also be given.

DRUGS AFFECTING THE CARDIOVASCULAR SYSTEM

Digitalis

Digitalis has no harmful effect on the fetus.

Hexamethonium

Hexamethonium may cause ileus in the newborn child.

Reserpine

Reserpine will cause a transitory non-infective nasal discharge in the infant, but neither reserpine nor hexamethonium is used very often.

Propanolol and atenolol

With propanolol and atenolol there may be fetal bradycardia and neonatal circulatory depression.

Antihypertensives

Methyldopa, bethanidine, guanethidine and hydralazine seem to have no harmful effect on the fetus. Both atropine and scopolamine accelerate the fetal heart rate, but the effect is transitory and not harmful.

ANTICOAGULANT DRUGS

Heparin

Heparin does not cross the placenta.

Oral anticoagulants

Oral anticoagulants reach the fetus. Warfarin may cause bony abnormalities if it is administered in early pregnancy, and in late pregnancy there may be retroplacental haemorrhage or bleeding into fetal tissues, with intrauterine death. Intravenous or subcutaneous heparin is therefore preferable, at least during the first trimester and the last four weeks of pregnancy.

ANTIBACTERIAL DRUGS

Sulphonamides

Sulphonamides compete with bilirubin for binding sites on serum albumin, and therefore increase any possible risk of kernicterus after birth.

Salicylates

Salicylates may act in a similar way to sulphonamides, so that it is wise to discontinue these drugs before birth if there is any probability of premature birth or if there is rhesus incompatibility.

Co-trimoxazole

Co-trimoxazole is a folate antagonist and therefore a possible teratogen.

Tetracyclines

The children of mothers taking tetracyclines during pregnancy may have greenish-yellow staining of their milk teeth, and there may be interference with their bone growth.

Streptomycin

With streptomycin there is a theoretical risk of damage to the 8th nerve of the fetus, but with ordinary doses this seems to be very rare.

Chloramphenicol

Chloramphenicol may cause postnatal collapse and hypothermia. The penicillins, erythromycin and most other antibiotics pass into fetal blood and the amniotic fluid, but seem to have no harmful effect.

Metronidazole

Metronidazole has not been proven to be teratogenic, but it is not usually prescribed in the first trimester (*see* p. 46).

HORMONES

Progestogens

Androgens such as testosterone should not be given to the mother during pregnancy as they may cause virilization of a female fetus. Synthetic progestogens, whose chemical structure is related to that of testosterone, given in cases of threatened or habitual abortion, have also caused virilization.

Allyloestrenol and dydrogesterone are safer than ethisterone or norethisterone, and hydroxyprogesterone hexanoate seems to be without risk (although it is of doubtful value for this purpose).

Diethylstilboestrol should not be given to pregnant women as it may cause vaginal septal defects in female fetuses, or vaginal adenosis which may rarely proceed to vaginal carcinoma 15 to 20 years later.

Adrenal steroids

Adrenal steroids may be given in physiological doses to pregnant women with Addison's disease without risk to the fetus. In a few uncommon diseases, such as lupus erythematosus, polyarteritis nodosa, status asthmaticus and thrombocytopenic purpura, steroids are used in larger pharmacological doses. Animal experiments have suggested that there may be some risk of fetal cleft palate, but human evidence is doubtful, and it is justifiable to use these drugs for severe maternal illness.

RADIOACTIVE SUBSTANCES

Radioactive isotopes of iodine, strontium and phosphorus cross the placenta and become localized in fetal tissues. Neither these substances nor any others which emit gamma rays should be used during pregnancy.

ANTITHYROID DRUGS

Drugs such as thiouracil or large doses of iodine may cause fetal goitre or hypothyroidism.

CYTOTOXIC AND ALKYLATING DRUGS

All of these, including methotrexate, busulphan, cyclophosphamide, chlorambucil and many others may harm the fetus. They are unlikely to be called for during pregnancy, but if there is a disease such as leukaemia in the mother it may be necessary to give such drugs in spite of the fetal risk.

SMOKING DURING PREGNANCY

Smoking during pregnancy is harmful to the fetus and will cause reduction in birth weight with an increase in perinatal mortality. It has been suggested that raised maternal carbon monoxide levels produce an increase in carboxyhaemoglobin which interferes with oxygen transport, but the ill-effects are more likely to be caused by nicotine which has a vasoconstrictive effect on maternal vessels in the placental bed. The adverse effect of smoking is greater if the mother is hypertensive.

ALCOHOL DURING PREGNANCY

Children born to mothers who are severely addicted to alcohol have a low birth weight and an increased neonatal and infant mortality. A few will have the fetal alcohol syndrome with a characteristic facial appearance, with a broad base to the nose, epicanthic folds, a long upper lip and a small lower jaw, with mental retardation. There is an increased incidence of other serious malformations. While no harmful effect has been shown from small doses of alcohol, on general principles even these must be undesirable in the early weeks of pregnancy.

OBSTETRICAL EXAMINATION

Any obstetrical examination should be preceded by consideration of the history, including the past medical record, the past obstetric history and the record of the present pregnancy.

ABDOMINAL EXAMINATION

By abdominal examination it is possible to ascertain:

the size of the uterus, and to note whether it corresponds with the period of amenorrhoea
the size of the fetus
the lie, presentation and attitude of the fetus
the relationship between the brim of the pelvis and the presenting part
whether the fetus is alive
the presence of abnormal conditions, such as excess of liquor amnii, twin pregnancy or abdominal tumours.

Inspection

By inspection an impression of the general shape and size of the uterus can be gained and fetal movements may be seen. If the occiput is anterior and the back of the fetus is to the front, the abdomen will appear smoothly convex; if the occiput is posterior, a flattening of the abdomen may be seen above the symphysis pubis. If the lie is transverse the uterus will be wider than usual, and the height of the fundus may be a little lower than with a longitudinal lie. If twins are present the uterus also appears wide but the height of the fundus will be higher than normal.

Palpation

The obstetrician stands on the patient's right side. A regular routine is followed:

The level of the fundus

The level of the fundus is determined by using the ulnar border of the hand and little finger and moving it downwards from the xiphisternum (Fig. 4.18(a)). Many obstetricians measure the distance between the upper edge of the symphysis pubis and the top of the fundus with a centimetre tape. From 14 to 34 weeks the distance in centimetres approximates to the weeks of gestation.

The presentation

As the majority of fetuses present by the vertex, the lower part of the uterus should be palpated next to establish whether the presentation is cephalic. This is done by placing both hands on the lower abdomen above the pelvic brim (Fig. 4.18(b)). The head is recognized because it is rounder and harder than the breech. Its mobility will depend upon its relation to the pelvic brim. If it is completely above the brim it is freely moveable (and is spoken of as floating above the brim) and the fingers of both hands can be made to meet below it; if the widest diameter has entered or passed through the brim the head is usually fixed and is described as engaged in the brim; if the head is deeply sunk in the pelvic cavity it may be difficult to feel it except with the finger tips.

The relationship between the head and the pelvis is described in 'fifths' (Fig. 4.19). A head that is completely free is described as 5/5; one that is beginning to enter the brim as 4/5, and one that has

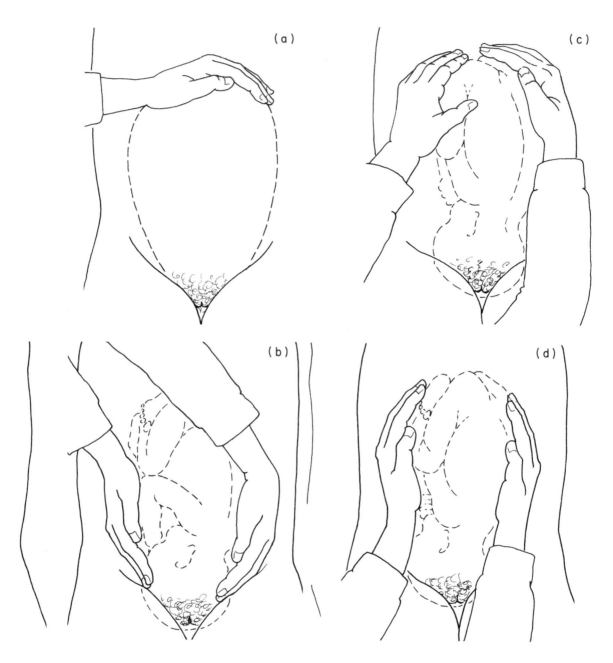

Fig. 2.4   Abdominal palpation. (a) determination of the level of the fundus of the uterus; (b) palpation of the lower pole of the uterus. In this case the head is well-flexed. The occiput is deep in the pelvis and would not be palpable, whereas the sinciput would be easily felt; (c) palpation of the upper pole. The breech is felt; (d) palpation of the sides of the uterus. The back is felt on the right and limbs on the left

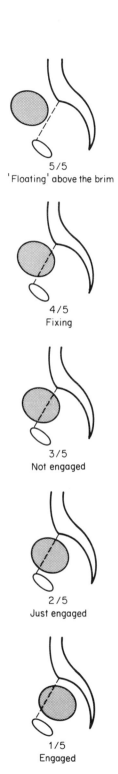

5/5
'Floating' above the brim

4/5
Fixing

3/5
Not engaged

2/5
Just engaged

1/5
Engaged

Fig. 2.5 Description of the position of the head in 'fifths'

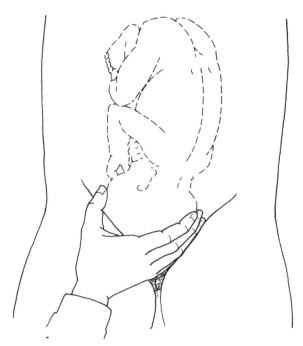

Fig. 2.6 Palpation of the lower pole of the uterus by Pawlik's method

a major part in the brim as 3/5. Once the widest diameter has passed the brim the notation 2/5 is used, and for a head deeply engaged in the pelvis 1/5. The fifths refer to the proportion of the head still palpable above the brim.

The degree of flexion of the head can often be made out by abdominal palpation. For example with a LOT position of the occiput the well-defined forehead (sinciput) will be felt on the right, but the occiput is less easily felt on the left as it is at a lower level, indicating that the head is well flexed. In such a case the anterior shoulder will be palpable near the midline (Fig. 2.4(b)).

If the head is above the brim of the pelvis it may be felt more easily by the single-handed grip shown in Fig. 4.20.

Palpation of the fundus

The fundus should then be palpated with both hands (Fig. 2.4(c)). If the breech occupies the fundus a broad mass will be felt; this is not as round or hard as the head. The breech is continuous with the fetal back, and a foot or knee can often be felt near it and may move under the hand. If the head occupies the fundus it is felt as a harder,

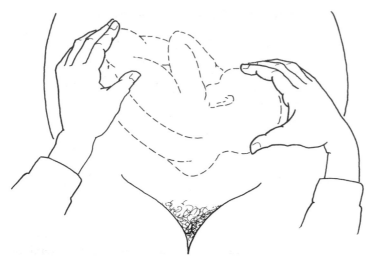

Fig. 2.7   Abdominal palpation of fetus lying transversely

rounder, smoother and more mobile mass than the breech. The head can be moved independently of the body, and it can sometimes be ballotted between the two hands.

Abdominal palpation

The sides of abdomen are then palpated to discover on which side the back lies. If the back is directed more to the front than to the back a broad smooth surface will be felt on one side of the abdomen, and on the other side a number of small knobs, which are the limbs (Fig. 2.4(d)). If these small parts are felt all over the abdomen the back must be directed posteriorly and to the side, and deep palpation may be necessary to feel it.

If the fetus is lying transversely the head is felt in one flank and the breech is felt in the other; if it is lying obliquely the head is often felt in one iliac fossa, and the breech higher up on the opposite side (Fig. 2.7).

Exclusion of cephalopelvic disproportion

In the last four weeks of pregnancy, if the head is presenting but is above the brim, an attempt is made to discover if it will engage, and thus to exclude cephalopelvic disproportion developing in labour. This may be done by moderate pressure on the head in a backwards and downwards direction. Another method is to raise the patient's head and shoulders, asking her to take the weight of her trunk on her hands or elbows, and the head will often enter the brim (Fig. 2.8). Perhaps the best method of all to test whether the head will engage is to examine the patient when she is standing.

At each visit the level of the fundus and the size of the fetus must be carefully noted. If the duration of pregnancy is uncertain repeated observations are most useful, and any suggestion that the fetus is small-for-dates or is not growing normally calls for investigation by ultrasound (*see* p. 61). If the uterus is larger than expected there may be an excess of liquor amnii or a multiple pregnancy. Twins may be diagnosed by palpation of more than two fetal poles, and often two heads are clearly recognized. Ultrasound will confirm the diagnosis.

Auscultation

The fetal heart sounds are listened for. They are best heard over the back of the fetus in vertex and breech presentations; it is only in face presentations that they are heard over the front of the fetus. In occipitoposterior positions, in which the back is directed to one side and posteriorly, the sounds may be heard either in the flank or near the midline.

In breech presentations the heart sounds will often be heard at a higher point in the abdomen than in vertex presentations, at the level of or a little above the umbilicus, unless the breech is

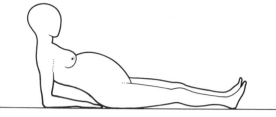

Fig. 2.8 Abdominal palpation. The patient is asked to sit up (or to lean on her elbows) to test whether the head will engage

deeply engaged, when they will be heard at the usual level.

VAGINAL EXAMINATION

A vaginal examination is often made at the patient's first attendance at the antenatal clinic to confirm the pregnancy and its duration, to determine the position of the uterus and to exclude other abnormalities such as ovarian cysts. The bony pelvis may also be examined, but the best time to assess the size and shape of the pelvis is at about the 36th week, by which time the soft tissues will be more relaxed and examination is easier. Further details of pelvic assessment are given on page 206.

However, most patients attending antenatal clinics are examined by ultrasound, which will confirm the duration of pregnancy, show that the fetus is alive, and exclude other abnormalities. If this is done it may be better not to examine the patient vaginally. A few women miscarry in early pregnancy and may blame vaginal examination for this.

Full aseptic precautions are required for a pelvic examination of any patient who may be in labour. During labour the most important observations will be the degree of dilatation of the cervix, whether the membranes are ruptured or not, the recognition of the presenting part, and the deter-

mination of its position and level in the pelvis.

Some obstetricians use the *Bishop score* to record the state of the cervix (Table 2.1). It enables different observers to relate their findings accurately. A score of less than 5 suggests that labour is unlikely to start without ripening of the cervix; a score of 7 indicates that labour should commence easily. This information is valuable if, for any reason, induction is contemplated.

The ischial spines are useful landmarks in determining the level of the presenting part during labour, and the degree of flexion or extension of the head can be found by palpation of the fontanelles. Feeling the posterior fontanelle indicates that the head is well flexed; feeling the anterior fontanelle indicates that the head is not well flexed, this is usually associated with occipitolateral or occipitoposterior positions.

RADIOLOGICAL EXAMINATION

With the development of ultrasound examination there is now hardly any place for radiological examination in obstetrics. Excessive irradiation of the fetus, particularly in the early weeks, may produce fetal abnormalities or cause abnormal mutations in the genes of the sex cells. It has also been suggested that even moderate exposure to irradiation *in utero* may increase the incidence of leukaemia in childhood, although this has not been universally accepted. It is therefore wise to avoid radiological examination as far as possible during pregnancy, and whenever the required information can be obtained by ultrasound examination that is to be preferred. Radiological pelvimetry may still have a limited place (*see* p. 206). Where this is indicated it should be done late in pregnancy, with as few exposures as possible.

ULTRASOUND EXAMINATION

See next section.

Table 2.1   Modified Bishop score

Score	0	1	2	3
Dilatation of cervix (cm)	0	1 or 2	3 or 4	5 or more
Consistency of cervix	Firm	Medium	Soft	–
Length of cervical canal (cm)	>2	2–1	1–0.5	<0.5
Position of cervix	Posterior	Central	Anterior	
Station of presenting part (cm above ischial spines)	3	2	1 or 0	Below

ULTRASOUND EXAMINATION IN OBSTETRICS

The introduction of ultrasound scanning has brought a new dimension to obstetric diagnosis and its use is now widespread and increasing. Ultrasound is technically defined as sound of higher frequency than that audible to the human ear but in clinical practice is limited to frequencies in the range from 1 to 10^7 cycles per second, i.e. 1–10 MHz. Obstetric ultrasound is usually performed in the range 3–5 MHz.

Current methods of examination employ reflected ultrasound to produce an image. The image is built up by energy reflected back from the transmitted beam from the transducer. The reflections come from organ interfaces, vessel walls and parenchymal tissue. The amount of energy reflected depends upon the orientation of the reflecting interface and the difference in acoustic impedance of the tissues at the interface. As the beam passes through tissue it is attenuated and the degree of attenuation determines the amount of energy reaching a given organ or interface. The ultrasound image is the result of the interplay of these two acoustic properties of tissue – reflection and attentuation. A tissue may be reflecting or non-reflecting, attenuating or non-attenuating. The same transducer is used both for transmitting and receiving; several different methods are used for detecting and displaying reflected echoes:

A-MODE

In A-mode the echoes are displayed as vertical spikes along the base line of a cathode ray tube with the height of the spike related to the amplitude of the detected echo. A-mode can be used in obstetrics to measure distances, as for example the biparietal diameter of the fetal skull (Fig. 2.9).

B-MODE

In B-mode the reflected echoes are represented by spots of light on the cathode ray tube. The brightness of each spot corresponds to the intensity of the reflected echo. B-mode is used for two-dimensional scanning.

B-scans can be produced in various ways: the original B-scanner was an articulated static scanner in which the image was obtained by moving the

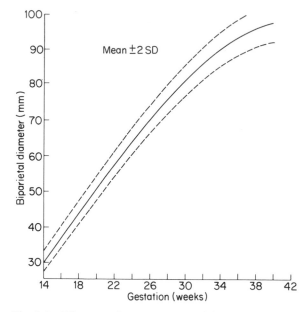

Fig. 2.9 Ultrasound measurement of the biparietal diameter of the fetal head

transducer over the body surface. By scanning a number of overlapping areas a compound picture was built up on the screen, each arc image being stored by the cathode ray tube (storage scope).

Real-time scanning

This form of B-scanning has replaced static B-scanning in routine obstetric ultrasound practice. Real-time images do not require a storage scope. They are perceived as continuous if the frame rate exceeds flicker-fusion frequency. The static scanner can cover a larger field of view but the moving image of the real-time scanner allows the observer the best chance of making an intelligent assessment of three-dimensional anatomy, of noting moving structures, and of selecting the most useful clinical anatomical cross section. Although real-time scanners do not have a storage scope, the digital memory (scan converter) allows a high quality freeze frame to be held on the screen. Two categories of real-time scanners are in common use for obstetric (and gynaecological) scanning:

Linear array

In this machine the ultrasound beam is derived from a number of transducer elements arranged in a line and firing sequentially. The linear format is particularly suitable for fetal imaging and the machines have the advantage of being small and relatively portable.

Mechanical sector

In this type of machine the transducer is oscillated round its own axis thus giving a large field of view. The resolution obtained with these scanners is very good, which makes them particularly suitable for the detailed scanning required to detect fetal cardiac abnormalities, for example, and, in gynaecology, the growth and development of ovarian follicles. Transvaginal sonography is a new development that will enable even more detailed examination of first trimester pregnancy and of the pelvic organs.

MEASUREMENTS USING ULTRASOUND

With care and experience very accurate measurements can be made of the fetus from early to late pregnancy. The accuracy of the measurements is limited by the physical limitations of the instruments as well as by observer error. At 3.5 MHz the resolution is no better than 1 mm, which for practical purposes means that measurements can only be made to the nearest whole millimetre. Electronic calipers on the display screen are now commonly used but although they make measuring easier, the same limitations of accuracy of measurement apply.

CLINICAL APPLICATIONS OF ULTRASOUND

The greater availability of ultrasound machines has led to the widespread use of diagnostic ultrasound in clinical obstetrics. In addition to ultrasonic fetal heart rate monitors of varying degrees of complexity, a simple linear array real-time scanner has become part of the normal equipment for both the antenatal clinic and the labour ward. Over 90 per cent of pregnant women in the UK have at least one scan, usually between 16 and 20 weeks gestation.

ULTRASOUND SCANNING IN THE FIRST AND SECOND TRIMESTERS

In all transabdominal ultrasound examinations in early pregnancy the best image is obtained when the patient has a fully distended urinary bladder. This is unneccessary with transvaginal probes.

Pregnancy diagnosis

The diagnosis of pregnancy can be made between five and six weeks after the last menstrual period (Fig. 2.10). At this time a gestational sac can be seen in the uterus and about one week later an embryo can be seen within the sac. It is usually possible at this stage to detect cardiac pulsation and to measure the crown–rump length. At the 12th week the placenta can be clearly identified and its position defined (Fig. 2.11).

Abortion

Bleeding in early pregnancy may cause destruction of the embryo. An early ultrasound scan in supposed threatened abortion will indicate whether or not the gestation sac and its contained embryo have survived and will thereby determine clinical management. In some cases the embryo dies either as a result of bleeding or because of some developmental defect giving rise to a so-called blighted ovum (Fig. 2.12). The finding of an empty gesta-

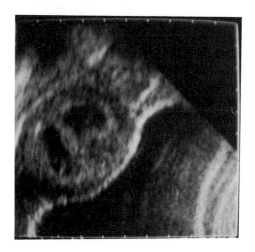

Fig. 2.10 Ultrasound scan of early twin pregnancy, 6 weeks

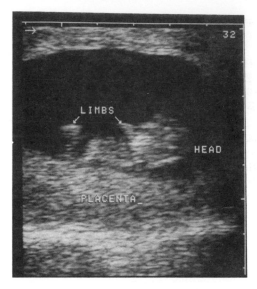

Fig. 2.11 Ultrasound scan of normal 10 week pregnancy

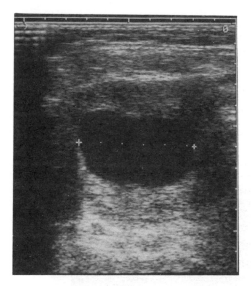

Fig. 2.12 Ultrasound scan of amniotic sac showing anembryonic pregnancy (blighted ovum)

tional sac after eight weeks indicates that the pregnancy is at an end although the products of conception may be retained in the uterus for some time (missed abortion). Twin pregnancy is a cause of first trimester bleeding and an ultrasound scan may reveal that one twin is aborting whilst the other survives.

Ectopic pregnancy

Transabdominal sonography has not been very reliable in visualizing tubal or other ectopic pregnancies. If an intrauterine gestation sac is seen in a patient with suspected ectopic pregnancy it virtually excludes a tubal pregnancy, since the two very rarely coexist (Fig. 2.13). On the other hand, if the uterus appears to be empty, an ectopic pregnancy cannot be excluded. Diagnosis of ectopic pregnancy is based on clinical examination, β-hCG assay and laparoscopy. In the future, however, transvaginal sonography is likely to become the main diagnostic technique.

Hydatidiform mole

The ultrasound appearance of this condition has a characteristic 'snowstorm' appearance and in a typical case enables the diagnosis to be made with confidence.

Multiple pregnancy

The diagnosis of twin pregnancy has been radically improved by ultrasound scanning. Two separate gestational sacs can be recognized before 10 weeks (*see* Fig. 2.10). After that, it is important to identify the head and body of each fetus in each sac. If one fetal head is deep in the pelvis it may be

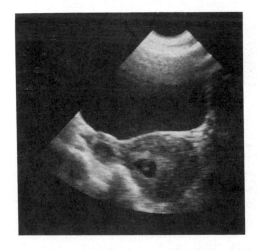

Fig. 2.13 Ultrasound scan of uterus containing normal gestation with ectopic pregnancy beside it

missed if the sonographer is not thorough in the examination. Because the ultrasound scan is only a slice through the area studied, care must be taken not to mistake two circles in different slices representing the head and thorax of a single fetus for two separate fetal heads. Similar difficulties may be met when there are more than two fetuses present.

Dating a pregnancy

One-third of all women attending the antenatal clinic either do not know for certain the date of their last menstrual period, have an irregular cycle or have been taking oral contraception. Measurement of the crown–rump length of the embryo is a good indicator of gestational age between six and 12 weeks. The biparietal diameter (*see* Fig. 2.9 and Fig. 2.14) of the fetal skull gives a very good indication of gestational age in the second trimester when the growth of the fetal head is rapid and variation in head size is small. In the third trimester the growth rate falls off and the biparietal diameter shows a much greater variation with the duration of pregnancy. For this reason ultrasound estimations of gestational age in the last trimester are of much less value to the clinician and need to be treated with caution. Sometimes the fetal head is

longer and narrower than normal (dolichocephaly) and this too can be a source of error in dating, although an experienced observer will note the longer than normal occipitofrontal diameter and will make due allowance for the narrower biparietal diameter. The biparietal diameter is by definition the widest transverse diameter of the head and failure to measure the head diameter at this point is another source of error, particularly if the head is deep in the pelvis. In spite of the possible sources of error there is no doubt that measurement of the fetal biparietal diameter gives a very good indication of gestational age and therefore of the expected date of delivery. An ultrasound examination of the fetus in the second trimester should give the expected date of delivery to within seven days (*see* Fig. 2.9). The fetal femur length is usually measured as well, as it correlates well with gestational age (Fig. 2.15).

Detecting congenital abnormality

Congenital abnormalities make a major contribution to perinatal morbidity and mortality. The early detection of fetal anomalies is one of the most important applications of ultrasound in pregnancy and there are strong arguments in favour of routine scanning of all pregnant women at 18 to 20 weeks gestation, when most of the major abnormalities

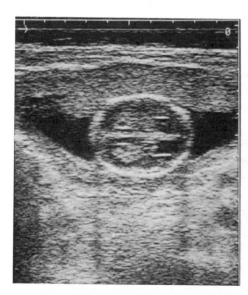

Fig. 2.14 Ultrasound scan of normal fetal head. The cerebral ventricles are seen, filled by the echogenic choroid plexus. The biparietal diameter can be measured at right angles to the midline echo

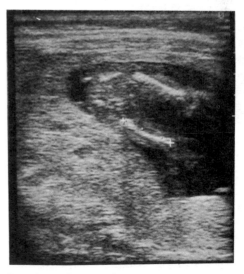

Fig. 2.15 Ultrasound scan of the femora of the fetus are shown and can be measured

can be detected. Considerable experience is required by the ultrasonographer before anomalies can be diagnosed with confidence and even with experienced observers, more than one examination may be needed.

Abnormalities of the central nervous system

Ultrasound scanning allows an early diagnosis to be made in cases of anencephaly (Fig. 2.16), hydrocephaly (Fig. 2.17), encephalocele (Fig. 2.18) and microcephaly. Spina bifida (Fig. 2.19) with or without hydrocephaly or meningomyelocele can also be diagnosed with a high degree of accuracy. Ultrasound is particularly useful when this abnormality is suspected as a result of serum alpha-fetoprotein screening, since, by this means, amniocentesis for assay of amniotic fluid α-fetoprotein can often be avoided.

Cardiac abnormalities

The heart chambers and valves can usually be visualized with real-time scanners and the heart rate counted. With experience many of the major abnormalities such as Fallot's tetralogy, left heart hypoplasia and atrioventricular valve atresia can be diagnosed. This is particularly important in the case of abnormalities which can be corrected surgi-

cally as the baby can then be delivered in a unit with facilities for paediatric cardiac surgery.

Abdomen and thorax

The diaphragm can be clearly seen and diaphragmatic hernias detected – another condition in which prenatal diagnosis makes early neonatal

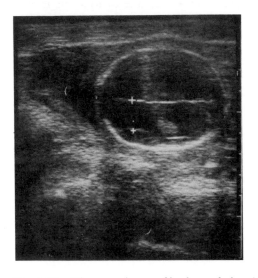

Fig. 2.17   Ultrasound scan of hydrocephaly with distended ventricles

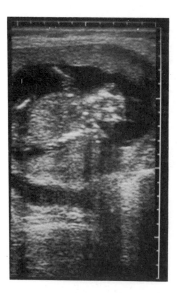

Fig. 2.16   Ultrasound scan of anencephalic fetus detected early in pregnancy

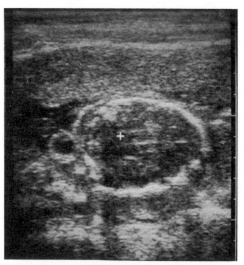

Fig. 2.18   Ultrasound scan of fetal head showing an encephalocele to the left of the figure

operative repair easier to arrange. Within the abdomen, hydronephrosis, polycystic or absent kidneys and urethral valves causing gross bladder distension can all be diagnosed by ultrasonic examination. Deficiencies in the anterior abdominal wall such as omphalocele and gastrochisis are also revealed by ultrasound. They may be associated with atresia of the bowel. Oesophageal atresia should be suspected when the fetal stomach cannot be visualized. Fetal ascites due to hydrops is also readily seen.

Other abnormalities

Abnormalities of the fetal limbs such as achondroplasia and osteogenesis imperfecta can be diagnosed in the second trimester. Excess (polyhydramnios) and deficiency (oligohydramnios) of amniotic fluid can be recognized subjectively, although precise quantification is not possible. As real-time equipment improves, imaging of the fetus will be easier and more subtle abnormalities will be detected by the experienced observer. Experience and skill will continue to be of very great importance in all ultrasound examinations made to detect fetal anomaly.

Guiding invasive procedures

Many genetic conditions can be diagnosed prenatally by analysing fetal samples. As well as ensuring that the fetus is alive and at the appropriate gestational age for the test, a real-time ultrasound probe held on the maternal abdominal wall can provide simultaneous guidance for a needle or biopsy forceps.

Amniocentesis

A fine needle is introduced transabdominally into a pool of amniotic fluid, avoiding fetus and placenta (Fig. 2.20). The commonest indication is for fetal chromosome analysis on the grounds of advanced maternal age, as the risk of Down's syndrome increases after 35 years. Amniotic fluid α-fetoprotein and acetylcholinesterase can be assayed for neural tube defects and many inborn errors of metabolism, such as Tay–Sachs disease, can be detected by enzyme assay.

Amniocentesis is usually performed at 15 to 17 weeks gestation and increases the risk of spontaneous abortion by 1 per cent. It may also be

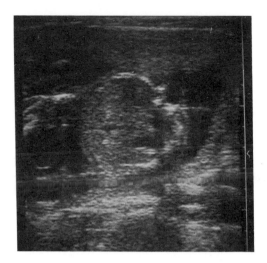

Fig. 2.19 Ultrasound scan of the fetal trunk is viewed transversely. The vertebral column is above and to the right and the cup-shaped bony defect of a spina bifida is seen

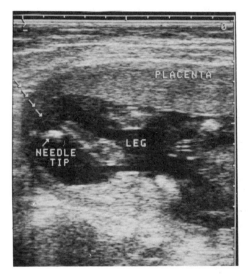

Fig. 2.20 Ultrasound scan used to assist amniocentesis. The needle track is indicated by the arrows. The upper edge of an anterior placenta has been avoided

performed diagnostically in later pregnancy for assessment of fetal maturity and bilirubin levels in rhesus isoimmunization, and therapeutically for removal of fluid in polyhydramnios (*see* p. 273).

Chorion villus biopsy (CVB)

The great advantage of this test is that it can be performed in the first trimester, usually at 10 weeks. Villi are obtained by needle aspiration or biopsy of the placenta, either transcervically or transabdominally (*see* p. 271).

As with amniotic fluid, prenatal diagnosis of chromosome aberrations and of inborn errors of metabolism is possible. In addition, villi are an excellent source of DNA and the increasing availability of gene probes is making more genetic diseases amenable to prenatal diagnosis. These include the haemoglobinopathies (sickle-cell disease, α- and β-thalassaemia) the haemophilias (A and B) and many cases of cystic fibrosis and Duchenne muscular dystrophy, as well as numerous others. The risk of spontaneous abortion is probably increased by about 2 per cent.

Fetal blood sampling

Fetal blood can be aspirated from the umbilical vein in the cord by ultrasound guidance from about 18 weeks onwards. It is used in the further evaluation of fetal anomalies by rapid chromosome analysis of fetal lymphocytes, and in fetuses at risk of blood group incompatibility, who can have a haemoglobin estimation and, if anaemic, a direct intravascular transfusion. A number of genetic diseases which cannot be diagnosed using villi can be detected with fetal blood samples. This procedure is available in only a few centres and, in experienced hands, has fetal loss rate of 1 to 2 per cent.

ULTRASOUND SCANNING IN THE THIRD TRIMESTER

The portability of modern real-time scanning machines allows them to be used in the antenatal clinic and labour ward.

Malpresentation

The diagnosis of malpresentation is usually easy by simple clinical examination. However, in an obese patient the detection of a breech presentation, for example, may be difficult and an ultrasound scan provides a quick and reliable way of resolving the problem.

Multiple pregnancy

Here again clinical examination may be difficult and if the patient has not had a scan earlier in the pregnancy the diagnosis can readily be made by ultrasound scanning, which will also reveal the lie and presentation of the fetuses.

Localizing the placenta in cases of antepartum haemorrhage

The placenta is readily seen with ultrasound and the placental site can be identified with considerable accuracy, which is very valuable in dealing with suspected placenta praevia (Fig. 2.21). Caution needs to be exercised, however, because there are certain inherent difficulties in precise localization. The exact site of the internal os may be difficult to visualize and may appear to be higher than it is because the full bladder may elongate the lower end of the uterus. With a posterior placenta, the fetal head may overshadow the lower margin of the placenta. Finally, and most importantly, the relationship of the placenta to the internal os changes as pregnancy advances so that the placenta moves upwards away from the internal os. For this reason, placentae which appear to be low-lying on scanning in the second trimester are rarely found to be so when the patient is rescanned in the third trimester. However, in spite of these difficulties an ultrasound scan is extremely valuable in determining the cause of an antepartum haemorrhage in the third trimester. The ultrasound findings coupled

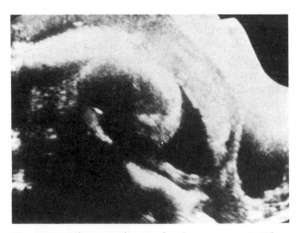

Fig. 2.21   Ultrasound scan of a placenta praevia. The placenta extends in front of the head onto the lower uterine segmented close to the bladder

with the clinical findings allow the diagnosis of placenta praevia to be made with confidence and clinical management undertaken accordingly. The detection of placental abruption causing antepartum haemorrhage is more difficult but a large retroplacental clot may be identified. In such cases, however, the clinical diagnosis is usually clear.

Placental morphology

Some abnormalities of placental morphology can be detected by ultrasound, for example the large placenta found in women with badly controlled diabetes and the hydropic placenta associated with fetal hydrops. The size of the fetus is related to the size of the placenta; a small placenta is characteristic of intrauterine growth retardation (*see* below).

Assessing the fetal growth pattern

The pattern of normal human growth *in utero* is incompletely understood, but for practical clinical purposes the important group of fetuses are those who show intrauterine growth retardation, a process that results in the birth of a baby whose weight is below the 10th centile for gestational age. These small-for-gestational-age babies are major contributors to perinatal mortality and morbidity, which is 10 times more frequent in growth-retarded fetuses. Growth retardation arises either from poor general nutrition of the mother or because the maternal blood supply of the placenta is reduced. General nutritional deprivation causes *symmetrical growth retardation* and the birth of a baby which is merely small. Poor placental perfusion, classically associated with pregnancy-induced hypertension, causes *asymmetrical growth retardation* in which a head-sparing effect is observed, the fetal head showing a lesser diminution in growth rate than the body. Asymmetrical growth retardation is due to preferential shunting of blood to the fetal brain, which develops at the expense of the fetal body. When born these babies have small bodies but relatively normal sized heads. Both types of growth retardation are likely to be associated with a high incidence of perinatal asphyxia and neonatal hypoglycaemia but the fetuses in the asymmetrical group are the more severely affected.

The clinical diagnosis of intrauterine growth retardation is not very accurate, but ultrasound measurements of the biparietal diameter and the circumference of the fetal head and the circumference of the fetal abdomen at the level of the liver give a much better assessment of fetal size. By comparing the fetal head and abdominal circumferences (the head–abdomen circumference ratio) the diagnosis of asymmetrical growth retardation can also be made. Because the fetal abdominal circumference bears a reasonably constant relationship to fetal weight, this measurement alone provides the clinician with a good estimate of what the baby would weigh if delivered immediately at the time the scan was performed. In clinical practice, once intrauterine growth retardation has been diagnosed a series of scans at two-weekly intervals is performed until it is clear that fetal growth is being seriously impaired and that delivery should be undertaken. The stage of the pregnancy at which this is done will depend upon individual circumstances and on observations of fetal activity and variations in the fetal heart rate pattern. Diminishing fetal activity and a non-reactive antenatal fetal heart trace are indications for early delivery of a fetus showing growth retardation.

At the other end of the fetal growth scale, developing macrosomy causing a large-for-gestational-age baby may be seen, for example in pregnancy complicated by maternal diabetes. Here the head–abdomen circumference ratio is reversed, the abdomen growing at a faster rate than the head as a result of disproportionate increase in the size of the fetal liver and trunk. It is clear, therefore, that by intelligent use of ultrasound and deviations from the normal pattern of fetal growth some of the associated potential disasters can be avoided.

Other uses of ultrasound in pregnancy

Fetal respiratory and other movements can be studied by using real-time scanning and blood flow velocity in the major fetal blood vessels can be studied using the Doppler effect. In general terms, fetal movements and good blood flow are indicators of fetal well-being, which can be modified by external influences. For example, fetal breathing slows considerably with hypoxia or after maternal ingestion of alcohol but is stimulated when the maternal blood glucose level rises. In the future, measurements of blood flow may be used to investigate placental function.

THE SAFETY OF ULTRASOUND

Ultrasound has been widely used as a diagnostic tool in clinical medicine for more than a quarter of a century. To date no studies have shown any deleterious effects of ultrasound on the fetus or the mother. A good deal of research has been carried out on animals and tissues, but the adverse effects that have been reported from some of these studies have occurred with ultrasound intensities, pulse lengths and exposure times far in excess of anything that is currently used, or is likely to be used, in obstetric diagnostic ultrasound. The search for possible hazards will continue, but in the meantime there is no reason to withhold the proven benefits of diagnostic ultrasound.

3

ABNORMAL PREGNANCY

ABNORMALITIES OF THE PELVIC ORGANS

RETROVERSION OF THE UTERUS

Pregnancy often occurs in a retroverted uterus and is nearly always uneventful. In the great majority of cases the uterus rises up normally into the abdomen at about the 12th week. In only a small minority of cases the uterus remains retroverted, and as it grows it comes to fill the pelvic cavity completely. The cervix is directed forwards, and even slightly upwards (*see* Fig. 3.1). The uterus is then said to be *incarcerated*. As the bladder base is attached to the supravaginal cervix the base of the bladder is distorted and the urethra is elongated. Retention of urine follows and the bladder becomes distended.

The acute retention is extremely painful and if it is not relieved by catheterization overflow incontinence will eventually occur, with frequent escape of small volumes of urine.

Diagnosis

If difficulty in micturition occurs between the 12th and 16th weeks of pregnancy the possibility of incarceration of a retroverted uterus must always be considered. On abdominal examination the distended bladder will be felt; it may contain as much as 3 litres of urine, and must not be mistaken for the pregnant uterus. On vaginal examination the posterior vaginal wall is found to be pushed

forward by a smooth elastic swelling which occupies the hollow of the sacrum. The cervix is found to be high up behind the symphysis pubis and directed forwards and slightly upwards; this confirms that the swelling in the pelvis is the uterus.

A fibromyoma in the posterior wall of the uterus might give rise to similar symptoms during pregnancy. If the tumour is soft and the cervix is

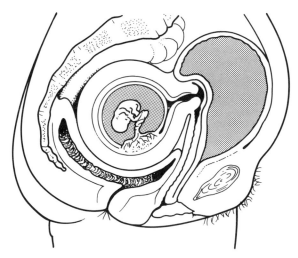

Fig. 3.1   Retroversion of the pregnant uterus

displaced forwards diagnosis may be very difficult. A pelvic ultrasound scan will help to resolve the difficulty.

Treatment

If a woman is found to have a pregnancy in a retroverted uterus before the 12th week there is no need to interfere as the uterus will probably right itself and rise up into the abdomen as it enlarges.

In the few cases in which retention occurs a catheter is immediately passed and the bladder is drained continuously. As the bladder empties the uterus nearly always rises up into the anteverted position and into the abdomen.

Only in extremely rare cases in which spontaneous correction of the position of the uterus does not follow catheterization will correction by manipulation under anaesthesia be required.

PROLAPSE OF THE PREGNANT UTERUS

Pregnancy may occur in a partially prolapsed uterus. As the uterus grows it eventually becomes too large to sink through the pelvic brim and usually, although not invariably, the cervix is then drawn up and no longer descends. Minor degrees of prolapse merely require support with a ring pessary until the uterus has grown well up into the abdomen.

Pregnancy in a completely prolapsed uterus is very rare. If the cervix remains outside the introitus it may become oedematous and fail to dilate during labour. The patient should be kept in bed for some days before labour, with the cervix within the vagina to allow the oedema to subside.

If a woman becomes pregnant after an operation for prolapse most obstetricians would advise delivery by caesarean section. If the cervix has been amputated it usually dilates more quickly than usual, but occasionally, because of scarring, it either tears or fails to dilate. In such a case caesarean section is carried out.

It is generally agreed that if stress incontinence has been successfully cured by operation caesarean section is advisable.

CONGENITAL ABNORMALITIES OF THE UTERUS AND VAGINA

The more gross uterine abnormalities are often accompanied by infertility, but lesser degrees of malformation do not prevent pregnancy occurring.

A woman with a double uterus may become pregnant in one or both sides. The risk of abortion or premature labour is increased, but labour is often normal. If pregnancy occurs in one uterus it is possible for the other one, which undergoes both myometrial and decidual hypertrophy, to obstruct the descent of the presenting part into the pelvis, and caesarean section may be necessary. The non-pregnant uterus is sometimes mistaken for a pelvic tumour such as an ovarian cyst.

With a bicornuate or septate uterus there may be repeated abortion. In other cases a malpresentation such as a transverse lie or a breech presentation may occur.

A vaginal septum may be present with or without a double uterus. Sometimes there is no obstruction to delivery, but in many cases the septum has to be excised or divided during labour.

UTERINE FIBROMYOMATA

The incidence of clinically detectable uterine fibromyomata during pregnancy is about 5 per 1000 in Caucasian women, but is much higher in Negroid women.

EFFECTS OF PREGNANCY ON FIBROMYOMATA

During pregnancy the tumours may undergo several pathological changes:

Increase in size and softening

There is hypertrophy of the muscle fibres of the tumour as in the rest of the myometrium, and there is also increased vascularity and oedema, so that it becomes larger and softer.

Necrobiosis (red degeneration)

This change is seldom seen in fibromyomata except during pregnancy. Rapid degeneration is caused by obstruction to the venous outflow from the tumour as it enlarges. The cut surface of the softened tumour has a reddish-purple colour.

The patient experiences pain at the site, and the fibromyoma becomes very tender. There is usually pyrexia and sometimes vomiting. This condition must be distinguished from other causes of acute abdominal pain in pregnancy, especially acute appendicitis, concealed abruptio placentae and torsion of an ovarian cyst which require active treatment – with red degeneration the symptoms and signs subside spontaneously in a few days.

Torsion of the pedicle

Torsion of the pedicle of a pedunculated subperitoneal tumour is a rare accident, but is more common during pregnancy than at other times.

EFFECTS OF FIBROMYOMATA ON PREGNANCY, LABOUR AND THE PUERPERIUM

Pregnancy

Miscarriage is sometimes associated with fibromyomata. It is only likely to occur with a subendometrial tumour.

Labour

Fibromyomata occur most commonly in the body of the uterus, and such tumours are drawn up out of the pelvis as the uterus enlarges, so that they do not obstruct labour. Cervical fibromyomata which remain in the pelvis prevent the head from engaging, may cause malpresentations and will obstruct labour.

The third stage of labour may be complicated by postpartum haemorrhage, especially with subendometrial tumours, and particularly if the placental attachment is over the tumour.

Puerperium

A subendometrial fibromyoma may become infected during labour, and separation of a necrotic tumour may cause late postpartum haemorrhage. After delivery fibromyomata regress as part of the general process of involution of the uterus, but they do not totally disappear.

Diagnosis

Fibromyomata which project are easily felt in the wall of the pregnant uterus, and are distinguished from fetal parts by their fixed position. They become more evident when the uterus contracts, whereas fetal parts become less obvious. They may be very difficult to detect when they have become softened and flattened in the uterine wall; however such tumours are very unlikely to interfere with labour.

If a woman who is known to have a fibromyomatous uterus becomes pregnant the signs of pregnancy are sometimes masked, or confusion may arise about the expected date of delivery because the uterus is larger than expected for the period of amenorrhoea. The tumours may make the swelling feel unlike the normal pregnant uterus in shape or consistency, or make it difficult to feel fetal parts. Confusion may occur if there is amenorrhoea from some cause other than pregnancy, such as the menopause. Conversely bleeding from threatened abortion may be attributed to menstrual bleeding if the signs of pregnancy are obscured.

In cases of doubt an immunological test for pregnancy is performed, and an ultrasound scan is carried out. This will show the presence in the uterus of a gestation sac containing a fetus, and the characteristic echo of the fibromyoma.

Treatment

Pregnancy

Most women with fibromyomata pass through pregnancy without difficulty.

If necrobiosis (red degeneration) occurs the symptoms (*see* p. 64) may be severe enough to require admission to hospital, but they almost always subside within a week or so without any treatment other than rest in bed and analgesic drugs. Myomectomy is unnecessary and carries a high risk of abortion and also of severe haemorrhage during the operation.

Torsion of a pedunculated subserous fibromyoma causes severe pain and vomiting and calls for laparotomy and removal of the tumour. Two rare conditions with which torsion of a fibromyoma may be confused are torsion of the pregnant uterus itself and intraperitoneal haemorrhage from a ruptured vein on the surface of a fibromyoma.

Labour

All pregnant women with fibromyomata should be delivered in hospital.

The great majority of these patients can safely be left to deliver vaginally. A small number will run into difficulties because a low-lying fibromyoma occupies the pelvis and obstructs the passage of the fetus (Fig. 3.2). The obstruction can often be anticipated before labour begins, but will certainly become obvious once it starts. Caesarean section solves the problem. No attempt should be made to remove fibromyomata at the time, since this may

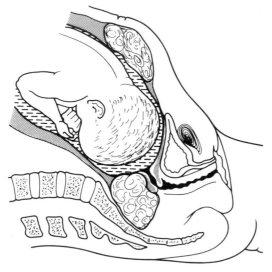

Fig. 3.2   Fibromyomata complicating pregnancy. The tumor in the anterior wall of the uterus has been drawn up out of the pelvis as the lower segment was formed, but the fibroid arising from the cervix remains in the pelvis and will obstruct labour

be hazardous and they diminish greatly in size after delivery. The decision about definitive treatment should be made three months after delivery when hysterectomy or myomectomy can be safely performed, if indeed any treatment is needed.

OVARIAN TUMOURS

Ovarian tumours are not commonly associated with pregnancy, the incidence being less than 1 in 1000 cases. Any type of ovarian tumour may occur, but simple serous cysts and benign teratomatous cysts are most often found. The most important consideration is that it is impossible to be sure that any ovarian tumour or cyst is not malignant. About 10 per cent of tumours in patients under 30 are malignant, and this proportion rises in older patients.

Torsion of the pedicle of an ovarian tumour occurs more often during pregnancy than at other times, and it may also occur during the puerperium. Rupture of a cyst or intracystic haemorrhage may occur, or necrosis from pressure on a cyst during labour, and infection and suppuration may follow.

Pregnancy is usually undisturbed by the tumour unless torsion or some other complication occurs. Labour is unaffected unless the tumour lies in the pelvic cavity when obstruction is probable. This is relatively more common with ovarian tumours than with fibromyomata because the latter usually rise up into the abdomen before labour begins.

Diagnosis

In the early months of pregnancy the uterus is easily distinguished by bimanual examination from the rounded and usually mobile ovarian tumour lying behind it in the rectovaginal pouch.

The chief condition which has to be distinguished from an intrapelvic ovarian cyst associated with pregnancy is retroversion of the gravid uterus. Contrary to expectation an ovarian cyst is not displaced to one side but lies in the midline behind the uterus. It is cystic and tense and a groove may be felt between the cyst and the cervix, which is directed downwards and backwards. A retroverted gravid uterus lies in the rectovaginal pouch, but the body of the uterus is soft and the cervix is directed forwards.

A twisted ovarian cyst with an early uterine pregnancy might be mistaken for a tubal pregnancy, but the correct treatment is laparotomy for both conditions. An ovarian tumour that cannot be recognized as a separate structure from the uterus might lead to an erroneous diagnosis of a fibromyoma or a bicornuate uterus. The diagnosis can often be clarified by an ultrasound scan.

Treatment

An ovarian tumour discovered during pregnancy should be removed as soon as it is diagnosed (except during the first 12 weeks) because of the possibility that it may be malignant. Moreover it is subject to the risks of torsion of the pedicle, rupture and intracystic haemorrhage. It is wise to wait until after the 12th week before operating, as there is a risk of miscarriage if the corpus luteum has to be removed with the ovary before the placenta has taken up its hormonal function. If the tumour proves to be innocent every effort is made to conserve ovarian tissue; the cyst or tumour is enucleated from the rest of the ovary.

If the diagnosis is not made until late in pregnancy, and if the ovarian tumour is not in the pelvic cavity, vaginal delivery is awaited and the tumour is removed in the early puerperium. If the tumour is in the pelvis, even if it is cystic, it is likely to obstruct delivery and caesarean section with removal of the tumour is necessary.

CARCINOMA OF THE CERVIX UTERI

CARCINOMA *IN SITU*

During pregnancy carcinoma *in situ* (cervical intraepithelial neoplasia – CIN) is found more often than invasive cancer of the cervix, as might be expected, since patients who ultimately develop invasive cancer may have had carcinoma *in situ* for some years beforehand.

It is the usual practice to take a cervical smear from patients at the time of their first visit to the antenatal clinic. If abnormal cells are found the cervix is carefully examined with a speculum to exclude obvious invasive cancer. If the cervix appears normal on ordinary inspection colposcopy should be performed to locate the areas on the cervix from which the abnormal cells have originated. Thereafter a colposcopically directed biopsy, taking only a small amount of tissue, can be carried out. If a diagnosis of dysplasia or carcinoma *in situ* is established, and invasive cancer excluded, treatment can safely be left until after delivery. Treatment is described in *Gynaecology by Ten Teachers*.

If any patient has not had a cervical smear examination during pregnancy this must be done in the postnatal clinic.

INVASIVE CARCINOMA

Invasive cancer of the cervix is a rare complication of pregnancy because the disease most often arises in the later years of menstrual life, when pregnancy is less likely to occur. Apart from early diagnosis by cervical smear, when there may be no symptoms, the disease is first discovered because of slight bleeding from the cervix, sometimes after coitus or vaginal examination. It quickly progresses in the same way as in the non-pregnant woman, with free bleeding and purulent discharge from the friable or ulcerated lesion on the cervix. When there is any doubt about the nature of such a lesion biopsy is essential.

If the growth is endocervical, intermittent bleeding will be the only symptom at first, and delay in diagnosis may occur because this is attributed to threatened abortion or antepartum haemorrhage.

Treatment

This depends on the stage of pregnancy at which the diagnosis is made. In early pregnancy therapeutic termination should be carried out and the cervical lesion should then be treated by radiotherapy or surgery in the usual way. In late pregnancy caesarean section should be performed and may be combined with a radical hysterectomy (caesarean-Wertheim operation).

It is difficult to know what to do when the diagnosis is made in midpregnancy before the fetus is viable. In such cases treatment may sometimes be postponed for a short time to allow the fetus to grow to a size and maturity at which it has hope of survival. Such a postponement should not exceed four weeks and can only be agreed to after consultation with the patient and her partner. The possibility that the delay may adversely affect the prognosis must be discussed. A compromise solution can usually be found, although in some cases this will involve sacrificing the fetus, for example by hysterotomy followed by radiotherapy or radical hysterectomy.

HYDATIDIFORM MOLE, CHORIOCARCINOMA AND OTHER ABNORMALITIES OF THE PLACENTA AND CORD

GESTATIONAL TROPHOBLASTIC DISEASE

During early pregnancy the conceptus may show abnormal proliferation of the trophoblast, which in the most severe cases forms a highly malignant new growth – choriocarcinoma.

On histological grounds three degrees of the abnormal process have been described:

Hydatidiform mole

In this condition there is usually no sign of a fetus and the chorionic villi show vesicular degeneration. The uterus is filled with a mass of grape-like vesicles (Fig. 3.3), varying in size from a pinhead to up to 2 cm in diameter. The vesicles are formed by cystic degeneration and accumulation of fluid in the mesenchyme of the villi, which show no fetal blood vessels (Fig. 3.4). The trophoblast is nourished by the maternal blood and there is proliferation of both the cyto- and syncytio-trophoblast.

Invasive mole

In some cases vesicular formation is much less evident but the trophoblast is more active, tending to invade deeply into the uterine wall, which it may sometimes penetrate and cause intraperitoneal haemorrhage. This type of mole has been called *invasive mole (chorioadenoma destruens).*

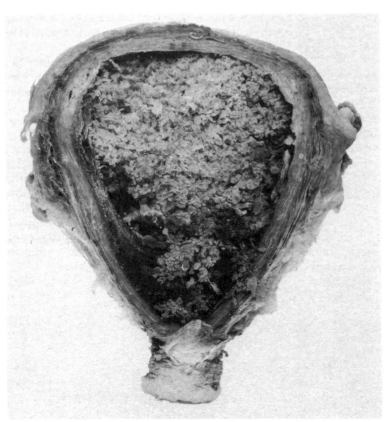

Fig. 3.3   Uterus containing a hydatidiform mole

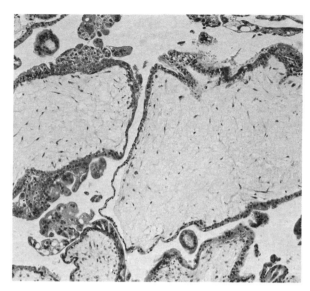

Fig. 3.4 Microscopical section of hydatidform mole. ×75

Choriocarcinoma

As a sequel or accompaniment to either of the preceding lesions *choriocarcinoma* may develop. This growth is extremely vascular, deep red in colour, with zones of necrosis. It consists of masses of syncytio- and cytotrophoblast, without villous formation. It invades blood vessels to become widely disseminated as metastases in distant organs, such as the lungs, brain, kidneys and spleen. Vaginal metastases are common. Spread may also occur by the lymphatics.

These three conditions cannot be sharply separated, and they represent a spectrum of trophoblastic activity from benign to malignant without precise lines of demarcation. Choriocarcinoma usually follows a molar pregnancy, but may rarely follow spontaneous abortion, delivery of a normal fetus, or an ectopic pregnancy. About 1 in 40 moles is followed by choriocarcinoma, but it occurs only in 1 in 160 000 term deliveries.

Aetiological factors and genetic studies

Gestational trophoblastic disease has a striking geographical distribution. It is more common in the Far East and parts of West Africa and South America than in western countries. For example,

the incidence in Taiwan is 1 in 82 gestations, in Indonesia it is 1 in 100 gestations, and in Europe and North America it occurs in about 1 in 2000 gestations. Registration of hydatiform mole in England and Wales gives an incidence of 1 per 1000 live births. Apart from the different socio-economic status of the women there is no obvious explanation for this.

The incidence of molar pregnancies is greater in women under 20 and those over 40 years of age.

Recently moles have been divided by morphological and genetic studies into two categories:

Complete moles

Complete moles show hydropic swelling of all the villi and there is no evidence of a fetus or of fetal blood vessels. The karyotype of these moles is 46, XX, but fluorescent banding techniques show that all the chromosomal material is of paternal origin. It is suggested that a defective or anucleate oöcyte is fertilized by a haploid sperm, which subsequently duplicates to restore the diploid number of 46.

Partial moles

Partial moles have normal villi intermixed with hydropic villi, and there may be a fetus with its blood vessels. Trophoblastic proliferation is less evident. Partial moles usually have triploid chromosomal structure, and it is suggested that they result from fertilization of one oöcyte by two sperm or a diploid sperm.

In all varieties of mole and in choriocarcinoma the trophoblast produces human chorionic gonadotrophin (hCG). In most cases of hydatidiform mole the amount of hCG secreted exceeds that produced in normal pregnancy. This is in contrast to the amounts of other hormones and proteins of fetal (α-fetoprotein), trophoblastic (human placental lactogen, schwangerschaftsprotein 1), ovarian (oestradiol, progesterone) and decidual origin, which are usually produced in quantities which are less than those produced in normal pregnancy. By the action of hCG both ovaries may become enlarged with multiple theca-lutein cysts.

Clinical features of hydatidiform mole

The first symptom is often uterine bleeding, usually beginning between the 12th and 16th weeks, but sometimes earlier. Excessive or persistent vomiting may occur. Hypertension and proteinuria are often present with large moles, and even eclampsia may occur. A curious, rare event is mild hyperthyroidism. The most likely cause of this is the enormous quantities of hCG produced; hCG has thyroid-stimulating hormone-like activity.

In about half of the cases the uterus is larger than in a normal pregnancy of the same duration, although in a few cases it is smaller. It may be tense or of normal consistency. There may be abdominal pain, which will be severe in cases of intraperitoneal bleeding. Fetal parts cannot be felt and fetal heart movements cannot be detected with ultrasound.

On vaginal examination watery, blood-stained discharge may be seen, and bilateral ovarian thecalutein cysts may be felt. Patients with moles often abort at about 20 weeks, when free bleeding occurs and vesicles will be seen.

A hydatidiform mole has to be diagnosed from threatened abortion of a twin or normal pregnancy. Quantitative assay of hCG in blood by radioimmunoassay may be diagnostic if levels are found exceeding those of a twin pregnancy, but this is not invariably the case. An ultrasound scan is a quicker and more reliable method of diagnosis, showing a 'snow-storm' appearance on the screen and the absence of any fetus.

Treatment of hydatidiform mole

If the mole is diagnosed when its extrusion has begun and the cervix is dilating the uterus should be encouraged to expel it. An intravenous infusion of Syntocinon is given (*see* p. 177) and, provided that the dose is increased gradually while the uterine response is observed, larger doses can be given than would be used during labour with a living fetus. Prostaglandins can also be used.

If a mole is diagnosed before spontaneous extrusion begins or is complete, it should be evacuated with a suction curette, using an infusion of Syntocinon or ergometrine to control the bleeding. Care must be taken not to perforate the uterus, but in spite of this risk the suction curette is preferable to hysterotomy.

Until recently, if the patient was near the menopause or already had the family she wanted, hysterectomy with the mole *in situ* was recommended, but with the ease of evacuation with the suction curette and the good results of treating choriocarcinoma, this would not now be recommended.

Prophylactic chemotherapy (*see* below) at the time of evacuation or expulsion of a hydatidiform mole is not generally recommended, because less than 1 in 40 moles will prove to be malignant (and these can be successfully treated) and chemotherapy is unpleasant for the patient.

Every patient must be followed up with regular radioimmunoassays of the blood levels of hCG, for example at fortnightly intervals for two months, then monthly for a year or longer. Provided that hCG levels are normal for two years after evacuation of a hydatidiform mole the risk of choriocarcinoma is virtually non-existent. All cases of trophoblastic disease will benefit from care in special centres where the doctors have accumulated experience of the disease.

Clinical features of choriocarcinoma

Most cases are now diagnosed during the follow-up of cases of hydatidiform mole by assays of hCG. Recurrence of growth in the uterus after evacuation or abortion of a mole, or growth following abortion or delivery, will cause bleeding which calls for curettage and leads to histological diagnosis. Vaginal metastases may appear as purplish-red nodules.

Symptoms of more advanced cases depend on the site of any metastases. For example, pulmonary metastases cause dyspnoea, haemoptysis, cough and pleural pain, and will be seen in a radiograph. Cerebral metastases will cause headache, neurological signs and eventual coma.

Treatment of choriocarcinoma

This tumour is notable as the first for which effective chemotherapy was discovered. With modern chemotherapy the prognosis, which was formerly hopeless, has been transformed, so that in Britain death from trophoblastic tumour after hydatidiform mole has become rare.

The main indications for chemotherapy after evacuation of a mole are high levels of hCG persisting in the first two months, the presence of detectable levels of hCG after six months, or persistent uterine bleeding. Various combinations of drugs are used. Repeated courses of chemotherapy are given until the hCG level becomes and remains normal.

These drugs cause severe damage to the bone marrow, with thrombocytopenia and agranulocytosis, and the consequent risk of anaemia, haemorrhagic complications and infections. If alopecia occurs it is temporary, but is none the less upsetting to some women. Special nursing precautions, antibiotic cover and administration of folinic acid after methotrexate may all be required. Surgery has little place in treatment, except for unusual complications such as intraperitoneal haemorrhage or a localized deposit which persists in spite of chemotherapy.

Chemotherapy can be selected for patients according to the risk of their becoming resistant to the therapy. This depends on factors such as age, the preceding pregnancy, the interval between pregnancy and diagnosis, the blood level of hCG, the size of the tumour and the site of metastases. Thus patients with a low risk of resistance tend to be young, have a hydatidiform mole preceding the choriocarcinoma (rather than an abortion or a term pregnancy), are diagnosed within four or six months after evacuation of the mole, have a blood level of hCG of less than 10^4 IU/L, have a tumour less than 5 cm in diameter and only one or two metastases, usually in the kidney or spleen.

These low risk patients can be treated with single agents of low toxicity, which will avoid alopecia.

High risk patients – those over 39 years of age, with choriocarcinoma following an abortion or a full term pregnancy after an interval of more than six months, blood hCG levels of more than 10^4 IU/L, tumours more than 5 cm in diameter and metastases in the liver or brain – have to be treated with a combination of effective agents, which show moderate or severe toxicity and will result in alopecia.

Chemotherapeutic treatment is summarized in Table 3.1.

Other chemotherapeutic drugs such as cisplatin, bleomycin and vinblastine may be required to achieve remission. Treatment is continuous unless the white blood cell count falls below 2000/mm³ or the platelets fall below 100 000/mm³.

The best results are obtained in special units, such as the ones in the Charing Cross Hospital in London, the Jessop Hospital in Sheffield and Ninewells Hospital in Dundee.

It has been customary to advise a woman who has had a hydatidiform mole to avoid pregnancy for two or three years, largely because of the fear of confusing an early pregnancy with recurrence of the mole or choriocarcinoma. There is no additional risk of another mole developing in a new pregnancy and, with ultrasound, confusion between a recurrent mole and a normal pregnancy is most unlikely. Consequently the advice to avoid a new conception can be modified to accord more with the woman's circumstances and wishes. The return of regular menstruation and persistently normal gonadotrophin levels over a six-month period should be a sufficient safeguard.

Table 3.1 Treatment of choriocarcinoma

Low risk patients
Methotrexate and folinic acid on alternate days for 8 days
Followed by 6 days rest
Courses continue every 2 weeks until hCG levels in serum are undetectable for at least 6 weeks

Medium and high risk patients
Etoposide, actinomycin D or methotrexate and folinic acid for 2 days
Followed by vincristine and cyclophosphamide a week later
Courses continue every 2 weeks until hCG in serum is undetectable for 8 to 10 weeks

OTHER ABNORMALITIES OF THE PLACENTA

ANOMALIES IN WEIGHT

The average weight of the placenta at term is about 500 g. The weight varies according to whether the umbilical cord has been clamped early or late, thus imprisoning less or more of the fetal blood. In cases of diabetes and haemolytic disease of the newborn the placental weight may increase to up to half the weight of the fetus.

SITE OF IMPLANTATION OF THE PLACENTA

The placenta is usually attached to the uterine wall near the fundus, to either the anterior or posterior surface. Anterior implantation may play a part in causing an occipitoposterior position of the fetus, as the fetal back cannot then be easily accommodated in the anterior position.

In about 1 in 250 pregnancies the placenta is implanted wholly or partially on the lower segment of the uterus (*placenta praevia*). This is a serious abnormality which may cause severe haemorrhage in pregnancy and in particular during labour (*see* p. 180).

BILOBATE AND TRILOBATE PLACENTA

Instead of a single disc the placenta may consist of two or three lobes, usually partly fused, but sometimes completely separate except for their vascular attachments. Such abnormalities are of no significance.

PLACENTA SUCCENTURIATA

This anomaly is not uncommon. One or more accessory lobes of placental substance are found on the chorion at a distance from the edge of the main placenta (Fig. 3.5(a)). They are united to the placenta by arteries and veins. A succenturiate lobe is of clinical importance because it is liable to be retained in the uterus after the placenta proper has been expelled, causing postpartum haemorrhage. The abnormality should be discovered when the membranes and placenta are inspected after delivery, when a round defect will be seen in the membranes, with a leash of vessels running from the edge of the placenta to end abruptly where they have been torn across at the edge of the defect. In such a case the uterine cavity should be explored immediately, and the succenturiate lobe removed.

PLACENTA CIRCUMVALLATA

This is due to a late outward proliferation of chorionic villi because the original area of the chorionic plate was unduly small (Fig. 3.5(b)). As a result the chorionic villi proliferate outwards into the decidua, beneath the ring of attachment of amnion and chorion. A white ring is seen on the fetal aspect of the placenta, and this bounds a central depression, from which the fetal vessels radiate and disappear under the white ring. This abnormality does not usually interfere with placental function, but it may be associated with antepartum or intrapartum haemorrhage, fetal intrauterine growth retardation and a slight excess of congenital abnormalities.

PLACENTA ACCRETA, INCRETA OR PERCRETA

In the third stage of labour the placenta normally

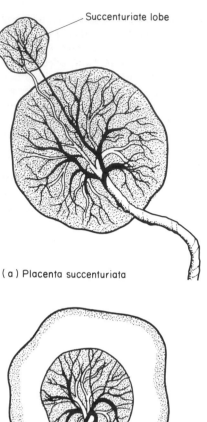

(a) Placenta succenturiata

(b) Placenta circumvallata

Fig. 3.5 Placenta showing haemangioma

separates through the stratum spongiosum of the maternal decidua. The superficial part of the decidua comes away with the placenta, and the deeper part remains on the uterine wall. Normally the chorionic villi only penetrate as far as this.

When the villi reach the uterine muscle and the spongy layer of decidua is absent there is no plane of cleavage between the placenta and its attachment to the uterus; the condition is called *placenta accreta*. When the villi penetrate the uterine muscle it is called *placenta increta* and when they reach the serosa it is *placenta percreta*. Placenta praevia, caesarean section and curettage are the most common predisposing causes. Sometimes the area of adhesion is limited to part of the placental site, but in rare cases the entire placenta is firmly attached. Morbid adhesion of the whole placenta occurs about once in 20 000 deliveries.

There is delay in the third stage of labour and the abnormality is only discovered when an attempt is made to remove the placenta manually and no plane of cleavage is found. If the whole placenta is adherent there can be no bleeding, but with partial adherence or after attempts at removal severe bleeding may occur. If adherence is only partial it is usually possible to remove the placenta, but there is a risk of leaving part of it behind.

In cases of complete placenta accreta it may be possible to remove the placenta piecemeal, but this is a dangerous procedure. Unless haemorrhage has been caused by attempts to remove the placenta or the uterus has been torn, when hysterectomy is inevitable, it is justifiable to leave the placenta *in situ* and await its separation by necrosis. Antibiotics should be given during this time.

INFECTION OF THE PLACENTA AND MEMBRANES

During normal pregnancy the uterine contents are protected from ascending infection by the cervical mucus plug and by intact membranes. Spontaneous premature rupture of the membranes may be followed by infection, a condition called *chorioamnionitis*, which is characterized by malodorous and bacteria-contaminated liquor, fetal tachycardia and maternal fever. The risk of infection increases with time and repeated vaginal examination. It may be followed by fetal pneumonia or maternal puerperal sepsis. Antibiotics may protect the mother from infection but do not cross the placenta in sufficient amounts to protect the fetus, who needs to be delivered.

THE PLACENTA IN HAEMOLYTIC DISEASE OF THE NEWBORN

In mild degrees of this condition no abnormality may be evident, although the placenta may be stained yellow with bile pigment. In cases of hydrops fetalis the placenta is oedematous, large, pale and friable, and often as heavy as the fetus

itself. There is abnormal persistence of the cytotrophoblast (Langhans' cells) of the chorionic villi; the reason for this is not known.

OTHER CHANGES IN THE PLACENTA

The placenta has a substantial functional reserve, readily adjusts to injury, repairs damages due to ischaemia and does not undergo ageing. The widely held view that ageing occurs progressively during the course of a normal pregnancy is due to a misinterpretation of the histological appearances of the normal processes of maturation of the villous tree and trophoblastic differentiation. Placental growth certainly decreases during the last few weeks of the third trimester, but this decline is neither invariable nor irreversible, as the placenta can still grow, even in hostile circumstances, and show a proliferative response to ischaemic damage.

Placental infarction

A fresh placental infarct is firm and dark red; in time it becomes harder in consistency and the colour changes progressively to become an amorphous, hard, white plaque. Whereas small infarcts are common and of no importance, extensive lesions, i.e. in excess of 10–30 per cent of active placental tissue, are associated with a loss of functional placental reserve leading to an increased incidence of fetal hypoxia, growth retardation and intrauterine death. Infarction is usually due to thrombosis of a maternal uteroplacental vessel and, if extensive, is secondary to maternal conditions, typically pre-eclampsia.

Fetal stem artery thrombosis

Macroscopically there is an area of pallor in the placenta, consisting of avascular villi supplied by an obliterated fetal stem artery. This lesion is not important unless 50 per cent of the placental villi are rendered avascular by multiple thrombotic obliteration of stem vessels.

Other lesions

Plaques, thrombi, calcification and cysts of the placenta are of no functional significance or clinical relevance. These macroscopic lesions, whether noted ultrasonically or postpartum, should not be considered as due to degeneration or ageing of the placenta.

TUMOURS OF THE PLACENTA

Apart from choriocarcinoma, tumours of the placenta are rare, and consist of masses of chorionic villi with hypertrophied blood vessels. Such vascular tumours are known as *haemangiomas* or *chorangiomas*. The tumour is usually single and the rest of the placenta is normal. Such a tumour is a rare cause of hydramnios, due to exudation of fluid from the surface of the tumour, if greater than 5 cm in diameter.

Very rarely metastases from a maternal carcinoma or melanoma may occur in the placenta.

ANOMALIES OF THE UMBILICAL CORD

ABNORMAL LENGTH

The usual length of the cord is about the same as that of the fetus, 50 cm at term, but considerable variations occur. Excessive length predisposes to descent of the cord below the presenting part and prolapse. The formation of loops round some part of the fetus may cause intrauterine death in the very rare cases in which the cord is pulled tight. During delivery the treatment for a loop round the neck is to slip it over the head after this is born, or if this cannot be done to divide the cord between clamps.

With an abnormally short cord delay in the second stage of labour, premature separation of the placenta or inversion of the uterus are rare accidents.

KNOTS IN THE CORD

These may be formed by fetal movements, the fetus passing through a loop which later forms a knot. Knots are rarely tight enough to obstruct the circulation, but they do occasionally cause intrauterine fetal death. Local protuberances of Wharton's jelly may give an appearance of knotting and have been described as false knots; they are of no importance.

ABNORMAL INSERTION OF THE CORD

The cord is usually attached to the centre of the placenta, but sometimes it is attached to the edge of the placenta (*battledore placenta*). This is of no importance.

In rare cases the cord is attached to the membranes at some distance from the edge of the placenta, and at this point the vessels may divide into branches which run on the membranes for some distance before reaching the edge of the placenta (*velamentous insertion of the cord*). This can be dangerous to the fetus if the vessels happen to pass across part of the chorion that lies below the presenting part (*vasa praevia*), as a branch may be torn when the membranes rupture.

SINGLE UMBILICAL ARTERY

This is an uncommon finding but it may be associated with other abnormalities of the fetus. The cut end of the cord should always be inspected after delivery, and if only one artery is seen the child should be carefully examined for any other defect.

ANTEPARTUM HAEMORRHAGE

The term antepartum haemorrhage is applied to bleeding from the vagina occurring at any time after the 28th week of pregnancy and before the birth of the child.

As defined above, antepartum haemorrhage may be described under three headings:

haemorrhage from a normally situated placenta.

This is called *abruptio placentae* or accidental haemorrhage

haemorrhage from partial separation of a placenta abnormally situated on the lower uterine segment. This is termed *placenta praevia*. Haemorrhage is unavoidable when the lower segment becomes stretched in labour haemorrhage from a lesion of the cervix or vagina such as an erosion, a polyp or a carcinoma. This may be called *incidental haemorrhage*.

ABRUPTIO PLACENTAE (ACCIDENTAL HAEMORRHAGE)

Varieties

Owing to the separation of a portion of the placenta from its uterine attachment, part of the wall of the intervillous space is breached and maternal blood escapes from the opened sinuses. This blood may track down between the membranes and the wall of the uterus and escape at the cervix (*revealed haemorrhage*, Fig. 3.6) or remain inside the uterine cavity (*concealed haemorrhage*, Fig. 3.7). In fact the distinction is more clinical than anatomical; in nearly all cases there is some external bleeding, but in concealed cases the degree of shock is out of all proportion to the external loss.

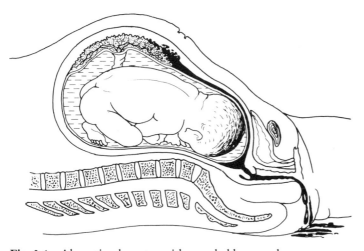

Fig. 3.6   Abruptio placentae with revealed haemorrhage

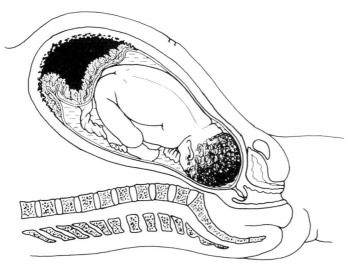

Fig. 3.7   Abruptio placentae with concealed haemorrhage

Cause and pathology

The reported incidence varies from 1 in 85 to 1 in 200 deliveries. In many cases no cause can be discovered, but about 25 per cent of the cases are associated with hypertension and proteinuria. It is not certain that the hypertension or proteinuria is the cause of the haemorrhage; proteinuria may follow rather than precede it.

It has been claimed that abruptio placentae is caused by folic acid deficiency. The disease is more common with advanced parity and in lower income groups. There is also said to be an association with megaloblastic anaemia, which is due to folic acid deficiency. Studies of folate levels and of the bone marrow have given some support to the theory. However, abruptio placentae is not especially frequent in Nigeria, where megaloblastic anaemia is common, and there has been little evidence that folic acid supplements during pregnancy reduce the incidence in this country.

A few cases of placental separation are caused by trauma during external version.

The bleeding in cases of abruptio placentae may be of any degree from a small retroplacental haematoma, which may not affect the fetus and which may only be discovered after the placenta is delivered, to a large collection of blood which distends the uterus and kills the fetus by separating a large part of the placenta.

In severe cases haemorrhages occur in the substance of the uterine wall and may extend to the peritoneal surface (Couvelaire uterus).

It is sometimes stated that such haemorrhage interferes with uterine contraction, and that this explains the continued bleeding which occurs in some of these cases, even after delivery of the fetus and placenta. This is improbable as the uterus is tense from spasm, rather than relaxed, before delivery. In concealed cases the whole uterus is tense and tender, but in revealed or less severe cases there is more localized tenderness over the site of haemorrhage. If postpartum haemorrhage occurs after placental abruption it is caused by hypofibrinogenaemia and failure of blood clotting rather than by atony of the uterus. Hypofibrinogenaemia may occur because thromboplastins are released into the maternal circulation, causing disseminated intravascular coagulopathy (DIC) (*see* p. 266 for a more detailed account).

There is some evidence to show that there is a uterorenal reflex, and that severe accidental haemorrhage of the concealed type causes spasm of the renal arterioles. This may be sufficiently widespread and prolonged to cause bilateral renal cortical necrosis or lower nephron nephrosis, which result in anuria.

Symptoms and signs

Abruptio placentae with revealed haemorrhage

With or without any obvious cause the patient notices blood coming from the vagina. The amount of blood lost varies, but is usually not great. There may also be slight abdominal discomfort and tenderness ove the placental site.

The initial diagnosis is between accidental haemorrhage and placenta praevia. Tenderness over the placental site, engagement of the fetal head (in late pregnancy) and fetal death or fetal distress suggest that the symptoms are due to accidental haemorrhage. However, in many slight cases the fetus is not adversely affected and in multiparae the fetal head may not engage until the onset of labour, even in normal cases. If the head is not engaged the placental site should be localized by ultrasound scan.

It is dangerous to attempt to exclude the presence of a placenta praevia by vaginal examination and the passage of a finger through the cervix. If the placenta should prove to be low-lying such an examination may cause very severe bleeding. In exceptional cases, in which the diagnosis is in real doubt and the degree of bleeding is such that investigation by ultrasound scan would take too long, the patient should be taken to the operating theatre and delivered by caesarean section.

Abruptio placentae with concealed haemorrhage

The symptoms and signs vary with the severity of the case. In the extreme cases the gravity of the patient's condition may be out of all proportion to the amount of blood effused into the uterus. Shock is due not only to the haemorrhage but also to the painful uterine distension. In spite of severe shock with a low blood pressure the pulse rate may not be raised, at least for a time, and this may be misleading.

The overdistension of the uterus causes severe and constant abdominal pain. The uterus may be larger than would be expected for the period of gestation reached and more globular in outline. It has a hard, wooden consistency and is extremely tender. The fetal outlines cannot be made out and the fetal heart cannot be heard.

Should the loss of blood be smaller the symptoms are correspondingly less severe. The patient complains of a sudden attack of abdominal pain and at the same time feels faint and suffers from nausea. She looks ill, her mucous membranes are pale, and the pulse rate is raised. No abnormality may be discovered on abdominal examination, except that palpation of the uterus elicits tenderness, usually localized to the placental site, and if a sufficient area of placenta has been detached the fetal heart sounds are often inaudible. A correct diagnosis is important as such a patient is likely to have a recurrent and more serious haemorrhage. Protein may be present in the urine.

In many cases the bleeding is partly concealed and partly revealed and the signs and symptoms are mixed.

The severity of a case with external haemorrhage must never be judged solely by the amount of blood lost *per vaginam* but by the general condition of the patient. A trifling external loss may be accompanied by serious concealed haemorrhage.

Diagnosis

Revealed haemorrhage

Reavealed haemorrhage in abruptio placentae simulates placenta praevia, and in many cases an immediate distinction is not possible. Placenta praevia is suggested by a history of recurrent attacks of bleeding, by the absence of hypertension or proteinuria, by a malpresentation or an unduly high presenting part. If the fetal head is engaged or investigation by ultrasound shows that the placenta is certainly situated in the upper uterine segment a firm diagnosis of abruption can be made.

The danger of vaginal examination, except in the operating theatre with all preparations made for caesarean section, has already been emphasized.

After delivery the diagnosis can be confirmed by examining the membranes; the hole through which the child is delivered is close to the placental edge if the case was one of placenta praevia.

Concealed haemorrhage

The diagnosis must be made from cases of intraperitoneal haemorrhage caused by advanced ectopic gestation, spontaneous rupture of the uterus, or acute hydramnios. These, although very rare complications of pregnancy, closely resemble abruptio placentae of the concealed variety. They must be diagnosed by the history and on the physical signs present in each case. Other conditions complicating pregnancy, such as red degeneration of a fibromyoma, torsion of the pedicle of an ovarian cyst, volvulus, intestinal obstruction, acute appendicitis or peritonitis from any other cause, may have to be considered during the early stages of a concealed haemorrhage. Some loss of blood *per vaginam* is nearly always present and this makes diagnosis easier. Ultrasound examination of the uterus has proved invaluable in the diagnosis of concealed accidental haemorrhage since the retroplacental clot can usually be visualized.

Prognosis

The most important factor in the prognosis is the degree of shock and its duration. The amount of blood lost will obviously be important. If the uterus starts to contract rhythmically, instead of remaining in spasm, the prognosis is improved, even if the external bleeding increases temporarily when the patient goes into labour. The sooner the uterus is emptied the sooner bleeding will be arrested and the risks of hypofibrinogenaemia or renal cortical necrosis will be reduced.

In cases of revealed haemorrhage the maternal risk is small, but in severe cases of concealed haemorrhage the maternal mortality may exceed 10 per cent.

The prognosis for the child is bad. The perinatal mortality is over 50 per cent. This is caused by asphyxia from placental separation, sometimes combined with fetal growth retardation or preterm delivery.

Treatment

All cases of antepartum haemorrhage should be admitted to hospital. In severe cases this is essential; in less severe cases the diagnosis is often uncertain and placenta praevia cannot always be excluded. A vaginal examination should not be made before the transfer of the patient to hospital. In cases with severe shock a blood transfusion and an injection of morphia should be given before moving the patient.

Since the term 'reavealed haemorrhage' includes cases which vary in severity from a slight loss of blood to a profuse flooding no single method of treatment will be applicable to all cases.

Revealed haemorrhage with slight bleeding

If the amount of bleeding is only slight and placenta praevia has been excluded by an ultrasound scan (*see* p. 82) there is no need to do more than put the patient at rest. In many cases no further bleeding occurs and the pregnancy continues to term. The eventual appearance of the placenta will show that part of it has been detached, being brown, shrunken, and more solid than the rest and having old blood clot adherent to it.

Revealed haemorrhage with more severe bleeding

This group includes cases in which the amount of bleeding is sufficient to be dangerous or there is any degree of shock. In most severe cases the fetus is already dead and need not be considered. The object of treatment is to empty the uterus, contract and retract it with as little bleeding as possible and without added risk to the mother. If the patient is in labour this is best achieved by allowing the uterus to empty itself. Caesarean section is seldom indicated if the fetus is dead. A blood transfusion should be given if the loss is more than slight or there are any signs of shock. If the patient is not already in labour that should be induced, by low rupture of the membranes, without delay. If regular contractions do not follow an oxytocin drip may be given; only in a few exceptional cases in which profuse bleeding persists should the uterus be emptied by caesarean section.

Many patients are already in labour, or labour soon follows induction. The second stage of labour may be shortened with the aid of the forceps or the vacuum extractor. The third stage should be conducted with care and an intravenous injection of oxytocin 5 units or ergometrine 500 micrograms should be given immediately after the birth of the head.

Caesarean section is not required in cases with slight bleeding unless there is evidence of fetal distress. Fetal blood sampling may be useful in these cases to assess the degree of hypoxia; some-times it will show that the fetus is so severely affected that section is not justifiable. However, caesarean section may be indicated when the fetus is alive, the patient is not in labour and bleeding is severe, but it should only be performed after maternal shock has been treated.

Concealed haemorrhage

Most cases of concealed haemorrhage are very serious, because the patient is collapsed as a result of the loss of blood and the painful distension of the uterus. The first essential is to treat the shock and not to attempt to deliver the child before this has been done. If the patient is first seen at home an emergency obstetric unit (flying squad) should be called and resuscitation commenced. The patient must be given an immediate injection of morphine, 15 mg. She should not be moved until severe shock has been treated by blood transfusion but transfer to hospital will be required, and should not be long delayed. If the patient's condition is poor and facilities for blood transfusion are not available, Haemaccel, Gelofusine or another plasma substitute may be used or, failing that, intravenous saline. A note is made of the girth of the abdomen, and the height of the fundus is marked upon the skin. Following these steps the condition of the patient is continuously observed. A further injection of morphine 10 mg is given if the pain is not relieved. In parts of the UK where obstetric flying squads are no longer in existence the patient should immediately be transferred to hospital by ambulance; provided the journey is short, little harm will result.

In a severe case several litres of blood will be needed. The pulse and blood pressure are not always reliable indices of need; the speed of transfusion is best judged by monitoring the central venous pressure with a catheter inserted through the external jugular vein.

As the state of shock passes off improvement usually occurs. Treatment will be influenced by the parity of the patient and by the duration of the pregnancy. The majority of these patients are multiparous women, and as the fetus is small and premature, an easy quick delivery is to be expected if labour is established. After the initial treatment for shock the membranes should be ruptured. It was formerly taught that the membranes should not be ruptured until the uterus had lost its wooden hardness, as it was feared that further loss of blood would occur from an atonic uterus. There is little ground for this fear and continued bleeding is more often due to hypofibrinogenaemia, and the danger of this or of renal necrosis is reduced by early rupture of the membranes and consequent reduction of intrauterine tension.

If the fetus is alive caesarean section is now recommended. The results in the past were poor, because the operation was performed in desperate cases, some of which had received inadequate transfusion, and in some of which DIC was present so that bleeding could not be checked, even by hysterectomy. The section must be performed before irreversible shock is established. Most cases respond rapidly to artificial rupture of the membranes. When the fetus is dead section should only be considered if the patients' condition is deteriorating in the absence of uterine contractions, especially in the case of a primigravida with a tight cervix.

The possibility of DIC as a result of concealed haemorrhage should be borne in mind. It should be suspected in any case of delayed or absent clotting. A clotting screen including fibrinogen estimation should be made and a critical level is considered to be 1.0 g/L. It can be treated by transfusing fresh frozen plasma which, unlike the blood issued by the transfusion service, contains fibrinogen in addition to all the coagulation factors. If fresh blood is available this will provide approximately 1 g in each 500 ml. However, the fibrinogen level is often less important than the circulatory condition. *See* page 266 for further discussion.

Treatment after the labour is over

The fact that the patient has been delivered after abruptio placentae and that there is no great amount of postpartum haemorrhage does not necessarily mean that she will do well. In the absence of efficient treatment some of these patients die a few hours after delivery from heart failure. The patients are not safe until recovery from shock is complete, as indicated by the general condition, the pulse rate and blood pressure. An amount of postpartum haemorrhage which would be trifling in the case of a robust woman may be of grave consequence in the case of a patient who has had severe antepartum haemorrhage, and it is always prudent to obtain a generous amount of cross-matched blood for these patients.

It is important to continue with blood transfusion until the patient's condition is restored to normal or until the total blood loss has been made good. Bleeding in the third stage must be controlled by ergometrine intravenously during delivery and intramuscularly afterwards.

RENAL CORTICAL NECROSIS AND LOWER NEPHRON NEPHROSIS

A rare but serious complication of abruptio placentae, particularly of the concealed variety, is renal failure with anuria or extreme oliguria. (Anuria may also occur as a very rare complication of eclampsia, septic abortion, or traumatic delivery and postpartum haemorrhage.)

Pathology

In fatal cases one of two pathological conditions is found, either renal cortical necrosis or lower nephron nephrosis.

In *renal cortical necrosis* both kidneys show uniform symmetrical necrosis of almost the entire cortex; only a thin layer under the capsule survives. The zone of necrosis involves nearly all the glomeruli and a large part of the tubular structure.

In *lower nephron nephrosis* the kidneys may appear normal to the naked eye, but microscopical examination reveals widespread necrosis and degeneration of the distal convoluted tubules and collecting tubules. The glomeruli are not involved.

The mode of production of these two pathological conditions has been much disputed, and it is very likely that they are only different degrees of one process. Renal cortical necrosis is caused by ischaemia; the blood flow through the cortex ceases. Working in Oxford, Trueta brought evidence to show that there is an arterial shunt in the kidney which regulates the blood flow through the cortex. When the shunt is closed the blood flows through the intralobular vessels to supply all the cortex (except a thin lamina which gains its blood supply from the capsule). When the shunt is open the blood returns to the veins by an alternative pathway which diverts it from the cortex. It is suggested that this shunt is brought into operation in cases of concealed haemorrhage by toxic substances which pass into the bloodstream, and perhaps also by nervous stimuli from the uterus along sympathetic pathways. Although the details of this theory are not universally accepted, it is at least certain that cortical necrosis is due to ischaemia. The changes are irreversible and lead to permanent renal failure which has to be treated by dialysis or renal transplant.

The cause of the changes of lower nephron nephrosis is less certain. They have been attributed to the direct action of a toxin, or alternatively to ischaemia. It is difficult to explain the escape of the glomeruli and the selective effect on the distal convoluted tubules on either hypothesis. It is believed that if there is only damage to the distal tubules spontaneous regeneration of these may occur.

Clinical features

The initial clinical features of anuria caused by cortical necrosis and lower nephron nephrosis are identical. After recovery from shock, or after delivery, the first danger sign is the passage of a few millilitres of blood-stained urine. Complete or nearly complete, anuria follows and only a small quantity of very dilute urine is passed. The patient remains well for several days, during which time the blood urea rises progressively. In fatal cases, after about ten days, drowsiness and twitching movements appear, and death from uraemia quickly follows the appearance of these signs. In other cases, spontaneous diuresis occurs after about a week, and rapid and apparently complete recovery occurs. It is believed that the cases in which the kidneys recover are those caused by lower nephron nephrosis.

Treatment

If there is evidence of DIC (*see* p. 266), with failure of the shed blood to clot and a lowered plasma fibrinogen level, heparin given intravenously may prevent deposition of fibrin in the glomeruli, which is one of the suggested causes for renal failure in these cases.

As there is no means of distinguishing the lethal cases of cortical necrosis from the cases of lower nephron nephrosis in which recovery may occur, the only possible course is to treat all cases alike, and hope that spontaneous diuresis will occur. Some patients have been lost by injudicious treatment, particularly by giving large volumes of fluid intravenously. Diuretics are useless and possibly harmful.

In anuric patients the only loss of water is in the breath, sweat and faeces, and this is less than 1000 ml per day. Unless there is additional loss by vomiting the total fluid intake should never exceed this. Since the metabolism of fat provides as much as 400 ml of water a day the fluid intake should be restricted to about 500 ml. Disturbance of electrolyte balance also occurs, but in the absence of normal renal function it is highly dangerous to give electrolytes, which can so easily be given to excess. The temporary disturbance of balance will neither interfere with spontaneous diuresis, nor will it be of a degree to endanger the patient before spontaneous diuresis occurs.

In order to provide energy and spare endogenous metabolism an intravenous infusion of glucose should be given into a large vein to avoid the common difficulty of thrombosis of small veins with glucose infusion. A catheter inserted into an arm vein may be advanced so that the tip lies in the superior vena cava. In addition to whatever the patient can take by mouth she is given enough carbohydrate and fat to provide a total of 1500 calories per day and 75 g of protein or amino acids.

Anuric patients are best treated in special centres where dialysis may be undertaken if necessary. Dialysis is indicated if:

there is overhydration as shown by pulmonary oedema
there are convulsions or coma
the blood urea level remains over 35 mmol/L
the blood potassium concentration exceeds 7 mmol/L
the serum bicarbonate concentration is less than 12 mmol/L.

Peritoneal dialysis is usually successful and allows some freedom in the diet. In some centres haemodialysis is preferred.

If diuresis occurs renal recovery is often surprisingly complete; otherwise the patient has to remain under the care of a renal unit for dialysis or renal transplantation.

PLACENTA PRAEVIA

A placenta is described as praevia when it is wholly or partly attached to the lower uterine segment. Haemorrhage is inevitable when labour begins.

DEGREES OF PLACENTA PRAEVIA

The degree of encroachment onto the lower uter-

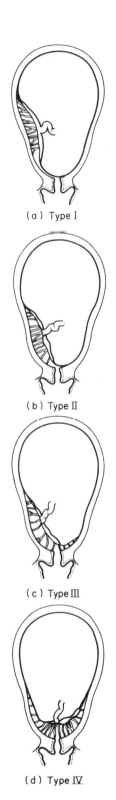

(a) Type I

(b) Type II

(c) Type III

(d) Type IV

Fig. 3.8   Classification of degrees of placenta praevia

ine segment is important because both treatment and prognosis are determined by it. Figure 3.8 illustrates the classification which is often used:

type I   the placenta is only partly attached to the lower segment. Its lower margin dips into the lower segment but is at a little distance from the internal cervical os. This is sometimes called a lateral placenta praevia

type II   more of the placenta is attached to the lower segment so that its lower margin reachs down to the internal os

type III   the placenta overlies the undilated internal os, but if a finger was passed through the cervix it would be able to reach the margin of the placenta

type IV   the placenta overlies the undilated internal os, but if a finger was passed through the cervix it could not reach the margin of the placenta. This type is often referred to as central or complete placenta praevia

This classification may be useful for descriptive purposes, but most unfortunately it gives the impression that the diagnosis of placenta praevia and its degree is made by passing a finger through the cervix. *This method of diagnosis can be disastrous and is to be avoided.*

Pathology

Placenta praevia occurs about once in 250 pregnancies, and is slightly more common in women who have had several children.

A placenta praevia is often irregular in shape and variable in thickness. It may cover a larger area than normal, and is often pathologically adherent in part to the lower uterine segment. These changes are explained by the comparatively poor blood supply which the placenta obtains from the less vascular lower segment. The cord frequently has a low marginal insertion.

The haemorrhage comes from maternal vessels which are opened up by separation of the placenta as the uterine contractions dilate the lower segment. The separation during pregnancy may be slight, but it is inevitably greater during labour, when severe bleeding occurs. Except in cases in which the placenta is torn there is no loss of fetal blood, but in severe cases fetal oxygenation will be impaired because of placental separation or compression during labour, or because maternal haemorrhage causes anaemia and hypotension, with reduced blood flow on the maternal side of the placenta. The cord vessels may be compressed in vasa praevia.

Symptoms and course of labour

During the last 12 weeks of pregnancy (and occasionally earlier) the patient notices slight haemorrhages from the vagina. These occur without evident cause, perhaps during sleep, but they may also follow hard exercise or any local disturbance such as coitus. There are usually repeated slight warning haemorrhages, but occasionally the first bleed may be a severe one, and in a few cases there is no bleeding until labour starts. There is no pain and the fetal movements and heart sounds are usually normal.

During labour severe haemorrhage is inevitable as the cervix dilates.

In the third stage of labour there may be postpartum haemorrhage because the placental site is larger than normal and lies on the lower segment which may not retract efficiently. Any cervical tear will bleed freely because of the increased vascularity.

Diagnosis

A history of repeated painless losses of blood in late pregnancy, small in amount at first but usually increasing, is strongly suggestive of placenta praevia.

On abdominal examination the fetal head is not engaged. It may be high and freely mobile; the breech may be presenting; or the lie may be oblique, because the placenta occupies the lower segment and prevents the head entering the pelvis. There is no tenderness and the fetal heart sounds are present.

On vaginal examination the presenting part may be obscured or be felt plainly through one fornix and indistinctly through the other, but a certain clinical diagnosis can only be made by feeling the placenta with a finger passed through the internal os. *This may be followed by furious bleeding*, and today such dangerous digital examination should always be avoided because the placental position can be determined by ultrasound.

In cases with slight bleeding it is safe to inspect the cervix by gentle passage of a speculum to exclude any incidental cause of bleeding. However, if a cervical erosion is found this does not exclude placenta praevia, and only if any cervical lesion is actually seen to be bleeding should it be accepted as a possible cause of the haemorrhage.

Hypertension or proteinuria are not found, except coincidentally.

Placental localization

Unless the patient is bleeding so profusely that immediate treatment is essential an attempt should be made to determine the position of the placenta. Several techniques have been tried in recent years but the only method now in common use is ultrasound scanning.

Ultrasound scanning

Ultrasound scanning is now freely available in all maternity units in Britain. It is without risk to the patient or fetus and is the method of choice. If a scan is performed at any stage of pregnancy for other reasons placental localization should always be undertaken at the same time, thus enabling many cases of placenta praevia to be diagnosed before any antepartum haemorrhage has occurred. A persistent malpresentation in late pregnancy, even in the absence of bleeding, requires ultrasound examination, when a placenta praevia may be discovered.

The characteristic mottled shadow on the screen may not outline the lower edge of the placenta accurately, but repeated scans can safely be performed if necessary. The placenta sometimes appears to be low-lying before the 32nd week, but re-examination later in pregnancy after the lower segment has formed may exclude this.

A fundal placenta is easy to outline, and this immediately excludes placenta praevia.

Prognosis

Maternal

The chief causes of death in cases of placenta praevia are haemorrhage and shock, and without efficient treatment the danger is great. The amount of bleeding will be least with a Type I (lateral) placenta praevia, but progressively greater with the more central types. Both antepartum and postpartum haemorrhage may occur. Some hazards arise from caesarean section, which is the necessary treatment, but in well-equipped units, with properly trained staff, these hazards are minimal. Sepsis is now rare; it used to be common when vaginal manipulations were carried out near the low-lying placental site.

The essential measure to reduce the risk of placenta praevia is to transfer any patient with slight antepartum haemorrhage to hospital at once, so that accurate diagnosis and preparation for treatment can be made before severe haemorrhage occurs. The maternal mortality in cases managed in this way is very low.

Fetal

Unless caesarean section is performed or unless the placenta praevia is of minor degree the outlook for the child is bad. Fetal death may occur from hypoxia caused by placental separation of compression, or by maternal hypotension and anaemia. Prematurity used to be a common cause of neonatal death, but with modern management it is less frequent.

Treatment

If there is any possibility of placenta praevia the patient must be admitted to hospital as soon as possible. In what is now an exceptional case, if the patient is first seen when bleeding severely in her own home she should be given morphine 15 mg intramuscularly and the doctor should send for the obstetric emergency team ('flying squad'), the members of which will be able to give a blood transfusion. *It is most important that no vaginal examination is made before transfer to hospital*, since such an examination may cause further serious haemorrhage. The patient's condition will determine whether she can be moved by ambulance immediately or only after blood transfusion.

In all cases with severe bleeding immediate active treatment is required and delay is perilous, but in the most common type of case seen today the patient is admitted when the bleeding has only been slight and there is time for investigation; it is usually possible to make a diagnosis by clinical and ultrasound examination. The chief cause of fetal mortality used to be prematurity, but it was found that if the bleeding was only slight and the fetus was some weeks premature, then the risk of keeping the patient in bed while the fetus grew was justifiable, provided that she was in a hospital

where treatment by blood transfusion and operation was available immediately should severe bleeding occur. This expectant attitude greatly reduced the fetal mortality without increasing the maternal mortality. If severe bleeding starts while the patient is in hospital caesarean section is performed immediately. The exact position of the placenta is of no importance and digital examination is dangerous and unnecessary.

In a few cases the diagnosis is still uncertain after ultrasound examination, and in these *few exceptional cases* when the pregnancy is near term it may be justifiable to make a pelvic examination, provided that it is done in the operating theatre with the patient anaesthetized and the instruments sterilized and ready for caesarean section. A finger is passed very gently through the cervix. If a placenta of Type II, III or IV is encountered, or if moderate or severe bleeding is precipitated, then caesarean section is performed. If the placenta is of Type I, and particularly if it is situated anteriorly, low rupture of the membranes is done, which allows the presenting part to descend and compress the lower margin of the placenta and so control the bleeding. If no placenta praevia is felt it is still wise to rupture the membranes, as the finger has now been inserted into the cavity of the uterus with a risk of introducing infection.

If the patient is shocked caesarean section should not be performed until this has been corrected by transfusion. Section should still be performed if there is severe bleeding and the fetus is premature or dead; the primary purpose of the operation is to control the bleeding by emptying the uterus and allowing it to retract.

If the placenta lies anteriorly a few obstetricians recommend upper segment caesarean section as there may be severe bleeding from large vessels in the lower segment and from the placenta during a lower segment operation, but it is nearly always found in practice that the lower segment operation can be safely performed, with the advantage of a much more secure uterine scar.

In all cases blood transfusion should be freely employed because, although the patient may recover from the initial haemorrhage, the possibility of further bleeding in the third stage must be anticipated.

VASA PRAEVIA

A rare cause of antipartum haemorrhage occurs

when there is a velamentous insertion of the cord (*see* p. 74) and the vessels lie on the membranes covering the internal os in front of the presenting part. When the membranes rupture these vessels may be torn and vaginal bleeding occurs. The blood lost is fetal blood and the fetus may become exsanguinated. The diagnosis is usually missed, but if suspected the blood should be tested at once for the presence of fetal red cells (Kleihauer-Berke or Kleihauer test) or fetal haemoglobin (AGE test). If the diagnosis is made the fetus should be delivered as quickly as possible.

POLYHYDRAMNIOS AND OLIGOHYDRAMNIOS

POLYHYDRAMNIOS

In this condition (which is often simply called hydramnios) there is an excess of liquor amnii. It is difficult to define exactly how much is excessive; the average volume of liquor at term is 800 ml, but a range of 400 to 1500 ml is accepted as normal. Probably only volumes in excess of 2000 ml would be noticed as abnormal on clinical examination. For theories about the mode of formation of amniotic fluid *see* page 14.

In most of the cases the excess fluid accumulates gradually (*chronic hydramnios*) and is only noticed after the 30th week. In a few exceptional cases hydramnios occurs earlier and more quickly (*acute hydramnios*), and many of these cases are associated with uniovular twins. The composition of the fluid in cases of hydramnios does not usually differ from normal.

Aetiological factors

Hydramnios occurs more often in multiparae than in primigravidae. It may have fetal or maternal causes.

Fetal causes

Hydramnios may occur with *twin pregnancy* of either type. Usually only one sac is distended. The association of acute hydramnios with uniovular twins has been mentioned.

Hydramnios often occurs with *anencephaly*. There may be some exudation from the exposed brain, but a more likely explanation is that the fetus does not swallow normally.

Hydramnios occurs with *oesophageal atresia*, when inability to swallow is certainly the explanation. In all cases in which there has been an excess of liquor the newborn infant must be examined to exclude oesophageal atresia.

Hydramnios may also occur with other fetal abnormalities, including spina bifida.

A rare cause is *chorioangioma of the placenta* (p. 74).

There may be excess of fluid in cases of *hydrops fetalis*.

Maternal causes

Hydramnios may occur with maternal diabetes. Not only is there an excess of amniotic fluid, but the placenta and fetus are large. There may be an excess of glucose in the liquor, but this is only found in a proportion of the cases and does not explain the hydramnios, which is probably caused by fetal polyuria. The polyuria is secondary to maternal and (therefore) fetal hyperglycaemia. Hydramnios is therefore most often seen when maternal diabetes is badly controlled.

Clinical features

The patient may notice that her abdomen is unduly enlarged and that the fetus is unusually mobile. If the uterus is very much enlarged she may have dyspnoea and indigestion. However, it is extraordinary how tolerant the patient may be of even an enormous accumulation of fluid, provided that it has formed slowly. In the rare cases of acute hydramnios there is abdominal pain and vomiting.

The physical signs depend on the amount of liquor. The abdomen is larger than expected for the duration of pregnancy, and the abdominal muscles may be stretched. It may be difficult to feel the fetus and the fetal heart sounds may be muffled or inaudible. A fluid thrill can be elicited.

The fetus is unduly mobile and the presentation is unstable. Oedema of the abdominal wall and vulva is sometimes seen. The tightness of the uterus varies, but in cases of acute hydramnios the uterus is very tense.

Diagnosis

Chronic hydramnios has to be distinguished from multiple pregnancy. This may be difficult, especially as hydramnios may complicate multiple pregnancy, in such a case the diagnosis of twins is easily missed. If the twin pregnancy is not complicated by hydramnios the essential clinical observations are the discovery of two heads and an unusual number of limbs. An ultrasound scan must be a routine in all cases of hydramnios to exclude mutiple pregnancy or fetal abnormalities such as anencephaly.

If pregnancy coexists with a large ovarian cyst the diagnosis from hydramnios can be difficult. Ultrasound scan will show two sacs, only one of which contains a fetus.

Acute hydramnios may simulate abruptio placentae with concealed haemorrhage, but in the latter condition the uterus is hard and tense and the fetal heart sounds are absent. In most cases of abruptio placentae there is at least a little external bleeding.

Effects on pregnancy and labour

Spontaneous preterm labour may occur. The membranes may rupture suddenly and there is a risk of prolapse of the umbilical cord. Because the fetus is unduly mobile malpresentations may occur. If a large quantity of liquor escapes suddenly the placental site may diminish in area, and this may lead to separation and antepartum haemorrhage. After delivery there is a risk of postpartum haemorrhage.

The perinatal mortality is greatly increased with hydramnios because there may be a fetal abnormality, and because of the possibility of preterm labour, cord prolapse and malpresentation.

Treatment

There is no known method of controlling the production or absorption of amniotic fluid, except that improved control in cases of diabetes may reduce the prevalence of hydramnios. Hydramnios without symptoms and without any evidence of fetal abnormality requires no treatment.

If ultrasound or radiological examination shows a gross fetal abnormality labour should be induced by rupturing the membranes and setting up a Syntocinon infusion after ensuring that the lie of the fetus is longitudinal. Routine ultrasound examination at 16–18 weeks should ensure that fetal abnormalities are detected before hydramnios develops.

In cases near term in which the patient is in serious discomfort labour should be induced. When there is a great deal of liquor under tension there is some risk of placental separation after rupturing the membranes, and some obstetricians would draw off part of the liquor by abdominal amniocentesis before the induction.

Abdominal amniocentesis is particularly suitable in cases in which the pregnancy is not sufficiently advanced for safe induction but the patient is in discomfort and there is no evidence of fetal abnormality. After localizing the placenta with ultrasound an epidural needle is inserted into the amniotic sac and fluid is withdrawn with an epidural catheter passed through the needle. Up to 2 litres of fluid may be removed, provided that it is only allowed to escape slowly. Although there is some risk of labour starting after amniocentesis the discomfort is relieved for a time. Unfortunately the fluid is often quickly replaced. The procedure may be repeated if necessary. There is always a slight risk of perforating a fetal vessel and causing bleeding into the amniotic sac.

OLIGOHYDRAMNIOS

This means deficiency of amniotic fluid, and is most often associated with poor placental function and fetal growth retardation.

Severe oligohydramnios is seen with obstructive lesions of the fetal urinary tract and with *renal agenesis*. In the latter the fetus has a typical facies (Potter's syndrome). The nose is hooked, the lower jaw is underdeveloped and the ears are set low. The amnion is studded with tiny white nodules. Microscopical examination shows these to be islands of degenerate squamous epithelium resting on a bed of flattened amniotic cells. It is thought that the squamous cells have been rubbed off by the dry skin of the fetus. There is usually pulmonary hypoplasia and the fetus invariably dies within 48 hours of birth.

In a few cases of oligohydramnios there is no evidence of renal or any other abnormality. The fetus has little room to move and if it presents by the breech in early pregnancy it will be unable to alter its position and version is impossible. Deformities of the limbs such as talipes and ankylosis of joints, may be caused by pressure, and amniotic adhesions may form bands which can constrict a limb.

If pregnancy continues beyond term there is a slight fall in the volume of liquor, which is not in itself of serious significance.

AMNIOTIC ADHESIONS

Amniotic bands may occur between the amnion and the head, body or limbs of the fetus. They are often associated with deformities, including craniofacial lesions and constriction rings or amputation of limbs. Possibly some of them result from early rupture of the amniotic sac, so that the fetus lies in a false cavity between the amnion and chorion.

HYPERTENSIVE DISORDERS OF PREGNANCY

The fact that some pregnant women had epileptiform fits was known to Hippocrates, who lived in the fourth century BC. The condition was called *eclampsia*, although the word does not refer to fits; the original Greek word meant 'flash out', in the sense of a sudden event. Little more was known about eclampsia until, in 1843, Lever (of Guy's Hospital) found that many of the women who had fits also had albumin in their urine. However, it was not until early in this century, when the sphygmomanometer was introduced, that it was recognized that eclampsia was associated with hypertension. The fact that albuminuria and hypertension could precede the onset of fits gave rise to the concept of 'pre-eclampsia' as a clinical condition.

For many years it was postulated that a toxin was liberated from the pregnant uterus, and the disorder became known as toxaemia of pregnancy. All efforts have so far failed to demonstrate any such toxin and the word 'toxaemia' is now avoided. The term 'pre-eclampsia' is criticized because only a small proportion of the patients develop eclampsia, and the term *pregnancy-induced hypertension* is now used. It will be easier to discuss the numerous theories of the aetiology of eclampsia and hypertension during pregnancy after describing their clinical and pathological features.

In these conditions signs precede symptoms. This means that early diagnosis is only possible if the pregnant woman is examined regularly, but it also means that early recognition and treatment of hypertension during pregnancy will almost always prevent eclampsia, which is a serious danger to the life of both mother and fetus.

The classic description of pregnancy-induced hypertension is that it is a condition occurring after the 20th week of pregnancy in which at least two of the three signs (hypertension, proteinuria and oedema) are present. The fact that oedema is found in about 50 per cent of normal pregnant women makes precise diagnosis difficult in some of the milder cases.

Further difficulties are that in some cases hypertension is pre-existing and therefore does not come into the above category, while in other cases the woman's blood pressure before pregnancy is unknown. Confusion has arisen in the past because of failure to classify hypertension during pregnancy accurately, and because of lack of agreement on definitions. The cases may be classified:

pregnancy-induced hypertension. This term includes eclampsia and cases formerly described as pre-eclampsia

chronic hypertension preceding pregnancy, of any aetiology

chronic hypertension with superimposed pregnancy-induced hypertension.

PREGNANCY-INDUCED HYPERTENSION

The signs of this condition usually appear over a

period of several days in the following order:

> fluid retention (or excessive weight gain)
> hypertension
> proteinuria.

However, they can appear in any order or all together in less than 24 hours. Some discussion of each of the signs is required.

Weight gain

During normal pregnancy the average weight gain is about 12 kg. Sometimes there is a loss of weight during the first trimester if nausea and vomiting are prominent. After the 12th week there is an average weight gain of about 0.5 kg per week until term, when the weight gain becomes less; indeed there may be a loss of about 0.5 kg in the week before delivery. There are great individual variations and the pattern may be distorted by dieting, overeating and vomiting. The weight gain is made up of the weight of the fetus, placenta and liquor, the increase in size of the uterus and breasts, the increased blood volume and expansion of the extracellular fluid, and fat deposition.

In pregnancy hypertension there is often, although not always, a large increase in salt and water retention in the extracellular space. This causes a sudden above-average weight gain. An increase of weight of 1 kg or more in a week should call for vigilance. As all the components of pregnancy weight gain depend upon the efficient functioning of the placenta, and as there is frequently a degree of placental insufficiency associated with hypertension, the total picture of weight fluctuations during pregnancy may be difficult to interpret. There is no evidence that women who are overweight before pregnancy or have an above-average weight gain throughout pregnancy are more likely to develop hypertension than slimmer women (although a fat arm may lead to an incorrect diagnosis of hypertension when the pressure is measured with a standard sphygmomanometer).

Oedema during pregnancy

A woman of average weight (55–60 kg) normally increases her extracellular fluid (apart from that in the fetus, placenta and liquor amnii) by over 2500 ml during the course of pregnancy. Osmotic equilibrium is maintained by the retention of sodium. This degree of fluid retention may cause slight thickening of the skin, rings on the fingers will be tighter and, if the carpal tunnel is restrictive, oedema of the sheath of the median nerve may cause paraesthesia of the fingers.

Excessive fluid retention eventually gives rise to oedema. This can usually first be detected over the lower subcutaneous surface of the tibia by gentle sustained pressure, but ultimately the feet and ankles are obviously swollen. Oedema of the feet and ankles may also be caused by pressure of the uterus on the pelvic veins, or by associated varicose veins. This non-significant dependent oedema is particularly common at the end of the day, especially when the woman has to spend much time standing, and during warm weather. Dependent oedema of moderate degree is so common that it is usually disregarded unless it is accompanied by other signs. Oedema of the fingers or face is more significant because gravity has little effect upon the accumulation of fluid in these places, but even here it does not establish a diagnosis of pregnancy-induced hypertension.

Blood pressure during pregnancy

Most younger women have a resting blood pressure of 110–120 mmHg systolic and 60–70 mmHg diastolic. There is wide variation in healthy women and the response to stress adds to the differences found at the first visit to a clinic or to the doctor. Ideally, to assess the changes observed during pregnancy, the pressure before pregnancy should be known, but as this is rarely the case it is necessary to take the readings made during the first trimester as the indicator of the normal state.

The control of blood pressure is affected by normal pregnancy. Pooling of blood in the legs and splanchnic area may result in transient cerebral ischaemia when the pregnant woman stands up suddenly or stands still for a time. The faintness that results is often regarded by lay folk as an indication of pregnancy. The pulse pressure is slightly higher during pregnancy than in the nonpregnant state because the diastolic pressure is lower. In the midtrimester some patients have a slight fall in both systolic and diastolic pressure, a change that reverts before term. In late pregnancy another factor causes variability; the pressure of the uterus on the large pelvic veins and the inferior vena cava brings about a diminished return of blood to the right side of the heart and induces a low-output hypotension. This most commonly occurs when the patient is lying on her back, especially if she is under an anaesthetic, and is termed the *supine hypotensive syndrome*.

There is some disagreement as to what may be regarded as a normal blood pressure during pregnancy. In most clinics 140/90 mm is taken to be the dividing point between physiology and pathology. Some will diagnose hypertension in pregnancy if there is an increase of 30 mm in systolic pressure or 15 mm in diastolic pressure over the baseline readings. The rise should be observed on two readings taken six hours apart.

The standards of hypertension used in general medicine are not appropriate in obstetrics. A pregnant woman with a blood pressure of 140/90 mm may be running into danger and at 160/110 she might develop eclampsia. Pregnant women are in a young age group, but during pregnancy the blood pressure may sometimes rise very quickly and the fetus may be at risk with relatively slight hypertension. The physiopathology of eclampsia differs from that of essential hypertension, whether benign or malignant.

If the blood pressure rises acutely, with the diastolic reading above 100 mm, the patient may complain of a severe and persistent frontal headache and may vomit. These are warning signals of the possibility of eclampsia. But of course many pregnant women develop headache for other reasons such as migraine, and in the absence of hypertension a headache during pregnancy is not to be taken as a complication of the pregnancy.

The patient who has an abnormally high blood pressure before pregnancy requires special consideration. In her case a rise in the diastolic pressure of 20 mmHg is usually required before a diagnosis of superimposed pregnancy-induced hypertension can be made.

Proteinuria during pregnancy

The term proteinuria is more accurate than albuminuria. Although at first the protein is largely albumin – the molecules of which are among the smallest of the plasma proteins – as hypertension worsens larger molecules, including globulins, appear in increasing proportions. Proteinuria is most easily detected with test paper strips although older methods, including boiling the urine, remain satisfactory. The test paper strips are very sensitive and indicate a degree of proteinuria which would not be detected by older methods. Nevertheless proteinuria during pregnancy is always potentially serious and demands investigation. Besides hypertension of pregnancy, the main causes are contamination from vaginal discharge, urinary tract infection and chronic renal disease.

Most patients do not take particular care when producing a urine specimen for the antenatal clinic or doctor's surgery, and often bring it in any jar that is at hand. Before accepting that proteinuria is present contamination must be excluded by obtaining a 'clean catch' midstream specimen, after cleansing the vulva with sterile water or saline.

Urinary infection can be excluded by examining the urine microscopically. When infection is present pus cells and bacteria can be seen. Bacteriological examination must also be used to confirm the diagnosis and to indicate the most appropriate treatment.

Proteinuria associated with chronic renal disease rarely presents a diagnostic problem because there is usually a history of the disease predating the pregnancy. Even if there is no such history it is likely that the proteinuria will be present throughout pregnancy, while pregnancy-induced hypertension is very uncommon before the third trimester.

After excluding these other causes of proteinuria it is reasonable to attribute it to pregnancy-induced hypertension. It is then always a sign of serious significance. The risk of intrauterine death of the fetus and of eclampsia is increased many times over when proteinuria occurs, even when there is only a slight increase in blood pressure.

A rarer type of proteinuria is *orthostatic proteinuria*. Orthostatic means 'standing straight', and the proteinuria only occurs after the patient has been on her feet for some time. At night in the recumbent position the proteinuria disappears. It is not peculiar to pregnancy, and is not uncommon in adolescents. In the standing posture the left renal vein is compressed where it crosses the vertebral column. This presumably raises the venous pressure in the left kidney; it has been shown that in this condition most of the protein in the urine comes from the left kidney. The diagnosis is most improbable in a fully ambulant pregnant woman. Unexplained proteinuria necessitates admission to hospital, but in some women the proteinuria promptly disappears; then the diagnosis of orthostatic proteinuria can be made by testing the urine before and after activity.

Sometimes other uncommon causes of proteinuria during pregnancy such as nephritis or disseminated lupus erythematosus, may need consideration.

Clinical features of pregnancy-induced hypertension

Pregnancy-induced hypertension with proteinuria occurs in 2–4 per cent of primigravidae and hypertension without proteinuria in 15–20 per cent. In second and subsequent pregnancies the incidence of hypertension, with or without proteinuria, is only about one-tenth as great as in first pregnancies. Even a previous abortion gives some protection against developing hypertension.

Those multiparae who develop the condition almost always have a history of a similar event in the preceding pregnancy or pregnancies. Unless there is some underlying vascular disease hypertension usually becomes less severe from one pregnancy to the next.

Pregnancy-induced hypertension is more common in women over 35, especially in relatively infertile primigravidae. Those who have essential hypertension are more likely to develop a further rise in blood pressure during pregnancy than normotensive women, but they do not invariably do so. However, in patients with hypertensive renal disease such a rise in pressure almost always occurs. It is more common in patients with diabetes mellitus, and almost invariably occurs when there is diabetic vascular disease.

There is an increased incidence of hypertension in association with multiple pregnancy, with polyhydramnios, with severe rhesus incompatibility and in cases of hydatidiform mole. The last association is of interest because the hypertension is frequently severe, occurs early in pregnancy (usually 16–20 weeks), and in the absence of a fetus.

One other condition deserves to be mentioned, although it is extremely rare. This is abdominal pregnancy, where the placenta has become attached to structures outside the uterus, but has succeeded in maintaining the fetus into the third trimester. In these cases hypertension frequently occurs.

Management of pregnancy-induced hypertension

Although the aetiology of pregnancy-induced hypertension is still obscure, empirical management has achieved considerable improvement in the prognosis for both mother and baby. It is possible that the severity of the disease has also declined in recent years. As a result the incidence of eclampsia in countries where there is comprehensive antenatal care has fallen from 1 in 1000 to 1 in 5000 births.

The most important factor in management is early diagnosis. Because hypertension becomes more likely as pregnancy nears term, antenatal attendances should be more frequent at this time. In the first 30 weeks of pregnancy visits are usually made monthly, from 30 to 36 weeks visits should be fortnightly, and after that, weekly. At each visit the patient is weighed, oedema is sought at the ankles and in the fingers, the resting blood pressure is recorded and the urine tested for protein. Excessive weight gain, moderate oedema, and a rise of blood pressure not exceeding 130/80 mmHg may be dealt with by advising rest at home. A check on the effectiveness of this advice must be made within a week.

If the blood pressure reaches 140/90 mm or the diastolic pressure rises 20 mm above the booking pressure the woman needs special supervision, with daily observation of the blood pressure and urine testing. Most obstetricians are now prepared to manage mild non-proteinuric cases at home, provided that the general practitioner or district midwife regularly checks the urine for protein. Worsening of the hypertension or proteinuria would necessitate immediate hospital admission.

The aim of treatment is to obtain a live baby, as mature as possible, while preventing injury to the mother. It is desirable to maintain the pregnancy until at least the 36th week, always providing that the placental function remains adequate and the mother's blood pressure is under sufficient control to minimize the risk of eclampsia, cerebral haemorrhage and abruptio placentae. Hypertension will not be cured until the fetus is delivered, and, however well controlled it may appear to be, it is usually necessary to keep the patient in hospital or under close supervision until this time.

The most important component of treatment is rest in bed. This will usually result in stabilization of the blood pressure and, because uterine blood flow is relatively greater when the patient is at rest, better fetal growth.

Sedatives are sometimes employed and these have a marginal effect upon the blood pressure.

Diazepam (Valium) should not be used for mild cases as it can have a depressant effect on the baby if it is born prematurely.

Hypotensive agents and diuretics should only be used in special circumstances. Reduction of the blood pressure to normal values can often be attained by the use of potent hypotensive agents, but this may be at the expense of placental function, which in many cases seems to depend on the raised blood pressure, in the same way as a damaged kidney may depend upon an increased blood pressure to maintain a tolerable function.

Routine observations in hospital will include records of the blood pressure at least twice daily, and more frequently if the condition is worsening. Oedema may be sought in the sacral region, but it is difficult to detect and checking the tightness of rings on the fingers is more profitable. A record should be kept of fluid intake and urinary output in all but the slightest cases, for reduction in urinary output almost always precedes eclampsia. Each urinary specimen should be tested for protein. The blood urea level should be checked on admission and periodically. Serum urate levels are of value in assessing progress of the disease and the prognosis for the fetus. Levels of 450 mmol/L and above are associated with a poor fetal prognosis and are an indication for delivery.

Regular palpation of the uterus to detect growth failure or diminishing liquor volume is helpful in judging placental function. These observations should be supplemented by ultrasonic measurements of the biparietal diameter of the fetal head and the abdominal circumference of the fetus. Serial measurements may indicate inpairment of fetal growth.

Doppler blood-flow measurements of the fetal circulation in the umbilical artery and of circulation in the placental bed give direct evidence of resistance to flow in the placental bed.

Another indication of fetal well-being is its activity. This can be assessed by the mother counting the number of fetal movements over a given time (a 'kick count'), by recording fetal breathing movements with ultrasound, or by observing the variation in fetal heart rate that accompanies fetal activity or occurs in response to uterine contractions.

In conditions in which the fetus may be compromised, such as pregnancy-induced hypertension, it is common practise to make daily simultaneous observations on the fetal heart and uterine contractions with a cardiotocograph (*antenatal CTG*).

Another method of fetal assessment is by the *biophysical profile*, which is based on real-time ultrasound observations of fetal breathing and movements, on tone in the fetus, on the quantity of the liquor amnii and on a non-stress test (*see* p. 131).

Sampling of fetal blood by cordocentesis, and estimation of pH or Po_2 may have a place in the severely compromised fetus.

A time may come in any pregnancy complicated by hypertension when the fetus is safer delivered and in a cot, even in the premature nursery, than in the unhealthy environment of the uterus. The purpose of all these investigations is to decide when this moment has arrived. In some cases labour starts prematurely, and in most cases there is a ready response to induction. In any event the patient should not be allowed to pass her expected date of delivery.

The worsening situation – imminent eclampsia

If the diastolic blood pressure remains above 100 mmHg in spite of rest in bed, or if proteinuria persists, and the duration of gestation is more than 36 weeks labour should be induced without hesitation. During labour the fetal heart rate should be continuously monitored.

If the fetus is very immature, between 28 and 33 weeks, hypotensive agents may be used to prevent further elevation of the blood pressure. However, the diastolic pressure should not be reduced to less than 90 mm, as this can reduce placental perfusion and lead to fetal death. Among the many powerful drugs on the market no one agent seems to be better than another. It is sensible to become familiar with one agent, and methyldopa is often chosen. If control of the blood pressure cannnot be achieved, or the amount of protein in the urine is increasing or heavy, or if there is evidence of placental failure, then early delivery is advisable, often by caesarean section.

In cases between 33 and 36 weeks judgment is exercised. The excellent care available in modern neonatal units has encouraged the decision to deliver the fetus early if there is any doubt about poor placental function or hazard to the mother.

Signs that an eclamptic fit is imminent include a continually rising blood pressure, increasing oedema of the face and hands, heavy proteinuria, oliguria, headache and disturbances of vision. Vomiting and epigastric pain, with tenderness over the liver, indicate hepatic haemorrhages or necrosis. Urgent action is required to prevent fits, to reduce the blood pressure, to promote diuresis and to deliver the fetus.

An intravenous injection of diazepam (Valium) 10 mg is given at once, followed by a slow infusion containing 40 mg in a litre of 5 per cent dextrose solution. This acts as a sedative and raises the threshold at which fits occur. Other effective sedatives which are sometimes used are chlormethiazole in a 0.8 per cent intravenous infusion, or intravenous infusions of magnesium sulphate (*see* p. 92).

The blood pressure can be most promptly reduced by intravenous administration of hydralazine (Apresoline). While monitoring the blood pressure closely, hydralazine 10 mg is injected intravenously over a period of 15 minutes. The initial dose is usually followed by a continuous slow infusion of 50 mg of hydralazine in a litre of Hartmann's solution. The rate of infusion is adjusted to keep the blood pressure just above 140/90 mm; if the pressure falls below this the infusion is stopped.

Frusemide (Lasix) 40 mg intravenously will produce a diuresis within minutes, this helps to reduce the blood pressure and appears to protect the kidneys from possible damage caused by a vascular shutdown. An indwelling catheter will avoid the discomfort of a full bladder or the disturbance of frequent micturition.

External stimuli are liable to trigger off a fit, therefore undue noise, bright lights and painful procedures should be avoided.

The method of delivery will depend upon the parity of the patient, the stage of pregnancy and the state of the cervix. In all but the most severe cases, and cases in which placental function is notably poor, vaginal delivery should be the aim. If delivery has to be effected before the 34th week, when induction is less certain, caesarean section may be considered, and it would be advised if there was not an immediate response to induction, or if labour was not progressing quickly.

During labour the maternal blood pressure must be recorded frequently. Painful uterine contractions may raise the blood pressure and trigger off a fit. Good control of pain is therefore essential and this can be best achieved with an epidural anaesthetic. The progress of the first stage of labour should be checked by vaginal examination at 2- to 3-hourly intervals, and the condition of the fetus monitored by continuous fetal heart rate recording.

The second stage should be short because of the risk of raising the maternal blood pressure. With an epidural anaesthetic a low forceps delivery or vacuum extraction is easy, and ensures the minimal risk.

The third stage of labour is potentially dangerous in the hypertensive patient because there is usually a transient rise in blood pressure when the uterus contracts down and the vascular space is reduced. This rise in pressure is greater if an oxytoxic drug is used, especially with ergometrine, which causes peripheral vasoconstriction. These patients seem to be particularly prone to this vasoconstrictor effect and it is therefore sensible to avoid the routine use of ergometrine in the third stage of labour. If anything is needed to prevent or treat postpartum haemorrhage Syntocinon, 5 units intravenously, is usually effective and its hypertensive effect is minimal.

Because of the possibility of postpartum eclampsia the blood pressure is carefully watched after delivery and the urinary output is recorded. Drugs should be withdrawn gradually over the course of three or four days, depending on the progress of the patient.

ECLAMPSIA

Eclampsia remains one of the most serious complications of pregnancy. It may occur before, during or shortly after delivery. The mortality varies with the number of fits, the quality of treatment and the speed with which it is made available. A maternal mortality of 2 or 3 per cent and a perinatal mortality of 15 per cent still occur, even in countries with modern obstetric services.

Eclampsia is characterized by the occurrence of major epileptiform convulsions in patients with signs and symptoms described above under imminent eclampsia. Four stages in the fits are described:

the aura. In eclampsia this is visual, with flashes of light and spots before the eyes

the cry, which is caused by spasm of the respiratory muscles and larynx; it is not usually noticeable

the tonic phase, during which the patient loses

consciousness, has generalized muscular spasm and becomes cyanosed. The fetus may show signs of hypoxia

the clonic phase, during which violent movements occur, the tongue may be bitten, and vomiting and the inhalation of vomit may occur. In severe cases recurrent fits occur and the patient remains deeply unconscious between them. The risks of hypoxia, inhalation of vomit and of cerebral haemorrhage caused by elevation of the blood pressure during the fits are considerable. Abruptio placentae, disseminated intravascular coagulation and renal necrosis are other serious dangers.

Treatment

The whole emphasis of this chapter has been on prevention of eclampsia by vigilance during pregnancy, during labour and soon after labour. It is especially important to recognize cases of worsening and fulminating hypertension so that further development can be prevented by delivery followed by full sedation for at least 48 hours.

If eclampsia does occur the aim is to prevent further fits. The greater the number of fits the worse is the prognosis for the mother and baby. Any stimulus may precipitate another fit, so the excitability of the central nervous system must be reduced by sedatives or anaesthesia and everything should be done to cut down external stimuli such as noise, bright light and discomfort, arising especially from a full bladder or a strained position in bed.

Heavy sedation is given immediately. Apart from those sedatives already described, magnesium sulphate may be given by slow intravenous infusion, initially 4–5 g over 20 minutes and then 1–3 g per hour. Because the patient is comatose or else heavily sedated there is a risk of both asphyxia and hypostatic pneumonia. A clear airway must be maintained and oxygen may be required. Provision must be made for aspiration of any vomit. False teeth must be removed, and a gag may be placed between the jaws. The patient may need restraint to prevent her injuring herself during the fits. An indwelling catheter will both prevent the stimulus of an overfull bladder and allow accurate observation of the urinary output.

Hypotensive agents, as already described on pages 90 and 96, may reduce the risk of cerebral haemorrhage or of abruptio placentae.

The patient will not be safe from the possibility of further fits until she is delivered, and the risk of hypostatic pneumonia is another reason to urge early delivery. The mode of delivery will depend to some extent on the prognosis for the fetus. If it is dead or very small caesarean section may not be justified, but with a fetus of reasonable size the risk of labour with a poorly functioning placenta may not be acceptable. If caesarean section is not chosen labour must be rapid and easy. Forceps or the vacuum extractor are often used for delivery, and with any additional obstetric problem section is advised.

Eclampsia may occur up to 48 hours or more after delivery. In this country postpartum eclampsia is now more common than antepartum eclampsia, perhaps because of relaxation of vigilance after delivery. It may be very severe and difficult to control. For treatment the patient is deeply sedated until the signs have improved.

These seriously ill patients are now often nursed in an intensive care unit, and deep sedation and positive pressure ventilation may help to reduce the risks of cerebral haemorrhage.

Remote prognosis of pregnancy-induced hypertension and eclampsia

After pregnancy-induced hypertension or eclampsia approximately one-third of women will be found to have residual hypertension. The question is whether these conditions caused the hypertension. At present it is held that these women would eventually have developed hypertension even if they never had a pregnancy. The evidence that supports this view is that the incidence of deaths from cardiovascular disease is the same at all comparable ages in nulliparous women and in women who have borne children.

Some women have hypertension in every successive pregnancy and most of these will later be found to have essential hypertension.

Pathology of pregnancy-induced hypertension and eclampsia

It is fortunately uncommon nowadays to have an opportunity to study the postmortem features of these conditions. The available evidence throws scant light upon the aetiology of the disease or of the mechanism by which the hypertension, oedema and proteinuria are produced. Most of the lesions observed in fatal cases result from the hypertension rather than provide an explanation for it.

Cerebral lesions

Because of the raised intracranial pressure the brain is oedematous and the convolutions are flattened. There are small haemorrhages scattered throughout its substance which may become confluent. Massive haemorrhage in the brain may be a cause of death. Haemorrhage and oedema may also occur in the retina.

Hepatic lesions

The lesions found in the liver in eclampsia are diagnostic of the disease. There is no other disorder which produces similar changes. Macroscopically the liver is enlarged and there are patchy focal red and yellow areas, of which the red are caused by haemorrhage and the yellow by necrosis of the liver cells. The red and yellow patches are visible under the capsule and throughout the cut surfaces. On microscopical section the haemorrhages are mainly grouped around the portal canals, but they may be so extensive that they completely disrupt the liver architecture. By interrupting the blood supply they cause necrosis in the periphery of the lobules with fatty change, which is responsible for the yellow colour. The extravasated blood shows many fibrinous thrombi.

The epigastric pain and liver tenderness which may occur in eclampsia probably arise from distension of the capsule. The interference with liver function is caused by destruction and damage to liver cells, and if this is severe it will result in jaundice. This is therefore a very serious sign. The damage to the liver may be so great that death occurs from hepatic failure.

Renal lesions

The primary renal lesion is in the glomeruli which show swelling of their cells and of the underlying basement membrane. The whole glomerulus appears to be so stuffed with its own swollen cells that it looks as if there is no room for blood to flow through the capillaries, but in fact a greatly diminished flow continues. It is generally held that the reduced renal blood flow is caused by vascular spasm, although the cause of the spasm is uncertain. Beyond the glomerulus the rest of the nephron which is supplied by the afferent arteriole is starved of oxygen. The result is necrosis of the proximal and distal convoluted tubules. This may be of any degree of severity from simple cloudy swelling up to death.

Depending on circumstances, large or small areas of the kidney may be involved. In extreme cases the cortex of the kidney may be destroyed almost entirely – a condition known as bilateral cortical necrosis (*see* p. 79). This is less common in eclampsia than in cases of abruptio placentae. In eclampsia the renal ischaemia is usually less severe and causes areas of patchy necrosis which affect the tubules rather than the glomeruli. Such lower nephron necrosis may be reversible, so that spontaneous recovery occurs. Whether the glomeruli or the tubules are chiefly affected, there is always some degree of renal failure, which in severe cases may progress to anuria.

These pathological changes explain the proteinuria by damage to the glomerular cells, and the oliguria by reduction of glomerular filtration. Sometimes the amount of glomerular filtrate may be very little diminished but the tubules are incapable of concentrating the fluid which reaches them.

Pathology of oedema

Oedema is due to an increase in fluid in the extracellular extravascular compartment of the body. Normally fluid flows out of the capillaries into the tissue space because of the hydrostatic pressure at the arterial end. Fluid flows back at the venous end of the capillary because of the high osmotic pressure brought about within the capillary by the outflow of fluid and the retention of protein molecules within it. One likely mechanism of production of oedema in pregnancy hypertension is the forcing out of fluid by increased blood pressure. Loss of protein in the urine might accentuate this effect.

Aetiology of pregnancy-induced hypertension and eclampsia

There are many theories of the cause of these conditions but none is entirely satisfactory.

Certain clinical observations must be fitted into any theory, however complex:

there is no instance of hypertension of this type

occurring outside pregnancy, although a number of other diseases have some similarities to it. It resolves completely when the pregnancy is over unless some structural damage has been caused by the hypertension

it occurs more commonly in first than in subsequent pregnancies

the incidence is high when there is pre-existing vascular disease or long-standing hypertension

it tends to be less severe in successive pregnancies unless there is pre-existing vascular disease

it occurs more frequently as pregnancy advances but its progress can often be slowed or even arrested. However, the only cure of the disease is the ending of the pregnancy

intrauterine death of the fetus is often associated with considerable improvement in the signs of the disease

it is not necessary for a fetus to be present. With a hydatidiform mole severe hypertension may occur early in pregnancy

it is more common in multiple pregnancy

it is more common in women who have diabetes mellitus, especially if there is diabetic arterial disease, nephropathy or retinopathy

it may occur in haemolytic disease with a hydropic placenta and fetus

the fetus is frequently light in weight for its period of gestation and shows signs of intrauterine malnutrition which has often preceded the development of the signs of pregnancy hypertension

hypertension sometimes appears or becomes worse after delivery, even to the stage of eclampsia. The occurrence of this has decreased since the risk of the pressor effect of ergometrine in these patients has been recognized.

Current theories of the aetiology of pregnancy-induced hypertension centre round three pathophysiological systems:

immunological mechanisms
altered vascular reactivity
coagulation disturbance.

Measurable differences can be observed during pregnancy in all these systems, and attempts have been made to find an explanation for pregnancy-induced hypertension based on these observations.

It is possible that there are different aetiological factors in different cases, and that we may be dealing with a number of linked conditions which share the physical signs of hypertension, proteinuria and oedema. In the present state of knowledge all that we shall attempt is to describe some of the changes that have been observed during pregnancy and discuss how they may be related to pregnancy-induced hypertension. Neither the observations nor the theories are simple.

Immunological mechanisms

Trophoblastic tissue contains HLA, ABO and tissue-specific antigens and immunoglobulins. Since half of these antigens are of paternal origin, development of maternal antibodies which would reject the placenta and fetus might be expected. Trophoblast seems to be capable of only low-grade antigenic activity, because surface coating with protective sialomucin and barrier antibodies occurs. There is also a reduction in maternal immune responsiveness, perhaps an effect of higher levels of hCG, hPL, progesterone and cortisone. Other maternal hormones and pregnancy proteins have been shown to be lymphocytic immunosuppressants.

It is known that from early pregnancy trophoblastic cells escape into the maternal circulation; this may occur to a greater extent in hypertensive pregnancy. Thus an excessive amount of antigen might be released into the maternal circulation and result in the formation of antigen-antibody complexes which are deposited in specific sites such as the renal glomeruli and placenta. Certainly immunofluorescent techniques have demonstrated deposition of immune complexes and IgM in renal glomeruli and spiral arterioles of the placental bed. This deposition might be responsible for the development of the hypertensive process.

The increased incidence of hypertension in first pregnancies is not explained.

Altered vascular reactivity

Renin is produced and stored in the juxtaglomerular apparatus of the kidney. It is also produced by the placenta and the fetal kidney. Renin acts on renin substrate to produce angiotensin I which is converted to the potent vasoconstrictor angiotensin II.

In normal pregnancy there is decreased response

to the vasoconstrictor effect of angiotensin II, while in hypertensive pregnancy the response is increased and there is an increase in circulating levels of angiotensin II. This reduced response to angiotensin II in normal pregnancy may result from a counterbalancing effect of prostacyclin (prostaglandin PGI_2), a potent vasodilator present in blood vessel walls. Prostacyclin concentrations increase in normal pregnancy. A mild increase in angiotensin II levels appears to cause a rise in blood pressure and an increase in uteroplacental blood flow, perhaps by stimulating increased production of the local vasodilator prostacyclin.

In severe pregnancy-induced hypertension there seems to be a reduced concentration of prostacyclin and its metabolites in maternal blood and in uterine and umbilical vessels. With reduction in prostacyclin activity there is less opposition to the vasoconstrictor action of angiotensin II and placental blood flow is *reduced*. A reduction in renal vascular wall prostaglandins might have a similar effect on renal blood flow, producing hypertension and renal damage.

The increased incidence of hypertension in first pregnancies is not explained, nor the reason for any reduction in prostacyclin activity.

Coagulation disturbance

Reduction in the number of circulating platelets, increase in fibrinogen degradation products and reduction in fibrinolytic activity have been observed in patients with severe pregnancy hypertension, suggesting that intravascular coagulation is occurring. Alterations have also been found in levels of factors VIII, IX and X. Fibrin deposition is a well-known histopathological feature of pregnancy hypertension. It has been postulated that the placenta may release thromboplastin, which causes disseminated intravascular coagulation, and that the fibrin deposition in the kidney and placenta results in the development of hypertension and placental insufficiency.

It is difficult to know whether the disseminated intravascular coagulation is cause or effect. Although some studies have suggested that alteration in the coagulation mechanism occurs *before* the development of hypertension, others have failed to confirm this. Early reports that treatment with heparin improves the outcome in early hypertension of pregnancy have not been confirmed, although the coagulation parameters are certainly

improved. It is possible that aspirin may be of prophylactic benefit.

CHRONIC HYPERTENSION PRECEDING PREGNANCY

Chronic hypertension preceding pregnancy may result from chronic pyelonephritis, chronic nephritis, polycystic disease of the kidneys, renal artery stenosis, coarctation of the aorta, phaechromocytoma or, most commonly, essential hypertension. Before making a diagnosis of essential hypertension the other possible underlying causes of hypertension must be excluded. For the obstetrician the importance of hypertension is that women starting pregnancy with a raised blood pressure are more likely to develop superadded pregnancy-induced hypertension than those who are normotensive. However this only occurs in a proportion of cases, and two out of three women who have a mild or moderate degree of essential hypertension at the start of pregnancy do not have a further rise of blood pressure and have babies of normal birth weight. However, hypertension caused by renal disease is more likely to progress.

If a pregnant woman is not seen until after the 12th week of pregnancy an accurate base-line pressure reading may not be obtained because of the tendency of the pressure to fall slightly in the middle trimester. This tendency is most marked in those who have mild hypertension of recent origin, and it is of good prognostic significance because the incidence of superadded hypertension is lower in this group of patients than in those hypertensive patients who do not show such a fall.

Management

A resting blood pressure of 140/90 mmHg or more during the first 24 weeks of pregnancy is usually deemed to be significantly raised, and at that time in pregnancy is unlikely to be due to pregnancy-induced hypertension.

If hypertension is found an effort must be made to discover any underlying cause of it, such as those mentioned above. The previous history may indicate the cause. The femoral pulses must be palpated; absence of pulsation would suggest the possibility of aortic coarctation. The urine is examined for protein and casts, and bacteriologically examined if any pus cells are found. The blood urea and serum urate levels may be estimated and other renal function tests may be required. Unfortunately, even if some underlying cause for the hypertension is discovered, specific treatment can seldom be given during pregnancy, and the management described here may be all that is possible until after delivery.

Proteinuria

Proteinuria is of serious prognostic significance when found with hypertension, for it implies that there is both renal and cardiovascular disease. Which of these is primary is not of immediate importance in obstetric practice, and fortunately most cases of essential hypertension have not progressed far enough to cause renal damage during the childbearing years. However, proteinuria may be due to chronic pyelonephritis, chronic nephritis or to relatively rare diseases such as systemic lupus erythematosus involving the kidney. This may be diagnosed by the discovery of LE cells in the blood.

The retina

The retina should be examined in all patients with hypertension, abnormal signs being nipping of the veins where they are crossed by the arteries, narrowing of the arteries, and occasionally haemorrhages or exudate. Such findings may show that the hypertensive disease is of long standing and preceded the pregnancy.

Mild essential hypertension

In all cases of mild essential hypertension (less than 150/100 mmHg) the patients must be seen more frequently than usual because of the risk of a further rise in blood pressure during pregnancy. A rise in diastolic pressure of 20 mm, or the appearance of proteinuria, is an indication for admission to hospital. Careful watch must be kept on the growth of the fetus both by clinical observation and with the help of ultrasound.

Moderate or severe hypertension

With moderate or severe hypertension (above 150/100 mmHg) the patient should be admitted to hospital for rest. The effect of rest gives a valuable indication of the prognosis, for if the blood pressure is thereby reduced a favourable outcome can

be expected. Such a patient may be sent home, but weekly checks of blood pressure and fetal growth must continue.

If the blood pressure does not fall with rest in bed and sedation, thought should be given to the use of hypotensive drugs. In using such drugs the prime consideration is the protection of the mother from the dangers of high blood pressure, such as cerebral haemorrhage and left heart failure. Artificial lowering of the blood pressure will only minimally improve the chance of survival of the fetus; indeed there is a danger that it may diminish the blood flow to the placenta and affect the fetus adversely.

Hypotensive drugs

The preference among the many hypotensive drugs at present is for methyldopa. It is started at a dosage of 250 mg twice daily and then slowly worked up towards a maximum dose of 4 g daily, depending on the response of the blood pressure. It has the special advantage that its effects are not dependent upon the patient standing up; with some other drugs a hypotensive effect is only seen when the patient is on her feet, and then the pressure may fall so precipitously that she feels faint. Several other hypotensive drugs are in use, including labetalol 100–200 mg twice daily and hydralazine 25–100 mg twice daily. A thiazide diuretic may also be given, together with a potassium supplement, to guard against depletion when this element is lost with sodium in the urine.

Some patients are already taking hypotensive drugs before they become pregnant; these drugs should be continued, adjusting the dose if necessary.

Treatment

Obstetric treatment in essential hypertension is exactly the same as for pregnancy-induced hypertension. It is essentially that of securing delivery at the best time to avoid serious maternal complications and to prevent fetal death *in utero*. When the diastolic pressure is between 90 and 99 mm the perinatal loss will be about 4 per cent; if it is between 100 and 109 mm, about 6 per cent and if it is above 110 mm, about 12 per cent. Much of this fetal loss occurs in the last few weeks of pregnancy, so that it is often best to secure delivery before term. The best time for this will depend on the particular case, but in general the higher the pressure the earlier the delivery should be. Renal and placental function tests, ultrasound measurements of fetal growth and fetal heart monitoring may all play a part in determining the optimum time for delivery. Assessment of the maturity of the fetal lung by measurement of the lecithin–sphingomyelin ratio in the liquor amnii may be helpful in deciding whether to induce labour.

The method of induction or delivery depends on the particular case. In a severe case If there is not a quick response to induction, caesarean section should be performed.

ABRUPTIO PLACENTAE AND HYPERTENSION DURING PREGNANCY

In about 25 per cent of cases of abruptio placentae moderate hypertension or proteinuria (or both) are discovered. It was at one time believed that pregnancy-induced hypertension or essential hypertension were common causes of abruptio placentae. However, in 90 per cent of cases of abruptio placentae there is no record of any *preceding* hypertension. It is certain that in some cases the hypertension and proteinuria *follow* the bleeding, perhaps as a result of a uterorenal reflex.

It seems likely that both events may occur, i.e. that hypertension may occasionally lead to placental separation, and that placental damage may sometimes cause hypertension.

INTERCURRENT DISEASES DURING PREGNANCY

PYELONEPHRITIS DURING PREGNANCY

In pyelonephritis there is inflammation of the renal pelvis and renal parenchyma.

Acute pyelonephritis has long been known as a common and apparently transient complication of pregnancy, but it is only relatively recently that it has been recognized that it is a potentially dangerous disease which, if it persists and becomes chronic, may progress to cause hypertension and ultimate renal failure. The obstetrician is in a particularly favourable position to prevent this, not only by effective treatment during pregnancy, but by securing for his patients proper subsequent investigation and care.

Aetiology

Bacteriuria

Acute pyelonephritis in pregnancy is sometimes just an episode in a long-standing disease process, which began in childhood or even during early infancy. Repeated attacks of urinary infection may occur throughout childhood, and often there is an exacerbation with the beginning of sexual activity

and during pregnancy. Infection in childhood may produce renal scarring with irregular narrowing of the renal cortex. The infecting organisms, usually coliforms, probably invade the bladder from the urethra and if the ureterovesical sphincter is incompetent they may ascend and proliferate in the upper urinary tract.

If women are examined early in pregnancy about 6 per cent of them will be found to have significant bacteriuria in two or more separate fresh midstream specimens of urine. A significant level is conventionally taken as more than 10^5 organisms per ml in a midstream specimen. This level was chosen empirically; it is believed that higher counts indicate that the bladder or higher urinary tract is colonized; lower counts may only indicate colonization of the urethra. (In a specimen obtained by suprapubic bladder aspiration any bacterial growth is regarded as significant.)

A few of the patients with bacteriuria have had evident infection in childhood, with recurrent clinical attacks, but in many the time of invasion of the upper urinary tract is unknown and the bacteriuria is completely asymptomatic. However, if asymptomatic cases are investigated by intravenous pyelography, particularly those cases in which the bacteriuria is not quickly eradicated by sulphonamides or ampicillin, many of the patients are found to have renal abnormalities such as chronic pyelonephritis or congenital malformations.

Women who are found to have bacteriuria are far more likely than others to develop acute pyelonephritis during pregnancy. If the bacteriuria responds to treatment during pregnancy the risk of acute pyelonephritis is largely prevented, but if the patients are not treated or if there is no response to treatments the incidence of pyelonephritis during pregnancy is as high as 30 per cent.

These facts show that all antenatal patients should be screened for bacteriuria, and those who have bacteriuria should be treated in an attempt to eradicate it. However, this will not eliminate all acute urinary infections in pregnant women because some attacks occur in patients who have no evident preceding bacteriuria.

To screen a large number of antenatal patients makes a heavy demand on the time of nurses in collecting the midstream specimens, and on laboratory facilities. One solution is to use dip-slides which have a thin coating of culture medium. One of the slides is dipped into each specimen of urine and the batch of slides is easily incubated. Subcultures are made from any positive slides and the fixed area of the medium on the side allows a rough colony count.

About 75 per cent of cases of bacteriuria are cured by a single course of ampicillin 500 mg 8-hourly for eight days or co-trimoxazole (Septrin) 480 mg 12-hourly for eight days. (Co-trimoxazole contains trimethoprim, a folic acid antagonist, and so during the first trimester a sulphonamide alone, e.g. sulphamethizole, may be chosen.) Most patients will be cured by one or other of these drugs. In resistant cases some other antibiotic may then be tried but in many of the cases in which the infection cannot be eradicated intravenous pyelography after delivery will show scarring due to chronic pyelonephritis, some congenital abnormality of the renal tract, or some other lesion such as a calculus.

Some have advised giving a long continuous course of treatment during pregnancy, but there is no evidence that this is better than a short course.

Changes in the renal pelvis and ureter in normal pregnancy

Intravenous pyelography which, in the past, was freely performed during pregnancy before the possible fetal hazard from radiation was recognized, shows that dilatation of the ureters and renal pelves occurs during pregnancy. In about 80 per cent of pregnant women there is marked stasis in the right ureter and also to some extent in the left ureter. The dilatation extends down as far as the brim of the bony pelvis; below this level the ureter often appears normal. The ureters often appear tortuous and may be kinked. The dilatation may be caused in part by pressure of the enlarged pregnant uterus on the ureter at the brim of the pelvis. The right ureter is more likely to be involved on account of the tendency of the uterus to incline towards the right side.

In addition to mechanical factors causing dilatation of the ureter there may be reduced tone in the ureteric musculature during pregnancy because although the ureter is dilated the intraureteric pressure is not increased. This atony is caused by the inhibitory effect of progesterone.

The infecting organism in pyelonephritis

An organism of the *Escherichia coli* group is present in nearly 80 per cent of cases. The organism has been obtained not only from the bladder, but directly from the kidney by ureteric catheterization. Other organisms are occasionally found, such as the *Streptococcus faecalis*, *Bacillus proteus* or *Staphylococci* spp.

The path of infection

Although it has been suggested that organisms may reach the kidney from the bloodstream or by the periureteric lymphatics it is more likely that they do so by upward spread from the bladder and by proliferation of organisms in the lumen of the ureter. Urine containing bacteria can enter the ureter if there is reflux at the ureterovesical junction and during pregnancy stasis of urinary flow makes upward spread more likely. The increase in urinary amino acid concentration in pregnancy makes the urine a favourable culture medium.

Symptoms

Acute pyelonephritis

The patient, usually more than 16 weeks pregnant, is suddenly seized with an acute attack of abdominal pain which is felt in the lumbar or iliac region of one or both sides. In 50 per cent of cases the infection is confined to the right side and in 16 per cent to the left; in 34 per cent of cases both kidneys are involved. The temperature rises suddenly to levels such as 39.5°C, and may be accompanied by a rigor; the pulse rate is rapid and often remains at about 120 per minute for several days. The patient may look ill and vomit repeatedly. There is tenderness over the affected kidney.

In severe untreated cases the urine is diminished in amount and of high specific gravity. It becomes turbid and contains pus and flocculent debris; the reaction is almost invariably acid. A pure culture of the coliform bacillus is usually obtained. The centrifuged deposit contains large quantities of these organisms, pus cells, epithelial cells, some red blood corpuscles and albumin. Macroscopic haematuria is occasionally seen.

Subacute pyelonephritis

In this form the symptoms are not so characteristic and the mode of onset is variable. There may be a gradual onset with malaise and increasing lumbar pain, frequency, vomiting, or symptoms suggesting pleurisy and pneumonia. The temperature is slightly raised and irregular; on palpation the kidney may be tender and feel enlarged. The attack in some cases is extremely mild; there may be pain but no other symptom, or the patient may have rigors without any apparent cause.

Diagnosis

The diagnosis is based upon the occurrence of a raised temperature, bacilluria, pyuria and tenderness in the situation of the kidney or down the line of the ureter.

When being examined the patient should be on her side (with the affected side uppermost) so that the uterus does not obscure the palpation of the kidney.

The diagnosis is confirmed by examination of a midstream specimen of urine. Part of the specimen is sent to the laboratory for bacteriological examination, including the testing of any organism found for sensitivity to the various antibiotics. The rest of the specimen may be examined immediately under the microscope for pus cells. The discovery of pus cells is sufficient for preliminary diagnosis and will permit treatment to be begun while the laboratory report is awaited.

The differential diagnosis may include:

other conditions causing acute abdominal pain during pregnancy, such as appendicitis, torsion of an ovarian cyst, red degeneration of a fibromyoma and concealed haemorrhage from abruptio placentae. The onset of pyelonephritis may sometimes be very acute with vomiting and possibly tenderness in the right iliac fossa, or even rigidity, so that the clinical picture may closely simulate that of appendicitis. However, in acute pyelonephritis the temperature is often higher (39°C or more) than is seen in appendicitis and rigors often occur, these are rare in appendicitis. Fetor of the breath does not usually occur and the tongue is cleaner than in appenditicis. If the urine is properly examined a mistake is unlikely

in cases of torsion of an ovarian cyst or of red degeneration of a fibromyoma a tender swelling can usually be felt. In abruptio placentae it is the uterus which is tender, there is often at least a little vaginal bleeding and the fetal heart may not be heard

cases of pneumonia or pleurisy occasionally give rise to diagnostic difficulty, for in these conditions pain arising from the right lower lobe or related pleura can be confused with renal pain. In all cases the chest should be properly examined. Epidemic myalgia affecting the diaphragm (Bornholm disease) may also cause confusion, but in all these conditions the urine does not contain pus cells

vomiting may be the predominating presenting symptom in cases of pyelonephritis, and dysuria may be absent. In any case of vomiting in pregnancy after the first trimester the urine should be examined for pus cells

the differential diagnosis of proteinuria is discussed on page 88. There is unlikely to be confusion in cases of acute pyelonephritis; it is more likely that chronic pyelonephritis will be mistaken for pregnancy-induced hypertension with proteinuria or for nephritis

a few cases present with pyrexia and little else and the urine should be examined carefully in any case of undiagnosed febrile illness

in chronic pyelonephritis anaemia frequently occurs and in cases of anaemia which do not respond to treatment this possibility should be remembered.

Treatment

The patient is put to bed in order to obtain rest and for the relief of pain. If one kidney is chiefly affected she will obtain more relief if she lies mainly upon the unaffected side, with the knees flexed to relax the abdominal muscles.

As soon as a specimen of urine has been obtained for bacteriological examination treatment is started with ampicillin, 500 mg 6-hourly. When the bacteriological report is available it may justify continuation of treatment with ampicillin; otherwise some other appropriate drug is chosen. If the correct antibacterial drug is given in adequate doses a clinical response is to be expected within two or three days, but treatment must be continued for at least three days after the fever and symptoms have subsided, and checked by repeated urinary cultures.

A large fluid intake will increase urinary flow and therefore reduce the time during which organisms can proliferate in the urine, but at the same time it will dilute any antibiotic in the urine. On balance, the advantage of an adequate urinary flow outweighs the disadvantage of diluting the antibiotic. If vomiting is severe, intravenous fluids may be needed.

Prognosis

Maternal prognosis

In the past, before sulphonamides and antibiotics were available, there were occasional cases of pyonephrosis and of multiple small abscesses in the renal parenchyma. Although such events are now rare, acute infection may be followed by further attacks which may continue for many years, and we have come to realize that sometimes chronic pyelonephritis may be an insidious, progressive and persistent disease, leading to gradual destruction of the renal parenchyma. Interstitial fibrosis occurs and the kidney shows irregular scarring and contraction. Histological examination shows patchy areas of fibrosis and of round cell infiltration in which both glomeruli and tubules may show ischaemic atrophy; other nephrons are distended from obstruction. The important sequel is hypertension, when further arteriolar changes occur in the kidney, and eventually uraemia may occur.

Follow-up after delivery

It is important that recurrent or persistent pyelonephritis should be treated effectively. In any suspicious case, and indeed in any patient who has had pyelonephritis during pregnancy, the urine should be examined repeatedly for pus cells and organisms. If these are found an intravenous pyelogram should be carried out after the pregnancy, but in fact impairment of structure or function will seldom be found until the disease has been present for some years.

If excretion of pus cells or bacilli continues, even intermittently, every attempt must be made to give adequate treatment with antibiotics or long-acting sulphonamides. In rare instances of severe unilateral disease nephrectomy may eventually be necessary to prevent or treat hypertension.

Fetal prognosis

If severe pyelonephritis with high fever is untreated abortion or intrauterine fetal death may occur. With less severe infection, and even in cases of asymptomatic bacteriuria, there may be fetal growth retardation or premature onset of labour, so that the perinatal mortality is increased. It is claimed that effective treatment will prevent this.

CHRONIC RENAL DISEASE DURING PREGNANCY

Chronic renal disease during pregnancy gives rise to concern because of fear that renal function may deteriorate, and because the fetus may be at risk.

In many cases the patient has already been investigated and there is an accurate diagnosis; chronic glomerulonephritis and chronic pyelonephritis are the most common lesions.

The same principles of management apply to all patients with chronic renal disease. First, there must be early assessment and investigation and for this the patient may require admission to hospital for observation and renal function tests, and to determine the effect of rest on her hypertension. A blood urea concentration of more than 5.0 mmol/L or a creatinine clearance of under 60 ml/min are taken as evidence of impaired renal function, although these can only be regarded as crude tests. Rarely it will be justifiable to carry out a single-film pyelogram or a renal biopsy during pregnancy, but usually these are part of the more extensive investigations to follow in the puerperium.

Frequent antenatal visits are essential, these will have to be weekly during pregnancy. The patient should be readmitted to hospital at the least sign of deterioration. Rest in bed for a large part of each day may be necessary. A high protein diet to offset the loss of protein in the urine and a low salt diet are recommended. In most cases it is advisable to admit the patient to hospital from the 30th week, and from this time on daily observations are made, as in cases of pregnancy-induced hypertension. The advice of a nephrologist may be required about the use of hypotensive drugs and diuretics.

The growth of the fetus is carefully watched with ultrasound (*see* p. 61). By such means the optimum time for delivery of the fetus can be chosen. It is unlikely to be later than 38 weeks and may have to be much earlier. The mode of delivery will depend on the circumstances of the case and caesarean section should be considered if the pregnancy has not reached the 35th week.

There is seldom any medical reason for terminating a pregnancy for chronic renal disease. There is no evidence that pregnancy causes any permanent deterioration in the renal or cardiovascular condition of these patients – a few will do badly, but probably these would have done badly if they had not become pregnant.

GLOMERULONEPHRITIS

Acute nephritis is a very rare coincidental illness during pregnancy and is treated as if the patient were not pregnant. If corticosteroids are given it must be remembered that they suppress normal adrenal activity and the patient may need supplementary doses of hydrocortisone during labour. They also cross the placenta and depress the fetal adrenals and there is therefore a low output of oestriol. In these cases the output of oestriol in the mother's urine is an unreliable index of placental function.

If a patient merely gives a history of a previous attack of acute nephritis and has no residual hypertension or proteinuria no problem is to be expected during pregnancy.

If, after nephritis, there is only a little proteinuria and slight hypertension which does not increase during pregnancy the prognosis is good for both mother and child. The urine may contain casts, but the precise diagnosis may only be made after pregnancy. However, in cases in which there is

exacerbation of the hypertension the fetus is at considerable risk.

In a few cases, and sometimes without a history of acute nephritis at the onset of the illness, the patient will present with massive proteinuria, oedema and low plasma protein levels, but with relatively little hypertension. In these cases of nephrosis the prognosis is already serious, but if the blood pressure rises during pregnancy the fetal risk is greatly increased.

On the whole the later stages of chronic nephritis are seldom seen by the obstetrician because the patients are too ill to become pregnant.

Occasionally a patient undergoing renal dialysis may become pregnant. The pregnancy is likely to be complicated by intrauterine fetal growth retardation and pregnancy-induced hypertension. The perinatal mortality rate is very high.

CHRONIC PYELONEPHRITIS

This condition may be distinguished by the history, from urine cultures and possibly by a pyelogram, a single film being taken. Renal biopsy later will confirm the diagnosis.

In these patients it is extremely important to maintain a constant watch for any exacerbation of urinary tract infection, which must be treated energetically and over a prolonged period. The outlook for the fetus is better than in cases of glomerulonephritis, but there is still an increased perinatal mortality and a tendency for the fetus to be small-for-dates.

LUPUS ERYTHEMATOSUS

Systemic lupus erythematosus may be mentioned here because of its hypertensive and renal complications. Its course during pregnancy is variable and unpredictable.

Intervillous coagulation may occur in the placenta causing fetal death, and (rarely) maternal pulmonary embolism may occur. These thrombotic complications are thought to be the result of impeded release of prostacyclin. It is a curious fact that the fetus may develop heart block, probably from endomyocardial fibrosis.

For treatment prednisone and aspirin are given, with the general care of hypertension and proteinuria already described.

VARIOUS OTHER RENAL LESIONS

POLYCYSTIC DISEASE OF THE KIDNEYS

A few patients with this congenital disease of the kidneys become pregnant. The problems are similar to those of chronic nephritis; the outcome depends on the degree of renal failure or of superadded hypertension.

RENAL TUBERCULOSIS

This offers no special problems to the obstetrician except those of diagnosis. It is rarely severe enough in women who become pregnant to cause any serious impairment of renal function or hypertension. It is treated with antituberculous drugs.

RENAL ARTERY STENOSIS

This is a rare cause of hypertension during pregnancy and will only be diagnosed after delivery, when investigations by intravenous pyelography and renal angiography are performed. Such investigations should be considered for all patients with unexplained persisting hypertension after delivery.

PREVIOUS NEPHRECTOMY

If the remaining kidney is normal there need be no concern during pregnancy.

PREGNANCY AFTER RENAL TRANSPLANTATION

An increasing number of women who have had successful renal transplants are becoming pregnant. The fact that the patient has become pregnant suggests that the function of the transplanted kidney is good. The rate of spontaneous abortion is increased, but if the pregnancy proceeds beyond the first trimester it is likely to end successfully in the birth of a live baby. The position of the transplanted kidney near the pelvic brim may prevent descent of the fetal head during labour and caesarean section is often performed. Although there is theoretical risk to the fetus from immunosuppressant drugs which the patient is required to take, in practice there does not seem to be an increased risk of congenital defects.

ANAEMIA DURING PREGNANCY

Physiological changes in the blood during pregnancy

During pregnancy the blood volume is increased by about 30 per cent, but there is a relatively greater increase in the volume of the plasma than of the red cells. This leads to a fall in the red cell count and in the haemoglobin concentration during pregnancy, although the total mass of haemoglobin in the body is increased by about 15 per cent. The increase in blood volume is maintained until shortly before term when there is a fall, but the original non-pregnant level is not reached until about six weeks after delivery.

Although haemodilution occurs, in many cases a more important explanation for the fall in haemoglobin concentration is relative iron deficiency. A haemoglobin level of 11 g/dl is regarded as the lower normal limit during pregnancy, but if the diet is adequate or if additional iron is given to pregnant women the haemoglobin concentration often does not fall below 12.5 g/dl.

The usual daily dietary intake of iron by a non-pregnant woman is about 10 mg, of which 10 per cent is absorbed. This balances the loss in the urine and faeces, from desquamation of the skin (amounting to about 0.5 mg daily) and from the menstrual loss. Menstrual loss varies greatly, but averages 12 mg per month.

If a woman is to maintain her iron balance during pregnancy she needs to retain about 800 mg of iron to provide 350 mg for the fetus, 100 mg for the placenta and 350 mg for her own increased haemoglobin mass. Since about 0.5 mg is still excreted daily, her total requirement over 280 days of pregnancy works out at 960 mg, or about 3.5 mg daily. The increased requirement is not spread uniformly over the whole of pregnancy, but rises from zero at 20 weeks to 8 mg daily at term.

There will be a loss of iron, from blood loss during delivery and in the lochia, of about 150 mg and a further deficit of about 150 mg during lactation, and these losses will use up the increased haemoglobin mass which has been built up during pregnancy.

During pregnancy a very good diet contains 15 mg iron daily and the ability of the duodenum and jejunum to absorb iron and the iron-binding capacity of the serum are increased to meet the added need. If the diet is less well supplied with iron the intake may be inadequate. About 30 per cent of the body iron (1000 mg) is in the cells of the reticuloendothelial system in the form of haemosiderin, and this forms a reserve. The serum iron level falls only when the iron stores are depleted. Not only may there be a deficiency of iron in the diet during pregnancy but many women start pregnancy with poor iron reserves. Several pregnancies in rapid succession will accentuate any deficiency.

Women who are taking a well-balanced diet with a high iron content do not need supplemental iron during pregnancy but those on less adequate diets need additional iron, which is often combined with a small dose of folic acid in a single tablet. Although simple ferrous sulphate, 200 mg three times daily, is the cheapest form of supplement, it tends to cause constipation and sometimes nausea. A slow-release preparation containing ferrous sulphate 150 mg with folic acid 0.5 mg is to be preferred, and has the advantage that the woman is only required to take one tablet a day. If ferrous sulphate causes gastrointestinal upset a good alternative is ferrous fumarate, 300 mg daily. It is best to postpone prophylactic iron administration until any nausea or vomiting of early pregnancy has passed.

Blood tests for anaemia during pregnancy

All women should have an estimation of haemoglobin level and simple examination of a blood film at the initial antenatal visit, and again at 30 and 36 weeks. More frequent examinations will be required if anaemia is found.

IRON-DEFICIENCY ANAEMIA

In Britain by far the most common type of anaemia during pregnancy is due to iron deficiency as a result of a poor diet, or of the woman failing to take the tablets which are prescribed for her. In many of the slighter cases the woman makes no complaint and anaemia is only discovered after routine examination of the blood. In a severe case the patient may look pale (although this is a most unreliable sign) and she may have noticed tiredness, breathlessness, palpitation or fainting. Apart from the adverse effect on the health of the mother during pregnancy, anaemia greatly increases the risk should haemorrhage occur unexpectedly during pregnancy or labour, and a determined effort must be made to treat anaemia before term is reached.

The patients have a low haemoglobin concentration and a low red cell count, with a low colour index and mean corpuscular haemoglobin concentration. In severe cases there is polychromasia, a low mean corpuscular volume and a low serum iron level. In practice not all these observations are made routinely, and in many cases the diagnosis is made by observing a satisfactory response to treatment with iron. But if there is not a quick response, or if the haemoglobin level is less than 9 g/dl, then a complete blood count is required.

In women from tropical countries iron-deficiency anaemia during pregnancy may result from worm infestation, and this may need investigation and treatment.

Treatment

There is usually time to treat the patient with oral iron. It is essential to make sure that adequate doses of an appropriate preparation are being swallowed. The ordinary doses may be doubled but nothing is gained by increasing the dose still further. There is a limit to the amount of iron that can be absorbed and with larger doses gastrointestinal symptoms may occur.

Women who do not respond, and in whom full investigation has not shown any other type of anaemia or any condition such as chronic renal disease, may be treated with parenteral iron.

Parenteral iron may also be used if pregnancy is advanced and time is short, but if the woman is very near to term blood transfusion will be the only way to raise the haemoglobin level quickly enough. In cases of very severe anaemia, such as may be seen in tropical countries, there is a risk of overloading the circulation by transfusion, and either packed cells must be given slowly covered by a diuretic such as frusemide. As a general rule no woman should be allowed to go into labour with a haemoglobin level below 10 g/dl.

Parenteral iron may be given by a deep intramuscular injection of an iron dextran compound (Imferon) or an iron sorbitol compound (Jectofer). Each of these contains the equivalent of 50 mg of iron per ml and the patient is given a daily injection of 2 ml until a satisfactory response is obtained. Iron dextran (but *not* iron sorbitol) may also be given by 'total dose' intravenous infusion, and this method may be useful for women with severe iron-deficiency anaemia who are unlikely to attend for a series of injections. The patient is admitted to hospital for six hours and 1 litre of normal saline containing the calculated dose of iron dextran is administered by slow intravenous drip. It is assumed that 250 mg of iron are required to raise the haemoglobin level by 1 g/dl, and the dose is calculated accordingly. Anaphylactic reactions to intravenous iron occasionally occur, so the initial drip rate should be very slow and the infusion closely supervised.

MEGALOBLASTIC ANAEMIA

Folic acid is required for normal maturation of red cells in the bone marrow. If there is a deficiency of folic acid the marrow fills with megaloblasts and the number of mature red cells in the peripheral blood is reduced. The blood may contain macrocytic cells and occasional nucleated red cells.

During pregnancy, because of increased fetal demand and inadequate absorption from the diet, anaemia due to folic acid deficiency may occur. It is relatively rare in this country but is much more common in some tropical countries. It occurs most often in multigravidae, in whom it may recur in successive pregnancies; it is more common in twin pregnancies.

The anaemia may develop rapidly in late pregnancy and is often severe, with a haemoglobin concentration of less than 9 g/dl. The diagnosis should be considered in any case of severe anaemia during late pregnancy, and also in any case in which there is no response to the administration of adequate doses of iron.

The clinical and haematological pictures are often confused because folic acid deficiency is accompanied by iron deficiency. Thus the macrocytes which are found in the peripheral blood in non-pregnant women with folic acid deficiency are rarely seen in pregnant women. Confirmation of the diagnosis is made by measuring the serum folate level or examining bone marrow obtained by sternal puncture, but it is often simpler to apply a simple therapeutic test by giving folic acid 20 mg orally daily, when there will be a rapid rise in the haemoglobin level in genuine cases.

Most obstetricians give folic acid prophylactically during pregnancy, in doses of 0.5 mg daily, with iron in combined pills. The fear that administration of folic acid might mask the diagnosis of pernicious anaemia is unfounded, as this disease is not likely to be found in women of childbearing age.

Tropical megaloblastic anaemia

Megaloblastic anaemia is a common complication of pregnancy in some tropical countries. These cases also appear to be due to folic acid deficiency but they are complicated by additional dietary deficiencies of protein or iron, by blood destruction by malaria or haemoglobinopathies or by blood loss from hook worm infestation.

HAEMOGLOBINOPATHIES

The normal haemoglobin molecule of the adult (HbA) has four polypeptide side chains, two alpha and two beta chains, so that the molecule can be designated $\alpha_2\beta_2$. In the normal adult about 2 per cent of the haemoglobin is of a different type (HbA$_2$) in which two of the polypeptide chains have a different amino acid sequence (δ), so that the designation of the molecule is $\alpha_2\delta_2$.

During intrauterine life fetal haemoglobin (HbF) is found, with two polypeptide chains differing from HbA, represented as $\alpha_2\gamma_2$. Fetal haemoglobin is more resistant to denaturation with alkali than adult haemoglobin, and this is the basis of the Kleihauer test (*see* p. 319). At term the blood contains 70 per cent HbF, but this starts to disappear after delivery so that by the time the infant is a year old only traces remain. However, if there is any disorder in which formation of HbA is impaired, such as the hereditary haemoglobinopathies described in the rest of this section, large amounts of HbF are found.

Abnormal haemoglobins

Over 100 variants of the haemoglobin molecule have been found. These have been given various designations, sometimes letters of the alphabet and sometimes with reference to places of discovery. There are two main types of abnormal haemoglobins which are encountered in pregnant women.

In the first there are alterations of the amino acid structure of the polypeptide chains. The glutamic acid of HbA is replaced by valine in HbS and by lysine in HbC. Haemoglobin S is related to sickle-cell disease and trait, and haemoglobin C to haemolytic anaemia. In the second type the amino acid sequences are normal but production of the α

or β chains is impaired, causing thalassaemia.

Most of the abnormal haemoglobins are inherited by Mendelian laws. The clinical manifestations depend on:

the types of haemoglobin present
their relative proportions, which in turn largely depend on whether the inheritance is homo- or heterozygous.

As the haemoglobins carry different electrical charges they can be distinguished by electrophoresis.

Haemoglobin S

Sickle-cell disease

Sickle-cell disease is usually fatal in childhood and is therefore relatively rare in pregnant women. It occurs almost entirely in Negroes who originated from central Africa. In sickle-cell disease the trait is inherited from both parents, so that the phenotype may be designated SS (homozygous). The importance of this haemoglobin is that whenever the oxygen tension in any part of the body falls the red cells assume a sickle shape and 'sludge' together, obstructing the circulation. Infarcts of various organs occur. There may be crises with severe thoracic or abdominal pain or pain in the long bones. Haemolysis of the abnormal cells occurs and causes anaemia. Renal damage may cause haematuria and pyelitis may occur. During pregnancy there may be hypertension. There may be enlargement of the liver and spleen and ulceration of the legs. Death may occur from thrombosis in a vital organ or from pulmonary embolism. If a woman survives to become pregnant severe crisis may occur and thrombosis of placental blood vessels may cause fetal death. The fetus may be small-for-dates.

Sickle-cell trait

Sickle-cell trait is common and usually harmless. Many Negroes inherit HbS from only one parent, so that less than half of their haemoglobin is of this type. The phenotype may be designated AS (where A stands for normal adult haemoglobin). There is often some HbF present. In this heterozygous state, which can be recognized by electrophoresis, the concentration of HbS is usually too low for serious sickling to occur in the tissues. However,

patients with sickle-cell trait are occasionally liable to pyelonephritis in pregnancy.

Haemoglobin C

This abnormal haemoglobin is also found in Negroes. Heterozygous inheritance (AC) is harmless but with homozygous inheritance (CC) haemolytic anaemia may occur. HbC is of more importance when it is combined with inheritance of HbS (see Mixed haemoglobinopathies, below).

Thalassaemia

Thalassaemia was so named because it was first thought to be restricted to Mediterranean peoples, but in fact it occurs more widely, especially in the near and far East. It is caused by defective formation of either the α or β chains. Both types may be of homo- or heterozygous inheritance, the former being termed thalassaemia major and the latter thalassaemia minor.

β thalassaemia minor is the variety which is most likely to concern the obstetrician. Only one β chain is affected and there is only mild hypochromic anaemia, with occasional splenomegaly. There is a raised level of HbA$_2$ and often HbF. It is important to realize that the anaemia is not due to iron deficiency; it is useless to prescribe iron, and prolonged iron administration could cause haemosiderosis. β thalassaemia is more serious if it is combined with inheritance of S or C haemoglobin (see below).

Patients with α thalassaemia major are unlikely to survive beyond childhood. α thalassaemia minor is of little obstetric importance, except if both parents are carriers, when the fetus may have homozygous α thalassaemia and fatal hydrops fetalis.

Mixed haemoglobinopathies

Mixed forms of disease are common. The effects produced depend on the chains involved. If both abnormal genes affect the same chains the effects are serious. In SC disease both β chains are abnormal and no HbA can be found; the patient is therefore as badly off as with homozygous SS disease. Similarly β thalassaemia with HbS or HbC results in severe anaemia. On the other hand combinations of S or C inheritance with α thalassaemia do not do this.

Management of haemoglobinopathies during pregnancy

With such complex problems and numerous combinations, some of which are very rare, the obstetrician will obviously need to seek expert guidance in diagnosis and treatment.

The increase of immigrant communities means that Britain, in common with many other Western countries, now has many women who may have haemoglobinopathies attending antenatal clinics; in some of these the effect of pregnancy may be serious. All women coming from countries where these disorders are common, such as Africa, the West Indies, Mediterranean countries and Asia, should have a blood electrophoresis examination at their first antenatal attendance.

Sickle-cell disease

It is usually advised that treatment with iron should be avoided as these patients have a high serum iron concentration and a low iron-binding capacity, so that administered iron may be deposited in the reticuloendothelial system causing haemosiderosis. Folic acid 15 mg daily should be given. In crises adequate oxygenation and hydration must be ensured, and heparin is given if bone pain or pulmonary thrombosis or embolism develops. Infections are vigorously treated with antibiotics and sodium bicarbonate is given to correct acidosis. It is particularly important to avoid hypoxia or circulatory depression if an anaesthetic is required for operative delivery.

Very severe anaemia, with haemoglobin levels of 5 g/dl or less, may develop in late pregnancy, and exchange transfusion may be required before labour. In less severe cases a cautious transfusion with packed cells covered by a rapidly acting diuretic such as frusemide may be given.

Sickle-cell trait

So long as adequate amounts of HbA are present there is unlikely to be any anaemia during pregnancy, but there is a slight increased susceptibility to urinary tract infection.

Thalassaemia

Heterozygotic thalassaemia minor is unlikely to require special treatment during pregnancy.

Mixed haemoglobinopathies

Combinations such as SC disease may cause severe anaemia and occasional crises during pregnancy, and would then require the same treatment as for SS disease.

Antenatal diagnosis of fetal haemoglobinopathy

Using fetoscopy or ultrasound-guided cordocentesis it is now possible to obtain a sample of fetal blood at about 16 weeks. It can be determined whether the fetus has inherited a serious haemoglobinopathy such as sickle-cell disease and selective termination is then possible. Fetoscopy carries a slight risk of abortion and loss of a normal fetus, but in cases with a high risk of inherited disease many parents would accept this in order to avoid the possibility of birth of an affected child. The risk of abortion or fetal loss is less with cordocentesis and this procedure is now preferred to fetoscopy.

HEART DISEASE IN PREGNANCY

Although most patients with heart disease go through pregnancy and labour successfully if their management is conducted efficiently, that there is an added risk is shown by the fact that heart disease is the commonest 'associated disease' to cause maternal death.

CARDIOVASCULAR CHANGES DURING PREGNANCY

There is a steady increase in blood volume from about eight weeks until about 35 weeks, when the volume is some 30 per cent greater than the non-pregnant volume. In the last five weeks of pregnancy the volume falls slowly and to a variable extent until delivery. After delivery there is a return to non-pregnant levels over four to six weeks.

The cardiac output follows the changes in blood volume, rising from an average of 5.5 litres per minute in the non-pregnant woman to an average of 7 litres per minute at 34 weeks. This output is maintained until term, and reaches a further peak at times during the second stage of labour. There is another transient rise as the uterus retracts down during the third stage; after that the output falls concurrently with the decrease in blood volume.

There must obviously be an additional flow of the same degree in the pulmonary circuit as in the general circulation. The increased general flow is largely distributed through the uterus, breasts and kidneys, but there is also some dilatation of peripheral skin capillaries. The maternal side of the placental circulation resembles an arteriovenous shunt, and it takes up an increasing part of the cardiac output in the last trimester of pregnancy. Thus even though cardiac output is increased the reduced systemic vascular resistance results in either a fall or no change in blood pressure.

Aetiology of heart disease in pregnancy

Rheumatic heart disease

Rheumatic heart disease remains the most common cause of heart disease during pregnancy in developing countries, although it is now becoming less common in the Western world. Mitral stenosis is the most common lesion found, and there may also be mitral regurgitation or aortic regurgitation; aortic stenosis is rarely seen.

Congenital heart disease

Congenital heart disease now accounts for about 30 per cent of cases. On the whole those patients who survive to the age of childbearing are those without cyanosis or gross disability, including cases of patent interatrial or intraventricular septal defect, patent ductus arteriosus, aortic coarctation, pulmonary stenosis, mitral valve prolapse and Marfan's syndrome. Cardiac surgery will often have been employed in these and other more complex congenital heart lesions. Other cases of congenital heart disease are rare in pregnancy, although the successful results of modern cardiac surgery bring more survivors to adult life.

Bacterial endocarditis

Bacterial endocarditis may occur as a complication of rheumatic valvular disease or of congenital lesions, and as a rare result of streptococcal puerperal infection.

Cardiac failure is a rare complication of severe and relatively acute hypertension (e.g. during eclampsia), but is hardly ever seen in cases of chronic essential hypertension during pregnancy.

Cardiomyopathy of pregnancy

This term refers to rare cases of myocardial disease of unknown aetiology occurring in late pregnancy or in the puerperium, and sometimes recurring in successive pregnancies, which causes congestive cardiac failure. There is tachycardia, gallop rhythm and reversible cardiac dilatation, but the exact pathology is uncertain, and it is doubtful if it is a single clear-cut clinical entity.

Cardiac arrhythmias

Cardiac arrhythmias are uncommon in pregnancy in the absence of pre-existing heart disease. Patients with supraventricular tachycardia may have more frequent episodes in late pregnancy, and patients with congenital heart block may show Stokes–Adams attacks for the first time during pregnancy. Pregnancy is well tolerated by patients with artificial pacemakers.

Coronary thrombosis

This is rare in pregnancy, but with a tendency to later childbearing and more smoking among women it may become more common.

Diagnosis

The heart should always be examined carefully at the first antenatal visit. The diagnosis of cardiac disease during pregnancy is sometimes difficult. Dyspnoea of slight degree and oedema of the ankles may occur in normal pregnancy. A soft systolic murmur without any other evidence of cardiac disease may have no signficance, but any diastolic murmur or harsh systolic murmur always suggests organic disease. It is often difficult to assess the size of the heart by clinical means during pregnancy. The axis of the heart is rotated in late pregnancy and this gives a false impression of enlargement. The electrocardiograph is also affected by the rotation and the shift of the electrical axis to the left is associated with the appearance of a Q wave in lead III. Echocardiography is the best method for investigating the pregnant cardiac patient. Radiography should not be used routinely, but may be needed to assess pulmonary venous congestion. The fetus must be protected from radiation with a lead abdominal shield.

Cyanosis, fibrillation or unequivocal evidence of

pulmonary congestion, such as haemoptysis or moist râles at the bases of the lungs, are always signs of serious organic disease.

Prognosis

Although the lesions present in particular cases are obviously important, especially in cases of congenital heart disease, the functional capacity of the myocardium is the most significant factor in prognosis, and for this reason it was formerly the practice to classify cases of heart disease in pregnancy thus:

> *grade I*
> no dyspnoea or limitation of activity
> *grade II*
> dyspnoea, with some limitation of activity
> *grade III*
> severe dyspnoea with limitation of even ordinary activity, but comfortable at rest
> *grade IV*
> dyspnoea even at rest, or history of cardiac failure.

However, cardiologists now seldom use this classification and prefer to assess the severity of heart disease during pregnancy on objective evidence obtained by clinical electrocardiographic and echocardiographic examination, supplemented if necessary by radiological studies.

Deterioration of even mild cases may sometimes occur during pregnancy, and respiratory infection will increase the danger. Careful assessment of all women with cardiac lesions should be made in early pregnancy by an experienced cardiologist, and he should continue to see the patients at intervals during pregnancy and the puerperium. The ideal plan is for such an assessment to be made before the pregnancy begins.

Management

The majority of patients with cardiac disease who become pregnant have only minor disability and will not require special treatment although, as indicated above, they should all be supervised during pregnancy by a cardiologist working closely with the obstetrician. Depending on the severity of the case, good antenatal care will include:

> adequate rest at home (ten hours at night and two hours horizontal rest in the afternoon)

with provision of help at home and transport to and from the hospital

avoidance of respiratory infection – shunning people with obvious colds and crowded places of entertainment – and immediate treatment of any respiratory infection

treatment of any dental sepsis, and if extractions are required penicillin should be given before and afterwards to reduce the risk of bacterial endocarditis

prevention and treatment of anaemia

admission to hospital for rest at any time if the cardiac condition seems to be deteriorating. For the more severe cases two or three weeks rest in hospital prior to labour is desirable

digitalis or other drugs may be needed for patients with arrhythmia or cardiac failure. Diuretics such as frusemide or chlorothiazide may be of help if there is fluid retention

special problems arise with patients who have had a valvular prosthesis inserted. Those with well-functioning prosthetic valves tolerate pregnancy well, but the need for anticoagulant treatment causes risk to the fetus. Oral anticoagulants are best discontinued during pregnancy as they cross the placenta and may affect the development of the long bones of the fetus, or they may cause fetal intracranial or other haemorrhage during labour. Heparin does not cross the placenta and is given instead of oral anticoagulants by subcutaneous injections, which the patient can learn to manage. With all anticoagulant drugs the risk of uterine haemorrhage is small as myometrial contraction will effectively control blood loss.

Cardiac surgery

In early pregnancy a decision may need to be made whether cardiac surgery is indicated or, if the lesion is unsuitable for operation, about termination of pregnancy. Open heart surgery is not performed during pregnancy but simpler procedures such as valvotomy can be carried out. Most patients, even those with quite severe disease, can tolerate pregnancy, so that termination is rarely essential. However, the longer term effects of bringing up the child need to be considered in deciding whether termination is to be advised in a particular case.

Cases of coarctation of the aorta run a slight risk of developing a dissecting aneurysm, but this risk does not justify caesarean section nor operation on the aorta during pregnancy.

Heart failure

Acute pulmonary oedema is most frequently seen in patients with tight constriction of the mitral valve; congestive failure is usually encountered in patients with gross cardiac enlargement, some of whom may be fibrillating. These patients need to be nursed in a propped-up position. Salt and fluid intake are restricted. Digitalis is indicated for congestive heart failure and especially if there is fibrillation. In acute pulmonary oedema morphine and oxygen are given, and venesection may be needed. Labour should never be induced in haste because the heart is in failure; in most cases improvement can be obtained before delivery.

Mode of delivery

Easy vaginal delivery should be the aim, and fortunately this often occurs. In the first stage analgesic drugs should be given in adequate doses, because tachycardia due to pain may be the starting point of failure. Intravenous infusions are best avoided, but if they are essential they must be used with care not to overload the circulation. The second stage should be short, and if this is proving not to be the case then prolonged expulsive effort is avoided by forceps delivery or vacuum extraction under pudendal block. If a general anaesthetic becomes necessary the services of an experienced anaesthetist should be secured, and every effort made to avoid hypoxia. Epidural anaesthesia should not be used except for very mild cases because of the risk of hypotension.

The sudden increase in blood volume caused by uterine contraction after delivery of the placenta may occasionally precipitate acute pulmonary oedema or heart failure and it is wisest not to use ergometrine or Syntocinon in the third stage unless postpartum haemorrhage occurs.

The indications for caesarean section are the same as for a patient with a normal heart, and it should not be undertaken except for a genuine obstetric reason.

Postnatal care

Even after a normal vaginal delivery heart failure can occur in the puerperium. The patient must have additional rest at this time, and may need a longer than average stay in hospital. In all but the mildest cases a course of penicillin should be given for the first 14 days postpartum to guard against bacterial endocarditis. The patient should be encouraged to feed her baby unless there is very severe heart disease.

Family planning and cardiac disease

Women with cardiac disease should limit their families to one or two children because the strain of pregnancy and labour are only the beginning of the additional physical and mental strain involved in the care of children. Except in mild cases the contraceptive pill is best avoided because of the risk of thromboembolism. The progestogen-only pill, the intrauterine device or the diaphragm are alternative methods of contraception for patients with severe cardiac disease. Termination of pregnancy may need to be considered if unplanned pregnancy occurs. Sterilization is a useful procedure once a patient has completed her family. It is best postponed for two or three months after delivery, when it can be performed laparoscopically.

PULMONARY TUBERCULOSIS AND PREGNANCY

The incidence of pulmonary tuberculosis during pregnancy is now so low in the United Kingdom that routine radiological examination of the chest in antenatal patients has been given up, but in communities with a significant incidence of the disease this investigation should be carried out, care being taken to shield the uterus from radiation.

Pregnancy does not adversely affect the course and prognosis of the disease, provided that the usual treatment is carried out. Termination is not necessary except in occasional advanced cases. The fetus is practically never infected *in utero*. Chemotherapy is the essential part of treatment. Long-continued treatment with streptomycin might affect the fetal VIIIth nerve, but the risk of this is small, so that streptomycin may be used if it is considered to be an essential part of the mother's treatment. Apart from this, pregnancy and labour are managed in the normal way.

The aim of treatment is to make the mother sputum-negative by the time the baby is born. If this is achieved the baby can be left with the mother in the ordinary way, and vaccinated with BCG. The mother must be warned that if the sputum is still positive at the time of delivery the baby will have to be separated completely from her until the BCG vaccination has built up resistance to the disease; this will take at least six weeks. If the mother is sputum-negative there is no objection to breast-feeding.

Long-term follow-up of these patients is important to ensure that the prescribed course of treatment is completed and that recurrence does not occur. Every effort must be made to improve the patient's diet and living conditions. Family planning advice is given so that further pregnancy is avoided for at least one year after completion of treatment.

OTHER RESPIRATORY DISEASES DURING PREGNANCY

PNEUMONIA

Lobar pneumonia is very uncommon with pregnancy today, but bronchopneumonia may complicate upper respiratory tract infections and viral pneumonia may occur. Vigorous treatment for bacterial infections with broad-spectrum antibiotics is essential. If the patient becomes seriously ill with high fever then abortion, premature labour or intrauterine fetal death may occur.

ASTHMA

Most cases are unaffected by pregnancy, but cases of emotional origin may be worse if pregnancy is resented, or better if it is welcomed. If cortisone is the only treatment which gives relief there is no contraindication, but it should not be used in the first 12 weeks because of a possible teratogenic effect. Inhalations of sympathomimetic or antihistamine preparations may be used.

EMPHYSEMA, BRONCHITIS AND BRONCHIECTASIS

During pregnancy the vital capacity is not reduced but pulmonary ventilation is increased, and patients with rigid rib cages may have severe dyspnoea. An antibiotic such as ampicillin 250 mg twice daily may be given regularly during the winter months to prevent superadded infection. If there is

severe dyspnoea assistance with forceps or the vacuum extractor in the second stage of labour may be required.

SARCOIDOSIS

This disorder appears to improve during pregnancy, but is likely to relapse afterwards.

CARBOHYDRATE METABOLISM IN PREGNANCY

GLYCOSURIA

Glycosuria often occurs during pregnancy as a result of a lowered renal threshold. The glomerular filtration of glucose is so much increased that reabsorption in the tubules is incomplete. The usual upper limit of glucose excretion during pregnancy is 140 mg/24 hours, but this is often exceeded and may reach 1 g/24 hours. The amount of glycosuria varies both from day to day and during each day. An early morning specimen of urine, excreted when the blood sugar level is low, is less likely to show glycosuria than a specimen collected after a meal. However, in pregnancy the situation is complicated because there is only a tenuous relationship between blood glucose levels and glycosuria as demonstrated by the glucose oxidase test strip (Clinistix). These strips appear to be less sensitive during pregnancy because of the presence of substances such as ascorbic acid in the urine which interfere with the reaction.

Glycosuria by itself does not have any significance, but it needs to be distinguished from glycosuria due to diabetes mellitus. Glycosuria found before the 16th week or occurring on two or more occasions in later pregnancy should be investigated by means of a standard 75 g oral glucose tolerance test. In cases of glycosuria in pregnancy it is uncommon to discover diabetes except when there are other indicators of diabetes, especially a family history of the disease in a parent or sibling, or a history of the birth of a baby weighing 4.5 kg or more.

GLUCOSE TOLERANCE IN PREGNANCY

During pregnancy the fasting levels of blood glucose are lower than in non-pregnant women by an average of 0.5 mmol/L. The peak levels of blood glucose after meals are higher, especially in late pregnancy. The tendency to postprandial hyperglycaemia occurs in spite of increased insulin production, so that there is in effect a decreased sensitivity to insulin. To maintain glucose homeostasis the pregnant woman must produce more insulin. Most women are able to respond to this demand, but a few are unable to do so and develop diabetes. The diabetogenic effect of pregnancy is increased by repeated pregnancies and by obesity. The need for increased production of insulin during pregnancy is seen in insulin-dependent diabetics, whose insulin dosage often has to be increased two- or threefold as pregnancy advances.

GLUCOSE AND INSULIN RELATIONSHIPS IN MOTHER AND FETUS

Glucose crosses the placenta freely; insulin does not. Hyperglycaemia in the mother is reflected by hyperglycaemia in the fetus. If there is persistent maternal hyperglycaemia in late pregnancy, as in diabetes, the fetal pancreas responds by producing an excess of insulin which cannot cross back into the maternal circulation and may therefore cause fetal hypoglycaemia.

DIABETES MELLITUS IN PREGNANCY

Most cases of pregnancy complicating diabetes are seen in women who are already diabetic at the start of the pregnancy. Most of these patients will already have been treated with insulin, but some of the older women with maturity-onset diabetes will have been treated with diet alone, or with diet and oral hypoglycaemic agents.

Some women develop diabetes during pregnancy and are called *gestational diabetics*. Of these, some remain diabetic at the end of pregnancy and the others revert to normal. Gestational diabetes is managed in exactly the same way as established diabetes.

There is a group of women who are not obviously diabetic but whose carbohydrate metabolism is not completely normal. In investigating pregnant women for possible diabetes the World Health Organization recommends that if the fasting blood glucose level is 8 mmol/L or more the patient should be classed as diabetic, whereas if the level is 6 mmol/L or less the diagnosis is excluded. For women whose fasting blood glucose level is between 6 and 8 mmol/L a standard 75 g oral glucose tolerance test is performed. If the 2-hour

blood glucose level exceeds 11 mmol/L the patient is regarded as diabetic; if it is less than 8 mmol/L she is not. Patients whose 2-hour blood glucose level lies between 8 and 11 mmol/L are described as having *impaired glucose tolerance*. (This term replaces the former terms chemical, asymptomatic and borderline diabetes.) Women with impaired glucose tolerance do not need treatment but must be carefully watched during pregnancy to see that they do not progress to become true gestational diabetics.

A *potential diabetic* is an individual who has an increased tendency to develop the disease during pregnancy, recognized by having had a heavy baby previously (4.5 kg or more) or because of a family history of diabetes in a parent or sibling.

Effect of pregnancy on diabetes

As noted above, the insulin requirement almost invariably needs to be increased during pregnancy to maintain control, and ketosis is more apt to occur because of the increased loss of glucose in the urine. Patients who are ordinarily treated by diet alone may need insulin during pregnancy.

Effect of diabetes on pregnancy

Unrecognized or badly treated diabetes leads to complications in both mother and baby.

Maternal complications

These include urinary tract infection, candidiasis of the vulva and vagina, pregnancy-induced hypertension, hydramnios and preterm labour.

Fetal and neonatal complications

These include an increased incidence of congenital abnormalities, intrauterine death in late pregnancy or death soon after birth from hypoglycaemia, and respiratory distress syndrome in the newborn. The infant is characteristically large (with enlargement of all the organs) and plethoric from polycythaemia secondary to intrauterine hypoxia, which gives rise to an increased incidence of hyperbilirubinaemia and neonatal jaundice. Hypocalcaemia is also often present. The risk of birth trauma is greater because of the large size of the fetus. The combined effect of all these factors is an increased perinatal mortality.

Management

The incidence of the complications listed above and the perinatal mortality rate can be greatly reduced by very careful control of maternal diabetes at every stage of pregnancy.

In the case of an established diabetic an assessment of her condition should ideally be made *before* the pregnancy occurs. Some diabetics with severe nephropathy or retinopathy may need to be advised against pregnancy; the perinatal mortality is especially high in cases with these complications. Good control of the diabetes during the months preceding conception and during the first trimester should reduce the incidence of congenital abnormality, which is now the most important single cause of perinatal loss.

A variant of haemoglobin A, known as HbA_{1c}, which is produced by slow glycosylation of HbA during the life of the red cell, may be a useful indicator of preceding average blood glucose levels. A level of HbA_{1c} above the normal proportion of 3–4 per cent of the total amount of haemoglobin suggests that there has been an abnormally high average level of blood glucose during the preceding two or three months. Diabetic women who have a high level of HbA_{1c} (more than 12 per cent) in early pregnancy have an increased tendency to fetal abnormality. When the level is raised in late pregnancy the fetus is more likely to be macrosomic. If the preconception HbA_{1c} index is high pregnancy should be postponed until better control of the diabetes has been achieved.

Close co-operation between obstetrician and diabetic physician throughout pregnancy is essential if a satisfactory outcome is to be achieved. The need to increase the insulin dosage progressively as pregnancy advances, to adjust the diet and to monitor blood glucose levels means that these women are best treated in specialized units with the ability to admit the patient at any time when control is less than perfect. For the intelligent and well-motivated patient control of blood glucose levels can be improved by employment of Dextrostix or BM stix and a blood glucose meter which she uses in her own home two or three times a week. Patients are often admitted to hospital between 36 and 38 weeks gestation and kept under constant supervision until delivery.

Obstetric management

Apart from routine antenatal care, an ultrasound scan of the fetus should be made at 18 weeks to establish maturity and exclude gross fetal abnormality. Thereafter fetal growth can be followed by repeated ultrasound examinations. Excessive fetal growth (macrosomia) can be detected from about the 30th week onwards by measuring the abdominal circumference. In late pregnancy daily observation by the mother of fetal movements and frequent cardiotocographic studies may help to prevent late intrauterine deaths. Although uncommon in a well-controlled diabetic pregnancy, fetal death may still occur as a result of fetal hypoxia due to changes in the maternal side of the placental circulation, the effect of HbA_{1c} on the passage of oxygen across the placenta and an increase in oxygen consumption by the fetus and placenta.

Premature delivery to avoid late intrauterine fetal death has been a standard procedure for many years, but is not necessary when very good control of the maternal diabetes has been maintained. Vaginal delivery should always be the aim, but obstetric complications, especially hypertension and disproportion, and concern about the adequacy of diabetic control lead to a relatively high rate of induction and caesarean section. During labour diabetic control is best maintained by the administration of glucose and insulin intravenously at a controlled rate by means of an infusion pump. Continuous fetal heart monitoring and fetal blood sampling are employed to detect fetal distress, which is more common in these cases.

As soon as the baby is delivered it should be handed over to a neonatal special care unit. Good control of maternal diabetes ensures normal maturation of the fetal lung and sharply reduces the risk and severity of the respiratory distress syndrome. Early feeding counteracts neonatal hypoglycaemia. If the infant's haematocrit (packed cell volume) is greater than 70 per cent then 10 per cent of the estimated blood volume is removed by venesection and replaced by an equal volume of serum. Hyperbilirubinaemia (p. 310) and hypocalcaemia (p. 308) may require treatment.

There is no contraindication to breast-feeding, and the majority of diabetic mothers feed their babies successfully.

Family planning

For diabetics this is an essential part of postnatal care. Most of the patients will be content with two or three children and once the family is complete sterilization is the most satisfactory long-term solution. For short-term family planning there is no contraindication to the use of the oral contraceptive pill or to the intrauterine device.

ACUTE SPECIFIC FEVERS

Although pregnancy does not alter the course of most specific fevers the fetal results may be serious. With high fever and toxic effects either miscarriage or premature labour may occur. Some organisms reach the fetus, including those of rubella, smallpox, vaccinia, chickenpox, typhoid fever, toxoplasmosis, Coxsackie virus disease, cytomegalic inclusion disease and listeriosis.

RUBELLA

Maternal viraemia results in direct infection of the fetus via the placenta. Fetal infection is as likely to occur with a subclinical infection as with severe infection of the mother. The result of fetal infection varies greatly, including fetal death, birth of a fetus with active rubella, congenital malformation, and in some cases no apparent damage. In some epidemics the incidence of congenital abnormality has been 50 per cent in the first month, 30 per cent in the second month and 15 per cent in the third month; with rare cases of damage after this.

The congenital defects produced vary according to the stage of pregnancy. Infection during the first and second months may produce congenital cataract or cardiac valvular lesions; during the third month deafness may result. Deafness and visual or neurological defects may not be recognized until later in childhood. One study showed that 23 per cent of children exposed to rubella *in utero* who were apparently normal at birth showed defects by the age of two.

The clinical diagnosis of rubella-like illness is difficult and a diagnosis of rubella is only correct in about 20 per cent of cases. It is therefore necessary to carry out immunological investigations whenever possible. The usual test is the haemagglutination inhibition test, which depends on the fact that serum containing antibody inhibits the agglutination of day-old chick erythrocytes by the virus. Haemagglutination inhibition antibodies appear soon after the rash and reach peak titres in six to 12 days. Absence of antibody immediately after exposure to infection indicates susceptibility; its presence indicates previous infection and immunity. Patients who present within two weeks of exposure and who have a rapid rise in antibody titres in blood samples taken one or two weeks apart may be assumed to have had a recent infection. In doubtful cases the patient's serum should be examined for rubella-specific IgM. This is a more complex test but the presence of this antibody is strong evidence of recent primary infection.

An effective vaccine is now available against rubella. This consists of living but attenuated virus. It is sad that numerous unborn children still suffer damage from this virus, although prevention of fetal rubella is possible. Since 1970 rubella vaccination has been offered to all girls aged 11 to 14 in the United Kingdom, but unfortunately it is still accepted on their behalf by only 84 per cent of parents. Vaccination is also offered to all women who are seronegative and are at special risk of exposure to rubella, such as nurses and teachers. Much is now being done by health authorities to try to increase the acceptance rate of vaccination. If living virus is used and if the recipient becomes pregnant soon after its administration there is a small risk the fetus may be infected. Adult women must be warned of this and instructed to use contraception for three months.

Pregnant women must be advised to avoid contact with any known case of rubella. In antenatal clinics every patient should have her antibody status determined at her first visit. This indicates those women who are immune because of previous infection, which may be useful information if any exposure occurs. The women who are susceptible should be vaccinated as soon as the pregnancy is over. Termination of pregnancy is justifiable if the patient has certain evidence of infection in the first trimester.

MEASLES

Measles is reported to affect the fetus *in utero*, but has not been proved to cause fetal abnormalities.

TYPHOID FEVER

Before the introduction of antibiotics typhoid

fever was a serious complication of pregnancy in that abortion, stillbirth or premature labour occurred in many cases. The bacilli have been demonstrated in the organs of the fetus.

SMALLPOX

Since this disease has been globally eradicated it is now unlikely to complicate pregnancy. Formerly the prognosis was grave for both mother and fetus.

CHICKENPOX

There is no evidence that this infection causes congenital abnormalities, but the child may be born covered with the rash.

SCARLET FEVER

This disease is caused by the haemolytic streptococcus which may also cause puerperal fever, and a scarlatiniform rash can occur in cases of puerperal streptococcal infection. If the disease occurs during pregnancy abortion may occur, but the fetus is not infected.

POLIOMYELITIS

Susceptibility to this disease may be increased during pregnancy. During the initial pyrexial illness fetal death may occur, but the virus does not cause fetal abnormalities and paralysis of the newborn is exceedingly rare. During labour special care is required only if respiration is impeded, and then forceps delivery is better than caesarean section. Immunization against poliomyelitis can safely be carried out during pregnancy.

CHOREA

So-called chorea gravidarum is Sydenham's (rheumatic) chorea occurring during pregnancy. If a patient who has recently had chorea becomes pregnant a recrudescence of the symptoms is common. Recovery is the rule and termination of the pregnancy is not required.

MALARIA

Pregnant women should not travel to malarious areas unless it is essential, but if their journey is necessary they should take appropriate prophy-laxis. During pregnancy severe exacerbation of latent malaria may occur, and disease which is already active may be made worse. Abortion, premature labour and low birth weight frequently occur, especially in cases of malignant tertian malaria. The appropriate locally-effective anti-malarial prophylaxis should be given to all pregnant women in malarious areas. The choice of agent will depend on the distribution of choroquine-resistant strains in the area. A combination of chloroquine 300 mg weekly and proguanil 200 mg daily is recommended for areas where chloroquine resistance is low; and chloroquine 300 mg and Maloprim (containing pyrimethamine 12.5 mg and dapsone 100 mg) weekly where resistance is high. If infection occurs the same treatment is given as to the non-pregnant.

INFLUENZA

A severe attack of influenza may have the same effect as any other severe fever in causing abortion or intrauterine fetal death. With infection in the first trimester the incidence of congenital abnormality, particularly neural tube defects, may be slightly increased.

TOXOPLASMOSIS

This is an uncommon disease caused by a small protozoon, *Toxoplasma gondii*, found in the intestines of cats. In England the incidence of congenital toxoplasmosis is lower than on the continent of Europe. The mother may only have a transient febrile illness but in about 50 per cent of cases the disease is transmitted to the fetus, in whom it causes encephalomyelitis and choriodoretinitis. The effect on the fetus is greatest when infection occurs in the second trimester. Most infected infants die, but those that survive for a time may have blindness, mental defects, hydrocephalus and calcification of the cerebral lesions. Diagnosis is difficult. New laboratory methods for assay of specific IgM antibody have been developed but at present it is not thought justifiable to use these for antenatal screening in the UK because of the low incidence of the disease. Fortunately one attack gives immunity and subsequent children are normal.

CYTOMEGALIC INCLUSION DISEASE

The group of cytomegalic viruses (CMV) are found in many animals and in the Western hemisphere most humans show antibodies to them after the age of 35. In the East the infection is acquired in early life and most children have antibodies. Although it requires very close contact to transfer the virus, an infected individual carries it permanently and is capable of passing it on. The clincal picture is extremely variable and often resembles that of glandular fever. Even if the effects in the mother are mild or subclinical the fetus may be badly affected. The majority of babies born after CMV infection during pregnancy progress normally, but those who are affected show abnormalities of the central nervous system, with a high incidence of mental retardation and deafness. Diagnosis is made by a complement fixation test and by radioimmunoassay for specific IgM antibody. There is no effective treatment or prevention. As the large majority of fetuses escape ill effects termination of pregnancy would not be justifiable on the basis of a serological result.

LISTERIOSIS

Infection of the mother with *Listeria monocytogenes* produces a flu-like illness with an elevated temperature and general malaise; it has been ascribed to the eating of soft, blue-veined cheese. In pregnancy transplacental spread to the fetus occurs followed by fetal death and abortion. The incidence in the UK is very low.

DISEASES OF THE ALIMENTARY TRACT

DENTAL CARIES

Decayed teeth and gingivitis are often observed during pregnancy or after delivery. The popular saying is 'For every child a tooth', and the fashionable belief is that the caries is caused by calcium deficiency. Since the enamel is not vascularized decalcification is not possible, but if dentine has already been exposed then decay may progress more rapidly. Dental inspection and treatment should be carried on in pregnancy. Fillings or extractions should be performed under local anaesthesia if possible and if a general anaesthetic is required 'gas' in a dental chair is more dangerous

in pregnancy than at other times. A proper anaesthetic, with every precaution taken against hypoxia, should be given.

HEARTBURN

During pregnancy the cardiac sphincter is relaxed and acid regurgitation may occur. Sometimes troublesome heartburn is due to a hiatus hernia. Relief may be obtained with alkalies in either tablet or liquid form. The symptoms are often worse if the patient lies flat.

PEPTIC ULCER

Symptoms nearly always improve during pregnancy, probably because the gastric acidity falls and there is an increased secretion of mucus. Perforation or haematemesis are very rare during pregnancy.

APPENDICITIS

Appendicitis is not common during pregnancy. The danger of the condition is enhanced because it is sometimes difficult to make an early diagnosis. If there is widespread peritonitis abortion may occur.

Abdominal pain on the right side during pregnancy may be due to pyelonephritis, extrauterine gestation, torsion of an ovarian cyst, red degeneration of a fibromyoma, biliary or renal colic, or appendicitis. A small right-sided haemorrhage from abruptio placentae may also simulate appendicitis. The most frequent error is to confuse pyelonephritis with appendicitis; in every case the urine must be carefully examined.

The symptoms of appendicitis are little altered during pregnancy, but the site of the pain and of maximum tenderness may be higher than usual because the caecum and appendix are displaced upwards.

Appendicectomy should be performed in spite of the pregnancy. A muscle splitting incision should be made at the site of maximum tenderness and every effort made to avoid handling the uterus.

INTESTINAL OBSTRUCTION

The most common cause of intestinal obstruction during pregnancy is a band resulting from adhesions following a previous operation; the obstruction occurs because of altered positions of the viscera brought about by the growth of the uterus. Other causes of obstruction during pregnancy are strangulated internal or external hernia, volvulus, intussusception and mesenteric thrombosis. Neoplasms of the bowel are rare.

The especial danger of intestinal obstruction during pregnancy is the delay that often elapses before the diagnosis is made, the symptoms so often being attributed to the pregnancy. The classic symptoms of pain, vomiting and constipation will be present but the physical sign of abdominal distension is masked by the pregnant uterus. A scar on the abdomen of a patient whose chief complaint is vomiting should always suggest the possibility of intestinal obstruction. Pyelonephritis, appendicitis, hyperemesis gravidarium, ureteric calculus and torsion of the pedicle of an ovarian cyst would all need to be considered in making the diagnosis.

When the diagnosis has been made laparotomy is performed without delay. Intravenous infusion of saline and gastric suction are started before the operation. Laparotomy for the relief of obstruction can be a difficult operation even without pregnancy and if the patient is near term and the bulk of the uterus interferes seriously it may have to be emptied by caesarean section before the operation for relief of obstruction can proceed.

HERNIA AND PREGNANCY

As a general rule herniae are not made worse by, and do not affect the course of, pregnancy. The growing uterus usually pushes the bowel away from the orifices of inguinal and femoral herniae and eventually blocks access to them. Rarely these types of herniae first appear during pregnancy, but fluctuant swellings which appear in the groin during pregnancy are usually found to be varicoceles.

In the case of umbilical hernia, if intestine is adherent to the sac it may rarely be dragged upon by the growing uterus, thus causing intestinal obstruction.

ULCERATIVE COLITIS

This disease is sometimes worse during pregnancy and is sometimes first diagnosed at that time. Women with active colitis should not become pregnant, but once the acute symptoms have subsided they may accept the risk of reactivation. The usual treatment, including steroids and prednisolone retention enemata, may be used during pregnancy but should be avoided if possible during the first trimester.

LIVER DISEASE IN PREGNANCY

INFECTIVE HEPATITIS

Pregnant women may suffer from both types of hepatitis, Type A, which is caused by a virus excreted in the faeces by a patient with the disease, and Type B, which is due to a virus spread by transfusion of infected blood or plasma or by injection with contaminated needles. The virus responsible for Type B can be identified by an antigen on its surface (Australia antigen). (Non-A non-B viruses may also cause hepatitis during pregnancy but are less common in Western countries.)

During pregnancy both types of hepatitis usually follow a similar course to that in non-pregnant women, and spontaneous recovery is to be expected. However, in a small number of cases, and more commonly in developing countries, liver damage is so severe that death occurs. Hepatitis during pregnancy does not cause fetal abnormalities, but abortion or premature labour may occur, as may intrauterine death in late pregnancy. At least half of the babies born to mothers who have had Type B hepatitis during pregnancy will show hepatitis B antigen in their blood, and a proportion of them develop hepatic lesions.

Medical and nursing staff may be infected with Type B virus contained in blood from a patient via any small cut or abrasion, or from contact with a Type B case, and patients with hepatitis are most safely nursed in a specialized liver unit.

TOXIC HEPATITIS CAUSED BY CHEMICAL AGENTS

Hepatic necrosis may occur a few days after prolonged or repeated administration of fluothane (Halothane) anaesthesia during pregnancy, and its use should be avoided at that time. In rare instances hepatic necrosis may also be caused by other substances including trichlorethylene and chlorpromazine compounds.

ECLAMPSIA

Hepatic lesions of a specific type may occur (p. 93).

ACUTE HEPATIC FAILURE DURING PREGNANCY (acute fatty liver of pregnancy)

This is a rare condition which occurs in late pregnancy. Acute fatty degeneration of centrilobar liver cells causes the rapid onset of vomiting, upper abdominal pain and jaundice. Most cases progress to coma and death in a few days. Intrauterine fetal death often occurs. Liver biopsy may be hazardous if there is a clotting deficiency, but will establish the diagnosis. The cause is unknown and there is no effective treatment, although a few cases have survived after early delivery. This condition does not seem to be the same as the acute hepatic necrosis which occasionally follows acute viral hepatitis.

RECURRENT CHOLESTATIC JAUNDICE OF PREGNANCY

Very slight jaundice may occur as a result of oestrogen-induced cholestasis. This causes pruritus and biochemical examination shows slightly raised levels of bilirubin, alkaline phosphatase and transferase in the serum. Women who are affected are unduly sensitive to oestrogens and develop this condition in every pregnancy or if they take oral contraceptives. No treatment is required and complete recovery occurs after the pregnancy or on stopping the oral contraceptive.

OTHER CAUSES OF JAUNDICE IN PREGNANCY

All the other causes of jaundice in non-pregnant women may occur during pregnancy and give difficulties in diagnosis. Examples are obstructive jaundice from gallstones, haemolytic jaundice from mismatched transfusion and jaundice from infection with haemolytic organisms.

SEXUALLY TRANSMITTED DISEASES IN PREGNANCY

GONORRHOEA

The disease may be contracted before pregnancy, at the time of conception or during pregnancy. Gonococcal infection of the fallopian tubes causes sterility if inadequately treated.

The symptoms and signs of gonorrhoea are not modified by pregnancy. Women with gonorrhoea may have very slight symptoms and if vaginal discharge is present it may be due to associated trichomonal or candidial vaginitis.

Gonorrhoea is unlikely to affect the pregnancy, although in a few cases the infection spreads to the uterine cavity and fallopian tubes after delivery. During labour the baby's eyes are in danger of being infected and the discovery of neonatal conjunctivitis is occasionally the first reason for suspecting the disease.

Careful investigation of any abnormal urethral or vaginal discharge during pregnancy is essential. Swabs for microscopical examination and bacterial culture are taken from the urethra and cervix. If it is not possible to plate these onto warm agar immediately, they are placed in Stuart's medium for transport to the laboratory.

Treatment

A single dose of amoxycillin or ampicillin 3 g combined with probenecid 1 g is given. If the patient is allergic to penicillin, or the organism is penicillin-resistant, there is a wide choice of effective antibiotics, but tetracycline should not be used during pregnancy. A single injection of spectinomycin 2 g or cefotaxime 1 g intramuscularly is often chosen. Cure must be established by repeated bacteriological tests and efforts must be made to treat the partners of patients. Serological tests for possible concurrent syphilis are made both before and after antibiotic treatment.

Gonococcal conjunctivitis of the newborn

See page 326.

SYPHILIS

The importance of syphilis in pregnancy is that the causative organism, *Treponema pallidum*, crosses the placenta and invades the fetus. Fetal infection is most likely when the mother is in the primary or secondary stage of the disease. Severe fetal infection will cause intrauterine death, followed by late abortion or premature delivery. With less severe infection the fetus may be born alive with congenital syphilis. The baby may be small-for-dates and show enlargement of the liver and spleen, purpura, thrombocytopenia and anaemia. At birth there may be bullous lesions on the skin (*syphilitic pemphigus*). After three or four weeks a widespread maculopapular rash may appear over the trunk and often the palms and soles, with mucous patches in the mouth and condylomata around the anus. There may be nasal infection and osteochondritis of long bones. Choroiditis may occur.

Sometimes there are no signs at the time of birth, but manifestations appear later in childhood.

Diagnosis

All pregnant women must have a screening blood test for syphilis in early pregnancy. The Kahn and Wassermann tests also give a positive reaction in cases of yaws, and more specific tests such as the TPI (*Treponema pallidum* immobilization) test or the FTA (fluorescent treponemal antibody) test are needed to confirm a suspicion of maternal syphilis. These tests are also performed on the newborn child if there is any possibility of congenital infection soon after birth at six and 12 weeks.

Treatment

If treatment is given early in pregnancy the fetal infection will be cured. Procaine penicillin 1.2 g is injected intramuscularly daily for ten days. In penicillin-sensitive patients erythromycin 500 mg four times daily for 14 days is an alternative treatment, but as this antibiotic may not cross the placenta the infant should also be given penicillin after delivery.

Neonatal infection

The baby should be barrier-nursed because any cutaneous or mucosal lesions are infectious. Procaine penicillin 100 mg is injected intramuscularly daily for 15 days, and the clinical and serological response is observed.

YAWS

Occasionally a positive test for syphilis will be found in a Central American, West Indian or African patient, who is in fact suffering from yaws. This endemic disease is acquired in youth from skin contact and is caused by an organism closely related to *Treponema pallidum*. It gives rise to a positive PDRL and FTA test for life. Yaws is a mild disease in temperate climates and does not harm the fetus. However, in view of the diagnostic difficulties it is usually wise to treat all seropositive patients as if they have syphilis.

HERPES GENITALIS

Herpetic lesions of the vulva, vagina and cervix are caused by sexually transmitted infection with type 2 herpes virus, and occasionally with type 1 virus from oral contact. Fetal infection may occur as an ascending infection during birth or when the membranes rupture, but the high incidence of abortion and of premature birth suggests that transplacental infection may also occur. Infected babies have widespread lesions in the central nervous system, the eyes, the skin and the mouth, with a high mortality and much morbidity in survivors. The diagnosis is made by cytological smears and viral cultures.

Because of the need to avoid fetal contact with the virus it is important to ensure that there are no active lesions in the birth canal at the time of delivery. Viral cultures should be made weekly from the 36th week. If active lesions are present or the cultures are positive, delivery should be by caesarean section before the membranes rupture.

CHLAMYDIAL INFECTION

Chlamydial infection (*Chlamydia trachomatis*) of the cervix may go undetected during pregnancy and may cause no complications. Infection of the infant's conjunctivae may occur during delivery (p. 326) and occasional cases of neonatal chlamydial pneumonia are seen.

HIV INFECTION (ACQUIRED IMMUNE DEFICIENCY SYNDROME (AIDS))

AIDS was first identified in 1981 in homosexual men in the USA. The causal agent, a retrovirus called human immunodeficiency virus (HIV), was discovered in 1983. By now there are, according to the World Health Organization, between five and ten million individuals of both sexes who possess antibodies in their serum against the disease. An unknown proportion of those infected, perhaps the majority, are likely to suffer from a failure of cell-mediated immunity or from AIDS, so that they eventually succumb to opportunistic infections. The disease is passed from one individual to another in semen during sexual intercourse (and especially during anal intercourse), by blood at transfusion during treatment with blood products (as in haemophilia) or by sharing contaminated needles when injecting drugs. Health care workers are at risk from needle-stick injuries, but these are very rare. Although there may be between 40 000 and 50 000 HIV-positive people in the UK, relatively few are women, and so far only about 150 women have progressed to frank AIDS.

The question of screening for HIV infection in the antenatal clinic is a contentious one; to screen all pregnant women would be costly in laboratory services and personnel. Its usefulness is being investigated by an MRC study.

Women at high risk of infection include:

sexual partners of men known to be HIV-positive
intravenous drug users
sexual partners of bisexual men
sexual partners of haemophiliacs
sexual partners of sub-Saharan Africans
prostitutes.

The pregnant HIV-positive woman is liable to infect her baby *in utero* or during birth or breast feeding.

Special care should be taken by attendants at birth and in the puerperium to avoid contamination with the blood of HIV-positive women and of those at high risk of infection who have not been proved negative serologically. The babies of both groups of women will need careful following-up after birth. Generally they should not be breast fed (*see* p. 250).

For a fuller account of HIV infection of AIDS *see Gynaecology by Ten Teachers*.

NEUROLOGICAL DISEASES DURING PREGNANCY

EPILEPSY

Epilepsy, or a history of it, occurs in as many as 1 in 200 pregnancies, and these patients need better consideration, with collaboration between the neurologist and the obstetrician. Women with epilepsy may wonder whether pregnancy will make their fits worse, whether the baby will be harmed by the epilepsy, or by drugs they are taking, and whether the baby will inherit the disease. A few women become pregnant because antiepileptic drugs interfere with the action of oral contraceptives.

The effect of pregnancy on epilepsy is extremely variable, but in a few patients fits which have been absent for a time recur, and in severe cases the frequency of fits may increase. During pregnancy drug treatment is continued, but patients should be seen frequently by the neurologist, who can adjust their drug dosage, often with the help of assays of blood levels. During labour drugs may not be absorbed and fits may recur.

With phenytoin (Epanutin) folic acid is antagonized, and there is a risk of fetal malformation. Sodium valproate may be substituted for it, but if phenytoin is used additional folic acid is given.

It is possible that a grand mal epileptic fit could be mistaken for an eclamptic fit. The two types of fit cannot be distinguished, and if a patient with hypertension or proteinuria has a fit, even if she is an epileptic, it is safest to assume that she has developed eclampsia and to treat her accordingly.

MYASTHENIA GRAVIS

Pregnancy has a variable effect on this disease. The dosage of neostigmine may need to be altered, but pregnancy and labour are usually uneventful. Uterine action is unaffected but forceps delivery or vacuum extraction may be required because of weak voluntary effort. Local or epidural analgesia should be used for this if possible, as these patients are unduly sensitive to general anaesthesia. Post-partum exacerbation of the disease is common and should be watched for. The newborn infant may be temporarily affected and hypotonic and motionless after birth. The myasthenia of the baby passes off after about ten days and treatment is only necessary if there is difficulty in breathing, sucking or swallowing.

MULTIPLE SCLEROSIS

The current view is that pregnancy has no effect on this disease and that any changes which occur during pregnancy would have taken place in any case. Spinal and caudal analgesia should be avoided at delivery. The question of termination of pregnancy sometimes arises because of the family problems of an incapacitated woman.

SUBARACHNOID HEMORRHAGE

Rupture of an intracranial aneurysm may occur during pregnancy, or a patient may become pregnant who has previously had this accident. Unless the haemorrhage occurs within six weeks of delivery, or there is hypertension, assisted vaginal delivery is preferable to caesarean section.

CEREBRAL THROMBOPHLEBITIS

Thrombosis of cerebral veins or dural sinuses may occur during pregnancy or the puerperium. A few cases are associated with pelvic infection, but often the cause is obscure. There may be general signs such as headache, fits and coma, often with fever and vomiting; or there may be focal neurological signs such as hemiplegia or aphasia. Anticoagulant drugs are given, and recovery may occur.

ACROPARAESTHESIA (CARPAL TUNNEL SYNDROME)

See page 46.

CRAMP IN PREGNANCY

See page 46.

ENDOCRINE DISORDERS IN PREGNANCY

ADDISON'S DISEASE

Addison's disease rarely complicates pregnancy. It presents the same features during pregnancy as in the non-pregnant state. Addisonian crises may occur at any time, but most often during early pregnancy – when vomiting may accentuate any electrolytic disturbance – during the stress of labour or during the early puerperium. The patient's replacement dosage of cortisone and fludrocortisone is continued during pregnancy and will often need to be increased if abnormal loss of sodium occurs. Frequent estimations of serum electrolytes are necessary to ensure adequate replacement therapy. To cover the stress of labour hydrocortisone 200 mg is injected intramuscularly at the onset, and 100 mg every six hours until delivery. Anaesthetics must be administered cautiously.

ACUTE ADRENAL FAILURE

Occasionally, as a result of septicaemia, haemorrhagic shock or amniotic embolism, haemorrhages in the adrenal glands cause acute adrenal insufficiency, so that the patient does not respond to normal resuscitative measures. If this occurs hydrocortisone is given intravenously in high dosage.

ADMINISTRATION OF CORTICOSTEROIDS DURING PREGNANCY

A woman who has been receiving treatment with corticosteroids (other than topical corticosteroids) for any condition before becoming pregnant may occasionally collapse under mild stress during pregnancy or labour; this possibility should be remembered when any patient shows an unexpected response to stress. The slow recovery of adrenal function after administration of corticosteroids means that any patient who has had such treatment during the 12 months preceding her pregnancy should be given hydrocortisone, as described above, during labour.

Although there is a very slight risk of corticosteroids given during pregnancy causing cleft lip or palate in the fetus, experience suggests that the risk can be ignored with doses of the order of 100 mg of cortisone or 20 mg of prednisolone daily.

PHAEOCHROMOCYTOMA

This is a very rare but exceedingly dangerous complication of pregnancy which is caused by a tumour of the adrenal medulla that produces an excess of noradrenaline and adrenaline.

Any stress, painful stimulus or mechanical disturbance of the tumour causes the release of these substances with resulting paroxysmal hypertension and tachycardia, during which cardiac failure may occur. In the attack there is pallor, sweating, headache and sometimes vomiting. Attacks may occur during pregnancy and simulate pregnancy-induced hypertension, but they also occur during labour or soon after delivery. Anaesthesia and operations are especially liable to precipitate an attack and a number of patients have died of so-called shock, the tumour only being found at post-mortem examination. It is the paroxysmal nature of the attacks which should arouse suspicion. It is not usually possible to palpate the small tumour, but the urinary excretion of catechol amines and of vanillyl mandelic acid is increased.

If the diagnosis is made during pregnancy it is best to deliver the patient by caesarean section when the fetus is sufficiently mature. Any hypertensive crisis is controlled by giving phentolamine intravenously. The tumour is removed later.

DISORDERS OF THE THYROID GLAND

The thyroid gland becomes larger and more vascular during pregnancy as a result of increased secretion of thyroid-stimulating hormone by the anterior pituitary gland. The amount of thyroxine-binding globulin in the blood doubles during the first trimester of pregnancy and as a result serum concentrations of total thyroxine (T_4) and of tri-iodothyronine (T_3) are increased. Free thyroxine levels are normal or slightly reduced. The basal metabolic rate is increased by up to 20 per cent, partly as a result of increased oxygen consumption by the uterus and fetoplacental tissues.

Non-toxic enlargement of the thyroid gland

Simple colloid goitres, as occur in districts where iodine is deficient, enlarge in pregnancy and, if the tumour is retrosternal, may press on the trachea. Surgical treatment can be carried out if necessary during pregnancy, but thyroxine should be given postoperatively to guard against hypothyroidism. In Hashimoto's disease the firm enlargement can be reduced without the need for surgery by administration of thyroxine.

Hyperthyroidism

Mild hyperthyroidism is not uncommon during pregnancy. If the overactivity of the gland is caused by an abnormal long-acting thyroid stimulator this will cross the placenta and cause neonatal hyperthyroidism. This subsides within three weeks.

Because of the raised basal metabolic rate and the enlargement of the thyroid gland which normally occur during pregnancy the diagnosis of mild hyperthyroidism may be difficult. Careful clinical assessment and assay of total and free thyroxine will be needed.

The treatment most commonly employed during pregnancy uses antithyroid drugs such as carbimazole and thiouracil. As these drugs cross the placenta there is a risk of fetal hypothyroidism. The risk can be avoided by keeping the mother euthyroid and giving a small dose of thyroxine such as 200 micrograms daily during the last trimester. This will cross the placenta and reach the fetus. Breast feeding is contraindicated as antithyroid drugs are excreted in the milk.

Hypothyroidism

Severe hypothyroidism causes infertility. Pregnancy may occur in mild cases but there is an increased risk of abortion. Treated cases of myxoedema who become pregnant require an increased dose of thyroxine.

PITUITARY PROLACTINOMA

Recent effective treatment of hyperprolactinaemia has allowed many patients, including those with prolactinomata, to become pregnant. Most of these tumours are confined to the pituitary fossa, but upward extension can compromise the optic chiasma. There is concern whether this might occur during pregnancy in patients who have had prolactinomata treated with bromocriptine, but bromocriptine causes considerable shrinkage of these tumours so that by the time pregnancy occurs the fossa contains only a small gland. Treated prolactinomata may be left alone during pregnancy, stopping the bromocriptine until after delivery and lactation.

DISEASES OF THE SKIN DURING PREGNANCY

Physiological changes are described on page 28. Almost any of the multitudinous diseases of the skin can occur during pregnancy, and conditions specifically related to pregnancy are rare. These include:

PRURITUS

Generalized pruritus may occur with cholestatic jaundice (p. 117), and a complaint of abdominal pruritus is not uncommon. Treatment is not very effective, but warm alkaline baths or the application of calamine lotion are often tried.

Pruritus vulvae may occur with infection by *Candida* or *Trichomonas vaginalis*.

PRURIGO GESTATIONIS

This condition was first described by Besnier, and consists of a papular eruption on the abdomen, thighs, buttocks and on the dorsal surfaces of the hands and feet. The lesions are small, discrete and very irritating. They resolve after delivery. Calamine lotion or phenol lotion (1 per cent) may be helpful, or oral antihistamines such as chlorpheniramine tablets (Piriton) 4 mg four times daily.

HERPES GESTATIONIS

This rare disease may recur in successive pregnancies. Severe pruritus is followed by the development of red erythematous patches on the abdomen and legs. These give way to rings of vesicles which appear in crops, and sometimes coalesce to form bullae which may become pustular or haemorrhagic. The patient is ill with fever, rigors and vomiting, and there is a striking eosinophilia. The clinical picture is similar to that of dermatitis herpetiformis.

Recovery is the rule, although there have been a few fatal cases. If the patient becomes severely ill abortion or intrauterine fetal death may occur. There is no specific treatment but corticosteroids may control the lesions, and systemic antibiotics are required for infection.

MALIGNANT DISEASE DURING PREGNANCY

Malignant disease is uncommon in association with pregnancy. If malignant disease is diagnosed during pregnancy the treatment of the disease becomes the first consideration. In only a few cases is surgical treatment or radiotherapy possible without affecting the fetus; in many cases the pregnancy must be brought to an end. In early pregnancy termination may be advised; in the second half of pregnancy a difficult choice sometimes has to be made between postponing early delivery in the interests of the fetus or of delivering a premature baby to allow treatment of the malignant disease to start. The patient's wishes and the nature of the disease will have to be taken into account.

Carcinoma of the cervix (p. 67) and carcinoma of the breast are the two lesions in which early treatment is especially important during pregnancy, although whether pregnancy has any adverse effect in these conditions is doubtful.

PSYCHIATRIC DISORDERS IN PREGNANCY AND THE PUERPERIUM

Pregnancy and motherhood change a woman's life-style profoundly. This is most apparent in a first pregnancy. While pregnancy affects each mother-to-be differently, three sorts of reaction can be recognized.

THE CONTENTED PATIENT

A few women feel better in pregnancy than at any other time in their lives; they just sparkle. It is thought that their happy mental state is due to an absence of premenstrual tension and depression, although there is no hard evidence to support such

an explanation; they are women who simply relish the prospect of motherhood.

THE PATIENT WITH COMMON ANXIETY

Most women with a stable personality enjoy the challenge of pregnancy although even they experience some anxiety and doubt about their ability to cope. This is most marked in the first trimester and again in the last few weeks before confinement.

These worries can easily be understood when the psychological stresses of pregnancy are considered. These include concern about the health of the unborn baby, fear of hospitals, physical examinations and injections. Apprehension is widespread about the delivery and the pain of labour and its control. Losing their figure and feeling less attractive may also worry some women, especially if they lack their partner's support. There is much heart-searching on the subject of an early return to work. Although there is considerable pressure on women to stay at home with their infant, a prospect which some women welcome, women realize that they will miss their colleagues' adult conversation and, not least, they fear a much reduced budget on which to manage. Loss of status and independence may also affect the professional woman. The mother who has nowhere to live is often distressed and will need help in taking the appropriate steps to secure accommodation for herself and her baby.

Management

During pregnancy the doctor should encourage the patient to discuss her problems; she should feel that the doctor has time to listen to her and once difficulties are clarified simple explanation will assist the mother-to-be to solve her own problems. This positive approach to reassurance is more effective than a bland 'don't worry'.

THE NEUROTIC PATIENT

The patient whose personality shows many neurotic traits may find it more difficult to adapt to her new role. She is more likely to develop symptoms of anxiety or depression. Overt psychiatric illness is present if symptoms interfere with her day to day activities. This neurotic illness is not specific to the pregnant state and includes anxiety neurosis, phobic states, obsessional states, depressive neurosis or a mixture of any of these conditions.

Clinical presentation

Neurotic patients may present in various ways. Tearfulness in the antenatal clinic is not uncommon, especially in women who do not understand their own feelings. Asking the woman why she is crying does not usually lead to a meaningful answer; time, sympathy and patience are needed to elucidate the problem. Women who have suffered a previous neurotic illness are usually more able to discuss their symptoms, which are not infrequently

hidden, and are only revealed by careful inquiry.

Psychiatric symptoms may present as somatic complaints such as vomiting, headache, backache, vaginal discharge or bleeding.

Management

Neurotic women need a lot of extra support. The patient's general practitioner can give invaluable support. This may be done by enlisting the help of the health visitor or social worker to assess the patient's needs.

It is important that the patient sees the same midwife and doctor at each clinic attendance, thus promoting good rapport. Extra time should be made available in which to discuss special difficulties.

If improvement does not occur the patient should be referred to a psychiatrist. Following a full history and examination of the mental state a diagnosis is made. Psychiatric treatment may take the form of:

psychotherapy
behavioural therapy, especially if obsessional symptoms are dominant
relaxation therapy, if the patient is suffering from an anxiety state or obsessional neurosis
drug therapy, which should only be given after the first trimester
Antidepressants or anxiolytic drugs, which may be used as appropriate.

THE PERSISTENT NON-ATTENDER

Some women are unable or unwilling to establish a relationship with their doctor or midwife. They ignore appointments and fail to answer letters. Some are disadvantaged or homeless, others have lost their trust in people in authority. The heavy smoker or the obese may also forego antenatal care, afraid of censorious lecturing. Alcohol or drug abuse is frequently the true reason for non-attendance.

DRUG DEPENDENCE

Although many women misuse drugs recreationally, relatively few become dependent. A large variety of drugs may be abused. From the obstetric point of view, opiates and alcohol are the most important. Fortunately, pregnancy is not common in the chronic heroin addict.

OPIATE DEPENDENCE

Three different groups should be considered:

> the street addict
> the stable addict under treatment in a drug-dependence clinic
> the addict who attends a drug clinic but is unco-operative.

The street addict

The woman often lives with a similarly addicted consort and both rely on street sources for their drugs. Powdered street heroin is currently becoming purer but may contain barbiturates or other drugs. The powder may also be diluted or 'cut' by impurities which range from chalk to glucose. The woman's drug supply is likely to be irregular and hence she lives by her wits. The need for a regular source of money to sustain her drug habit dominates her thinking. Little cash is left for food, accommodation or other necessities. She tends to inject drugs, running the risk of infection and further jeopardizing her poor general health. Responding to the climate of anxiety regarding AIDS and hepatitis B, some women have stopped taking their drugs by injection. Others have made a partial concession by not sharing needles or syringes.

The effect on the fetus is potentially serious. Premature labour, growth retardation and neonatal withdrawal symptoms are common sequelae of the street addict's life-style and drug misuse.

The stable addict under medical care

This woman presents with few problems as her general health and nutrition are usually adequate. She is more likely to accept medical advice since she wants to do the best for her baby. She is likely to agree to a regime of slow drug withdrawal until complete abstinence is reached.

The baby should be unharmed but remains at risk. If drugs are freely available, relapse may be precipitated by stress and the demands made by a newborn baby.

The uncooperative addict

Such a patient is likely to be involved in buying and selling drugs and is not committed to renounce dependence. Her fetus is likely to be compromized.

Clinical features of drug dependence

There is no difficulty in diagnosis if the patient is referred from a drug dependence clinic. However, suspicion should be aroused when attendance at the antenatal clinic is poor, when injection marks are seen on the legs, arms, groin and even occasionally the neck, or when the patient presents with drug withdrawal symptoms. When experiencing withdrawal symptoms the patient may lie curled up on the couch complaining of:

> abdominal cramps
> photophobia
> anxiety
> sweating
> diarrhoea or vomiting
> lacrymation and rhinorrhoea.

Management

In early pregnancy psychiatric advice and referral to a drug dependence clinic will be required. The aim is abstinence while prescribing reducing doses of methadone. Emotional support for the patient during this period, and especially after abstinence has been achieved, is vital.

In late pregnancy even slow withdrawal of drugs may cause withdrawal symptoms in mother and fetus. The lowest dose of methadone which prevents this may have to be continued. Assessment of her true opiate needs is very difficult. Specialist advice is essential and hospital admission may be advisable to monitor withdrawal symptoms. Inpatient care also provides an opportunity of screening for other medical problems and to correct the addict's poor general state of health and nutrition.

Withdrawal symptoms in the newborn infant may occur up to several days after delivery; they include a shrill cry, irritability, tremors, respiratory distress and feeding difficulties. A paediatrician should be consulted to supervise the infant's therapy. In view of the possible late onset of symptoms, early discharge from hospital is not recommended. Social support and regular monitoring of the infant is essential.

Breast feeding is beneficial in theory but after discharge from hospital there is a real danger of return to uncontrolled drug-taking. For this reason breast feeding should be discouraged.

In the United Kingdom notification of an opiate-dependent person to the Medical Officer, Drugs' Branch, at the Home Office, Lombard Street, London SW1, is mandatory.

ALCOHOL ABUSE

Even small daily amounts of alcohol, such as one or two glasses of wine, may lead to physical harm. The unborn child is exposed to the hazard of growth retardation and increased perinatal mortality. Some may develop the fetal alcohol syndrome and other malformations if the mother is truly addicted. The fetal alcohol syndrome is manifest by mental retardation and a characteristic facies.

Management

This demands a sympathetic attitude, open discussion of the problem and energetic counselling to encourage the patient to accept the need for complete abstinence. Progress should be reviewed frequently. Blood alcohol levels and mean corpuscular volume estimations will help to monitor compliance with treatment.

SMOKING AND PREGNANCY

This habit is deleterious for the mother and her fetus and can be managed on similar lines to alcohol abuse. Babies born to mothers who smoke tend to be underweight and the perinatal mortality is increased.

SCHIZOPHRENIA IN PREGNANCY

Schizophrenia is a common psychiatric illness which affects almost 1 per cent of the general population; it is therefore occasionally encountered in pregnancy. The illness is characterized by disorders of perception (hallucinations) mood (anxiety, elation, depression) thinking (delusions) and behaviour. Treatment with phenothiazines is very effective and, provided maintenance therapy is continued, the patient is likely to remain mentally well throughout the pregnancy. However, relapse in the puerperium is common.

It is important to continue the patient's maintenance therapy, even in the first few weeks of pregnancy, and to liaise with the patient's psychiatrist. The mother-to-be needs extra support from her doctor, midwife and social worker as she may be slower than average to establish a useful relationship with clinic staff. For the same reason continuity of care is important. She will also need encouragement to socialize with other young mothers; her attendance at antenatal classes is therefore particularly important. It is helpful to establish early rapport with the patient's partner and to encourage a supportive, but not too intense an atmosphere at home.

MENTAL HANDICAP IN PREGNANCY

This condition is characterized by a deficiency of intellectual functioning. All degrees of handicap may be encountered.

Mental handicap in a stable environment

If her partner or parents are able to offer good support the patient may cope quite well. Verbal skills may be adequate and her problem may not be appreciated until it is found that she cannot read or answer questions which she does not understand. As a slow learner she will need additional help to manage her baby and she should not be allowed home until she can cope. The help of the health visitor or social worker should be sought.

Mental handicap in an unstable environment

This poses a much more difficult problem. If the woman's social competence is also low she is unlikely to cope with the demands of a newborn baby, whose safety is the most important consideration. In spite of the difficulties, some handicapped mothers desire to care for their baby although their social workers may consider this unrealistic. In such cases admission to a mother and baby home may be possible; there, professional staff are available to teach parenting skills and the mother's competence to look after the baby will be carefully assessed. For some, separation from the baby becomes inevitable, causing great distress. Support and counselling is vital while the infant's future is decided by the Social Services Department. Adoption or long-term fostering are the alternatives, to be avoided if possible.

VOMITING IN PREGNANCY

Vomiting during the first few weeks of pregnancy is a common event and only rarely a problem. The persistent vomiting of *hyperemesis gravidarum* is rare and poses a risk to the health of both mother and child. The pathogenesis is not clear. Psychological explanations of the condition are largely anecdotal and unhelpful. The change in the mental state occurs secondary to ketosis and to dehydration. Anyone who has been seasick can understand how these women feel (*see* p. 45).

A totally different picture is seen in *hysterical vomiting*. The patient is likely to complain of vomiting after every meal and of not being able to keep a drop of water down. However, she manages to look well physically and her weight is appropriate. Both the patient and her partner are convinced that there is a physical explanation for her symptoms. Psychological exploration may not succeed because of denial of underlying emotional conflict. It is important not to make this diagnosis unless secondary gain can be demonstrated. The differential diagnosis includes hyperemesis gravidarum, hydatidiform mole, red degeneration of a fibroid, increased intracranial pressure, an acute abdominal emergency or severe urinary infection.

DENIAL OF PREGNANCY

This represents a mental mechanism providing temporary escape from an unwanted pregnancy.

PSEUDOCYESIS

This is a rare disorder in childless women who desire children. Amenorrhoea and abdominal swelling may be present but the positive signs of pregnancy are absent.

INSOMNIA

This is a common symptom in pregnancy, especially in the last few weeks before delivery. A sleep deficit is easily built up and adds to the mother's difficulties in labour and in the early weeks of caring for her baby. The cause of sleeplessness may be difficult to find. It may help to ascertain the sleep pattern and to discuss any specific fears or anxieties. The use of bedboards, extra pillows or hot drinks may also be helpful. A short-acting benzodiazepine such as temazepan 10–20 mg at night may be needed for two to three weeks, although the long-term use of benzodiazepines should be avoided, as the danger of dependence is real.

PUERPERAL DISORDERS

Many mothers and most of their doctors know that psychiatric illness after childbirth is common. Postnatal depression and anxiety states are well known although the different types of depression are less well recognized. The current policy of very early discharge following delivery makes early diagnosis more difficult. However, the obstetrician is given a second opportunity to assess the mental health of his patient at the time of the postnatal examination or in the contraception clinic.

POSTNATAL DEPRESSION

Three main types of postnatal depression are recognized:

maternity blues (mild depression)
depression of intermediate severity:
  neurotic depression
  atypical depression
psychotic depression.

Maternity blues

A very common condition which affects 60–70 per cent of all newly confined women. It is characterized by tearfulness, insomnia, fatigue, fears, anxiety and despondency; some women complain that they cannot think straight. Mild depression starts on the third to fifth day after confinement, lasts for one to three days and resolves spontaneously. It responds quickly to explanation, reassurance and a night sedative for one or two nights.

Depression of intermediate severity

Neurotic depression

Neurotic depression is much more prolonged and occurs in women who have always found it hard to cope with stress. Pregnancy may trigger uncomfortable memories of childhood or raise doubts about femininity or of a woman's biological role. A past unsatisfactory relationship with her own mother or a poor rapport with her partner are precipitating factors. Having a baby is never a good recipe for cementing a marriage. A mother who normally finds life stressful is liable to experience even more severe difficulties after delivery when faced with the reality of motherhood.

The patient feels miserable and tearful and is unable to cope with her responsibilities; depression is often associated with anxiety. The mood disturbance is not constant as she can be cheered and she tends to feel worse towards the end of the day. Appetite is poor but overeating may be perceived as comforting. There is often difficulty in getting to sleep but, in spite of her exhaustion, she ruminates about her problems.

These women need practical help and support. Help should be enlisted from the health visitor and social worker. Psychotherapeutic intervention may be required.

Atypical depression

In contrast to neurotic depression, this type of depression occurs in previously competent and stable women. It is fairly common and may affect one in ten of recently confined women. The illness may vary in severity from mild to severe and is puzzling for the patient and her consort. The main complaint is not of depression but of an inability to cope with the baby and household. The onset is slow and insidious, unlike mild depression (*see* p. 126). Neither partner understand what is happening. A previously competent wife and mother complains that she is always tired and irritable and that everything seems too much of an effort. The anticipated happy experience of having a baby is spoilt. Anger, often overtly expressed, is common and may be directed against the partner, the doctor or even the baby. In spite of the young mother's exhaustion insomnia occurs, with night feeds exacerbating the problem. Even when the baby sleeps through the night, the mother's sleep pattern does not return to normal. Energy and drive are at a low ebb and she has little or no interest in herself, her baby or her family; loss of libido is invariably present. Feelings of guilt are a frequent feature, the young mother believes she is letting down her partner, her baby and her other children.

The clinical picture may vary considerably from day to day and this inconsistency adds to the partner's confusion. One day his wife may be smiling and happy but the next she is desperate and crying again. The house is in chaos; she may tell him that she is an utter failure and that suicide is her only way out. Self-destructive thoughts may be translated into action, especially in a relatively severe illness which has not been recognized.

Early diagnosis is important to prevent unnecessary suffering and to preserve the family equilibrium. The obstetrician may not make the diagnosis until the postnatal examination. Frequently the mother's distress has not even been noted by her doctor.

A simple question enquiring about how she feels may be quite sufficient to encourage the mother to report her difficulties. The doctor then has to explain that she is suffering from a well recognized illness. Ideally, the partner should be present and the couple interviewed together. Reassurance that this type of depression occurs in nearly 10 per cent of women can be very helpful and relieves guilt feelings.

A non-sedative antidepressant such as lofepramine 210 mg/day in divided doses or imipramine 75–150 mg/day is appropriate. The patient must understand that her medication should not be abandoned as soon as she feels better in two or three weeks time; antidepressants need to be continued for some months after complete symptomatic recovery. Relapse tends to occur if drugs are stopped too early or are withdrawn abruptly. A close watch should be kept on the patient's progress by her family doctor.

The mother who has expressed suicidal ideas needs admission to a psychiatric unit, preferably taking her baby with her.

Psychotic depression

Puerperal psychotic depression is the most severe form of postnatal illness and may be associated with other manifestations. The incidence is low, occurring in only one to two per thousand deliveries. The psychosis may present with symptoms of elation (mania), depression, schizophrenia or a mixture of these. The clinical features may vary from hour to hour. Little is gained by classifying puerperal psychoses.

Clinical features

The onset is usually very acute within the first week after delivery. Occasionally there is a delay of two to four weeks. Sleepless nights may precede morbid anxiety and a changing mental state. The woman's behaviour becomes unpredictable and rapid mood changes varying from depression to mania may be observed. Schizophrenic symptoms such as paranoid ideas, hallucinations and delusions may be present. Confusion and disorientation are common, giving the illness an organic flavour in the absence of organic disease. The patient's thought content may reveal preoccupation with the baby although lack of interest is also sometimes noted. Less frequently the mother reveals open hostility to the infant or perhaps expresses the belief that the baby is not her own. Suicidal thoughts may be prominent, especially if a depressive mood is associated with a delusional guilt. The distressed mother may even plan to kill the baby (infanticide) prior to taking her own life. When asked, she will usually reveal these plans. A suicidal mother must never be left alone.

A seriously disturbed mother in an obstetric unit tends to upset other patients and alarm staff. This can be prevented if a psychiatric opinion is arranged as soon as the premonitory signs of insomnia and morbid anxiety are noted. Most patients will require admission to a psychiatric unit and, if possible, the baby should accompany her so that close contact between the patient and her baby can be maintained. With the effective yet discreet supervision available in this type of unit, even disturbed mothers can play an active role in caring for their infants. The fostering of mothering skills and indeed of parenting skills is of prime importance and the partner is encouraged to spend as much time as possible with mother and baby. As the patient improves and gains confidence she gradually takes over the complete care of her baby. Together they may leave hospital for increasing periods of time. A successful weekend at home is a good guide to progress.

Sometimes improvement is associated with the emergence of new symptoms, feelings of guilt, anger or inadequacy and unless the mother has an opportunity to discuss these problems her recovery may be delayed. The partner's attitude is an important factor in her recovery; if he feels angry or resentful because his life has been disrupted by her illness he is less likely to be supportive.

Chlorpromazine is used to control irrational behaviour, hallucinations and delusions. Tricyclic antidepressants alone or in combination with chlorpromazine are given when a depressive mood dominates the clinical picture. Elation or hypomania may respond to chlorpromazine, haloperidol or lithium carbonate.

CHRONIC FATIGUE

Many mothers complain of feeling constantly exhausted in the first few months after delivery. If organic causes, e.g. anaemia, can be ruled out then the baby is usually responsible for this state of affairs. Many babies cry excessively, even when all has been done to make them comfortable. Others demand frequent night feeds, depriving their mothers of an adequate period of uninterrupted sleep.

Chronic fatigue leads to irritability so that enjoyment of the infant is impaired. Occasionally baby battering occurs in this setting, when the mother feels trapped and there is no relief in sight. A review of the mother's daily activity and the baby's feeding regime will usually confirm the diagnosis. It is important to distinguish chronic fatigue from atypical depression (*see* p. 127). The mother will need practical help to let her catch up on her sleep deficit. Her partner, family or friends can often provide relief but regular domestic help may be indicated. If no improvement occurs she should be referred for psychiatric assessment.

LOSS OF LIBIDO

This is common after childbirth as an isolated symptom. The couple can be reassured that although loss of libido can be quite prolonged, return to normal is the usual outcome. The aetiology is not clear. Perineal discomfort, ignorance regarding an episiotomy and fear of conception may all play a part.

NEUROTIC DISORDERS

Anxiety states, phobic states or obsessional illness may all occur in the puerperium. Preoccupation with the infant may colour the symptomatology. The treatment for neurotic conditions after delivery is the same as in pregnancy (*see* p. 123).

THE PREVENTION OF POSTNATAL PSYCHIATRIC ILLNESS

There is no proof that prevention is possible but the woman at risk needs extra care during pregnancy and the puerperium. This will encourage early diagnosis of her problems and enable prompt treatment before the family equilibrium is disturbed.

The following factors make postnatal psychiatric illness more likely:

psychiatric illness following previous childbirth
the history of a non-puerperal depressive illness
a strong family history of depression
a history of lack of support by the woman's partner or family
a history of marital stress
isolation, which may be cultural, or due to a recent house move
recent loss of a parent or other distressing event.

It is of great advantage if the antenatal patient can be seen by the same doctor, obstetrician or midwife at each attendance. Advice can then be given on:

good parenting
restricting unimportant tasks and planning tasks
avoiding house moving just before or after delivery
additional rest
organizing domestic help and on planning domestic chores
priorities in housework (e.g. clean curtains are less important than baby care and feeding the family)
vitamin B6, 100 mg per day orally for one month prior to delivery and continued for a further month, may stop postnatal depression developing. It has the advantage that both patient and doctor feel they are taking a positive step towards prevention
progesterone by intramuscular injection daily for one week followed by a Cyclogest suppository 400 mg two to three times daily for several weeks is prescribed by some clinicians. However, the evidence for low progesterone levels is lacking. It is suggested that some patients are sensitive to the normal fall of progesterone after delivery.

STILLBIRTH AND NEONATAL DEATH

Death *in utero* during labour or loss of a newborn are devastating experiences for the mother. The labour ward staff are also affected. The mother should not be nursed in the postnatal ward; alternative accommodation should be found and early discharge, where appropriate, is ideal. Both parents should be seen together and be given all the available information to explain their loss. Careful timing of this interview is important. Most parents wish to have a while alone with their baby; holding it in their arms, they can establish an identity with the infant, whom they can name and mourn. A photograph taken at this time may be treasured at a later stage.

The parents will always want to know why and how it happened. This can lead naturally to the need for a post-mortem examination. The more they understand, the less guilty they will feel.

Practical help includes advice on hospital burial arrangements and on registering the death. Many units are able to offer a religious service in the Chapel and have a Book of Remembrance.

On discharge, the parents should be warned that the mourning process will take months. Explaining the death to older children, family, friends and colleagues at work is a daunting experience; practical guidance is much appreciated.

It is important to emphasize the supportive role of the general practitioner. The lost baby cannot be replaced by a new pregnancy. It may take three to six months of adjustment before the parents are ready to plan an addition to their family.

Bereaved parents may wish to ask many questions over the next few weeks. An early appointment should be made prior to discharge to give them this opportunity. An unhurried interview, perhaps arranged in the gynaecological clinic, may be appropriate. Full notes, the post-mortem report and results of all investigations must be available to make the consultation meaningful for both parents and doctor.

THE FETUS AT RISK IN LATE PREGNANCY

During pregnancy and labour the fetus may be at risk of damage or death from many causes.

However it has become the custom to talk of the fetus at risk in the more limited sense of at risk from acute or chronic placental insufficiency. Acute placental failure may result from placental separation by haemorrhage (abruptio placentae) or it may come at the end of a phase of gradually declining placental efficiency. In the latter case acute failure may only become manifest during labour when the uterine contractions interfere with blood flow. This failure is commonly called fetal distress. It is discussed in Chapter 5, page 216.

The importance of acute hypoxia, which may cause sudden fetal death during labour, has been appreciated for a long time, but recognition of the long-term damage which may result from chronic intrauterine malnutrition and lead to the birth of a small-for-dates baby is more recent.

PLACENTAL INSUFFICIENCY DURING PREGNANCY

During pregnancy the fetus depends on the placenta and the umbilical vessels for transport of oxygen and nutrients from the maternal blood, and for excretion of carbon dioxide and the products of metabolism. Because of the constancy of the mother's internal environment the composition of the blood reaching the placenta is unlikely to vary much except in desperate conditions of maternal circulatory failure or asphyxia, or in cases of gross metabolic disturbance such as severe diabetes or renal disease. Even if the maternal nutrition is poor the maternal blood will show little alteration, and this explains the fact that a normal sized child may be born in such circumstances, and that the fetus of a mother with poor iron reserves is not anaemic as long as her serum iron concentration is maintained. Fetal ill-health therefore seldom arises because of alteration in the biochemical quality of the maternal blood – the ability of the placenta to act as an organ of transfer is the important consideration.

Restriction of the maternal blood flow through the placenta can have a serious effect upon fetal growth and development. Placental tissue may be lost by infarction or the separation from the uterine wall that occurs when abortion threatens or when there is a small retroplacental haemorrhage. Spasm or thrombosis of small decidual vessels may also have the same effect. In a few patients who give birth to babies who have obviously suffered from chronic placental insuf-

ficiency the placenta is small for no apparent reason.

If pregnancy is prolonged beyond term the placenta sometimes becomes inadequate for the needs of the large, still growing fetus. Significant structural changes in the placenta are seldom found in such cases. There may be calcification of the decidual plate, but the intervillous circulation is not impaired by this. Although intrauterine death before the onset of labour is rare in cases of postmaturity, fetal distress may occur during labour.

Intrauterine death may occur in cases of diabetes but the cause of this is uncertain. The fetus is often very large, but so is the placenta, and placental failure is not an adequate explanation.

In cases of haemolytic disease the placenta is large and oedematous, with persistence of Langhans' layer of cytotrophoblast in the villi, but the fetus probably dies from cardiac failure caused by the severe haemolytic anaemia rather than from placental insufficiency.

TESTS OF PLACENTAL FUNCTION

There is much still to be discovered about placental function, but the practical need for the obstetrician is to obtain some warning of placental insufficiency so that the fetus at risk of intrauterine death may be delivered before this occurs. Conversely, such a test might be reassuring and prevent the unnecessary hazard of premature delivery. Unfortunately there is no absolutely reliable test for placental function. Clinical judgment must still be used. Indeed clinical assessment of the patient is usually the basis for requesting the more sophisticated physical or biochemical tests of function.

Three important clinical indicators of placental function are the pattern of maternal weight gain, and the growth of the uterus and fetus.

The maternal weight

This should normally increase by about 0.5 kg weekly after the first trimester, provided that the patient is not dieting or vomiting and has no other disorder causing malnutrition. The components of this weight gain include the fetus, placenta, liquor, uterus, breasts and the fat store. In addition there is the increase in blood volume and extracellular fluid. These very diverse components are all dependent directly on placental function, or indirectly on it by way of the hormones it produces. Thus failure to gain weight adequately should be regarded as an indication to carry out some other placental function tests.

Uterine growth

This is not always easy to assess and the variation between observations may be considerable. Nevertheless simple measurements of the height of the fundus above the symphysis pubis have more to recommend them than the common practice of assessing fundal height in relation to the umbilicus or xiphisternum. The fundal height should increase by about 1 cm weekly from the 16th week of pregnancy, and with an average sized fetus should equal the number of weeks of gestation plus or minus 2 cm. Measurements of abdominal girth are much less satisfactory indicators of uterine growth. In the case of both measurements the variability is lessened appreciably if the same person sees the patient at each antenatal visit. If the uterus seems to be growing slowly this is another reason to perform other placental function tests.

Fetal growth

The most reliable measurements of the fetus are obtained with ultrasound. Serial measurements of the biparietal diameter of the fetal head are comparatively easy to obtain. It should be remembered that the head of the fetus is a privileged area in so far as the greatest part of the cardiac output with the most highly oxygenated blood is diverted there. It is therefore the last part of the fetus to suffer from malnutrition. If earlier signs of poor growth are to be sought it is better to measure the abdominal circumference at the level of the liver and to relate this to the size of the head. This technique calls for more sophisticated apparatus and expertise on the part of the operator.

Fetal activity

The most important indicator of placental function is the well-being of the fetus. A valuable sign of a healthy fetus is vigorous activity. The mother may be able to give some indication of this by keeping a 'kick count'. She can be asked to note how frequently the baby moves in a given period, perhaps 30 minutes. Alternatively she can be asked to note how long it takes for the baby to move ten times.

A more sophisticated way of assessing fetal activity is to produce a continuous record of the fetal heart rate over a period of 30 minutes or more. This is done with a cardiotocograph and is often called a non-stress test. A change in rate with fetal activity and variability of the rate from beat to beat are associated with fetal health. The heart rate may change with a uterine contraction but the normal rate is restored as soon as the contraction passes off.

A still more elaborate method of fetal assessment is the biophysical profile. This is a score based on real-time ultrasound observations of fetal breathing and body movements, tone, quantity of amniotic fluid, and on a non-stress test. Lack of movements and amniotic fluid suggest the fetus is in danger of hypoxia, but inactivity in the fetus may also be physiological. Prolonged observation over more than 30 minutes may be necessary and even then there is a high false-positive rate. This test has therefore not been widely adopted in the UK.

Doppler studies

The reflection of ultrasound waves from the wave produced by the pulse of blood moving along a blood vessel can be detected and compared with the energy output of the source. This provides a measure of the speed of passage of the pulse wave. If the vessel diameter is measureable then the flow of the volume of blood per minute may be calculated. As this is of poor reproducibility the shape of the Doppler wave form, which should show forward flow during diastole as well as systole, is analysed. High diastolic flow indicates low resistance and impaired diastolic flow indicates high down-stream resistance. This is the basis of Doppler blood flow studies of the arcuate arteries in the placental bed and the umbilical arteries in the cord. The former is a reflection of the afferent supply of oxygen and nutrients from the mother to the fetus; the latter is a measure of fetal well-being which is still being evaluated.

Placental function tests

Attempts have been made to judge the functional activity of the placenta by measuring one or more of its hormone or enzyme products in maternal blood or urine. Blood levels of oestrogens and progesterone vary with placental function, but diurnal variations and variations due to activity and posture are so great that they are unreliable indicators of fetal well-being. The excretion of oestrogens (particularly oestriol, *see* p. 12) in the maternal urine during a 24-hour period gives a more consistent indication of placental function. The normal range of values for excretion is considerable, and isolated observations are of little value, but repeated observations may show an obvious trend.

Other tests which are less frequently employed include serum levels of placental lactogen (hPL) and of heat-stable alkaline phosphatase.

POSTMATURITY

Postmaturity means the prolongation of pregnancy beyond its normal duration. It is important because surveys of perinatal deaths have shown that the risk of intrauterine death increases, particularly in pregnancies continuing more than two weeks beyond term. However, there is no agreement on the normal limits of duration of pregnancy. The difficulty in making any definition is that the precise date of conception in any particular pregnancy is unknown, and even with regular menstrual cycles of normal length the date of ovulation is only approximately known. In women with irregular or prolonged cycles calculations based on the date of the last menstrual period are bound to be inaccurate.

Apart from the uncertainty about the date of ovulation, it is improbable that all fetuses will mature in precisely the same number of days. The cause of the onset of labour at term is uncertain (p. 151).

Diagnosis

General statistical statements based on large numbers of cases can easily be made, showing that delivery takes place over two weeks after the expected date of delivery in more than 10 per cent of cases (*see* Fig. 2.2, p. 38) but in any particular pregnancy the diagnosis of postmaturity is often uncertain.

In cases in which the date of the last menstrual period is absolutely certain, and in which the previous menstrual cycles were of normal length, the diagnosis of maturity can reasonably be based on this. If the menstrual history is uncertain an attempt can be made to assess maturity by scrutiny of the antenatal records to discover whether the size of the uterus was determined by bimanual examination at an early visit by an experienced obstetrician. Between the 8th and the 14th weeks an accurate assessment of the uterine size can generally be made. Ultrasound measurements of the crown–rump length of the fetus up to about the 14th week and of the biparietal diameter of the fetal head up to about the 28th week, give a reliable indication of the duration of gestation. The date at which the mother first felt fetal movements may be of interest, but as this can range from 16 to 22 weeks, depending on her previous obstetric experience and her obesity, this is hardly reliable enough evidence on which to base any important decision.

Other tests for the assessment of maturity, including radiological examination of fetal ossific centres and chemical and cytological examination of liquor amnii, have now been superseded by ultrasound observations (*see* p. 57).

Clinical significance

The delayed onset of labour might in theory have two disadvantages:

after term, as the uterine blood flow diminishes and degenerative changes progress, the placental function may become inadequate for a large fetus that is still growing

there may be mechanical difficulties during labour because of the increased size of the fetus, and perhaps a uterus which is slow to begin labour may also prove to be inefficient during labour.

The risk of the fetus dying in the uterus from hypoxia before the onset of labour has probably been exaggerated, although this does occasionally occur. However, there is good evidence that the risk of fetal distress and fetal death during labour is greater in postmature than in normal cases. In part this is due to more difficult labour because of the larger size of the fetus and incoordinate uterine action, and in part to the more frequent occurrence of oligohydramnios. The skull of the postmature fetus is more ossified, so that moulding is less easy. A particular hazard for the neonate is meconium aspiration.

The risk of hypoxia in postmature cases is increased if there is also hypertension, and perhaps in the case of an elderly primigravida.

Medico-legal significance

Postmaturity may be of medico-legal importance, as a husband may question the paternity of a child born more than 44 weeks after he left his wife. In law each case is decided on the evidence and there is no legal definition or set upper limit for the normal duration of pregnancy. In one astonishing decision a child born 346 days after the last cohabitation was judged to be legitimate, but in another case a child born after 360 days was adjudged illegitimate on appeal.

Management

Postmaturity is often a cause of worry, and sometimes of expense and inconvenience, to the mother. Pressure is often put upon the obstetrician to induce labour. While this is often justifiable in cases in which the menstrual history is certain, in other cases there is a risk that the fetus may, after induction, prove to be premature rather than postmature. The clinical evidence must be carefully reviewed before deciding to induce labour. Uncertainty over gestational age is eliminated by early ultrasound dating and is a very strong argument in favour of routine scanning of all pregnant women in the second trimester.

Since many women and their relatives tend to worry when the date given to them as the expected date of delivery has been passed, it is most desirable that every mother should be told that the calculated date is only an approximation, and that normal labour may start up to two weeks later.

Each case of suspected postmaturity should be dealt with according to its special circumstances. There is no justification for making a rule that all cases must be induced at some stated week of pregnancy; the risks of indiscriminate induction might well exceed those of postmaturity. There will be more anxiety in the case of older primigravidae, or patients with hypertension. Induction might well be recommended if the fetus is evidently large, and for patients in whom there is a risk of disproportion if the fetus continues to grow. There can be little justification for induction until the woman is at least two weeks overdue except in cases with hypertension or some other reason to suspect placental insufficiency.

Labour may be induced in cases of postmaturity by insertion of vaginal prostaglandin pessaries (p. 275). If labour does not quickly follow, amniotomy is performed. When the fetal head is well down in the pelvic cavity and the cervix is soft and taken up, labour follows induction without delay. Very careful monitoring of the progress of the labour and of the condition of the fetus are required. Particular attention is paid to whether or not amniotic fluid is draining, and to thick meconium. If there is evidence of fetal hypoxia during the first stage of labour, preferably confirmed by examination of a sample of fetal blood obtained by scalp puncture, caesarean section may be necessary. In the second stage clinical signs of fetal distress call for forceps delivery without delay.

INTRAUTERINE DEATH OF THE FETUS

In addition to cases in which the fetus dies during delivery as a result of asphyxia or difficult labour, others are seen in which it dies *in utero* before labour starts. This is usually followed by expulsion of the fetus from the uterus within a few days. However, in exceptional cases the dead fetus is not expelled from the uterus at once, but is retained for several weeks.

Causes

In some cases the cause of death is obvious; but in others it is obscure because autolysis of the tissues of the fetus and placenta occurs, and as a result postmortem findings are difficult to interpret. The causes of intrauterine fetal death may be classified under the following headings:

Pregnancy-induced hypertension, essential hypertension and chronic renal disease

Fetal hypoxia is produced by reduction in the maternal blood supply to the placenta because of spasm, and sometimes thrombosis, of the maternal vessels. Added to this there may be separation of the placenta (abruptio placentae) or extensive clotting of maternal blood around the chorionic villi.

Diabetes mellitus

If maternal diabetes is poorly controlled fetal death *in utero* often occurs.

Postmaturity

This is an uncommon cause of fetal death before labour (*see above*).

Abruptio placentae

Cord accidents

True knots in the cord or constriction of the cord round a limb are very rare causes of fetal death.

Haemolytic disease

In such instances the fetus is usually hydropic.

Unexplained placental insufficiency

Apart from the cases of hypertension and renal disease already mentioned, in a few patients unexplained placental insufficiency occurs in successive pregnancies. Further investigation may reveal anticardiolipin antibodies in maternal blood. The fetus does not grow at the normal rate and intrauterine death may occur. The placenta is found to be small but appears to be normal in other respects. In the absence of any explanation for some of these cases, the only advice which can be offered is intensive fetal monitoring and rest in bed during most of the pregnancy, with the hope that this will increase the uterine blood flow. Delivery before the time at which previous deaths occurred is wise, either by induction of labour or caesarean section. Tests of fetal well-being may give some guidance in deciding when to advise delivery.

Fetal malformation

With gross malformation intrauterine death sometimes occurs.

Infective diseases

Any disease that causes high fever and toxic illness may cause fetal death.

Untreated syphilis and rare fetal infection with herpes virus or other viruses may cause death. Severe rubella is sometimes fatal to the fetus.

Pathological anatomy

The fetus is usually born in a macerated condition.

Its skin is peeling and stained reddish-brown by absorption of blood pigments. The whole body is softened and toneless; the cranial bones are loosened and easily moveable on one another. The liquor amnii and the fluid in all the serous cavities contain blood pigments. Maceration occurs rapidly, and may be advanced within 24 hours of fetal death. Necropsy, although frequently unrewarding, is advised in all cases.

Symptoms and diagnosis

The woman may notice that the fetal movements have not been present for several days, and the breasts may diminish in size. In cases of hypertension the blood pressure sometimes falls. The following signs may be found:

After the 24th week the fetal heart sounds can normally be heard with a stethoscope; failure to hear them on careful auscultation will be strong presumptive evidence of fetal death. Ultrasound apparatus can detect the fetal heart beat as early as the eighth week of pregnancy, and if a careful and repeated search shows no evidence of cardiac activity, fetal death is almost certain.

The uterus may be found to be smaller than the duration of pregnancy would warrant. A more accurate sign is to note how much alteration takes place in the size of the uterus during a period of observation. For this the bladder must be empty and the level of the fundus accurately noted. The patient is examined week by week. If no uterine enlargement is observed in four weeks this strongly suggests that the fetus is dead. In some cases the uterus not only ceases to grow but gets smaller because of absorption of the liquor amnii.

Sometimes secretion of colostrum from the breasts occurs a few days after the death of the fetus.

Ultrasonic examination or a radiograph will show overlapping and disalignment of the skull bones (Spalding's sign (Fig. 3.9)) and occasionally the presence of gas in the fetal heart and great vessels (Roberts' sign). Spalding's sign is not usually present until a week after fetal death, but gas formation may be seen after only two days. Immunological tests for pregnancy are usually negative within a week after the death of the fetus, but sometimes a weakly positive test persists for a time, presumably because some chorionic tissue is still active. The excretion of oestriol in the mother's urine falls sharply.

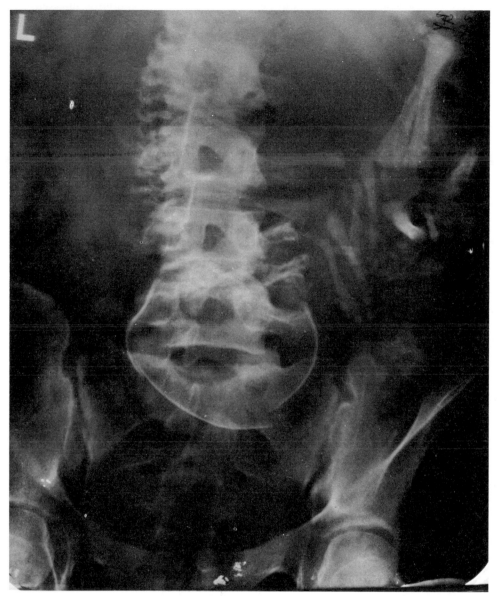

Fig. 3.9 Intrauterine death of a fetus. Spalding's sign is present. There is marked overlapping of the vault of the skull

It will be seen that fetal death is difficult to diagnose from a single clinical examination of the patient, and urgent sonography is usually requested. Very little importance should be attached to the patient's statements about fetal movements; false hope will lead to confusion of intestinal with fetal movement.

Management

In the majority of cases labour soon follows death of the fetus, but sometimes labour does not occur for several weeks. In these cases there is no urgent call for interference, unless the complications of hypofibrinogenaemia and DIC occur (p. 266). If the patient becomes greatly distressed when she knows that the fetus is dead the labour can be induced, but amniotomy is unwise because of the risk of anaerobic uterine infection from growth of bacteria in the dead placental and fetal tissues if labour does not follow quickly.

Labour may be induced with vaginal prostaglandin pessaries or gel or extraamniotic injections of prostaglandins (*see* p. 275). It is also possible to induce labour by the intra-amniotic injection of prostaglandins and a hypertonic solution of urea (p. 276). Such patients should have follow-up, bereavement counselling and, where appropriate, genetic counselling.

MULTIPLE PREGNANCY

In Caucasian women twin conceptions occur spontaneously about once in 90 pregnancies, triplets about once in 10000 and quadruplets about once in 500000. The spontaneous occurrence of the higher multiples up to octuplets has been reliably recorded.

The spontaneous incidence of twins is greater in the Negro race, reaching 1 in 30 in some West African tribes, and lower in the Mongol race (1 in 150). A tendency to multiple pregnancy is inherited, and it occurs more frequently in certain families. A woman who has given birth to twins is said to be 10 times more likely to have a multiple conception in a subsequent pregnancy than a woman who has not previously had twins.

The incidence of twin pregnancies rises slightly with increasing maternal age up to 40, and (independently) with increasing parity. All these factors of race, familial tendency, parity and age affect binovular rather than uniovular twins.

Multiple pregnancies have frequently occurred after induction of ovulation, including septuplet and octuplet pregnancies. The risk is slight with clomiphene but considerable with ovarian stimulation with gonadotrophins. These patients must be monitored carefully by measuring the oestrogen response and by scanning the ovaries with ultrasound. An injection of hCG to release the oöcytes is only given when it is certain that there are only one or two ripe follicles. Multiple pregnancy may also follow assisted conception when multiple oöcytes or fertilized ova are replaced.

In spontaneous multiple pregnancies the normal sex ratio at birth, with a slight preponderance of males, is altered to a female preponderance.

Varieties of twins

Twins may be binovular or uniovular (Fig. 3.10).

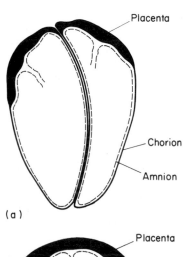

(a)

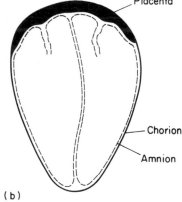

(b)

Fig. 3.10 The arrangement of the placentae and membranes in twin pregnancy. (a) probably binovular twins. The placentae are separated and each fetus has its own amnion and chorion. (b) probably uniovular twins. Each fetus has its own amnion, but the chorions are fused and the placentae are anastomosed. (Depending on the race, there is an 80–94% chance that these twins are binovular)

Binovular twins

Binovular twins are developed from two separate ova which may or may not come from the same ovary. This variety of twins is three times more common than the uniovular variety. The children may be of the same or of different sex, and are not more alike than is usual with members of the same family. As they are developed from separate ova and separate spermatozoa their genetic material will differ. They have separate and distinct placentae. Sometimes these are loosely joined at their margins but there is never any anastomosis between their blood vessels. Each fetus has its own amnion and chorion.

Uniovular twins

Uniovular twins are developed from a single ovum which, after fertilization, has undergone division to form two embryos. Division may occur in the early stage of segmentation, or later when two germinal areas are formed in one blastodermic vesicle. Uniovular twins are always of the same sex and are often remarkably alike in their physical and mental characters. The arrangement of genes in the chromosomes is identical, and inherited characteristics such as blood groups are necessarily the same. Uniovular twins which arise from very early division each have a complete set of membranes (chorion and amnion); those which arise by later division have only one chorion but usually have separate amniotic sacs.

Monoamniotic twins are rare; this type is associated with a higher fetal loss from cord entanglement. The umbilical cords are usually separate, but the fetal circulations often communicate by anastomoses in the placentae. This communication may cause unequal development of the fetuses, and occasionally death of one fetus. If one fetus perishes early in pregnancy it is retained until term, when the small fetus is discovered compressed flat on the membranes (*fetus papyraceous*).

When the process of division of a single germinal area is incomplete some form of *conjoined twins* may occur. Many varieties have been described; they may be joined by the sternum, the pelvis or the head, and the degree of union varies from fusion of skin and soft tissues to formation of a double monster in which head, trunk, viscera or limbs may be shared or duplicated.

Diagnosis of twins

With twins all the early symptoms of pregnancy such as morning sickness may be more pronounced, and pregnancy-induced hypertension is common. If the patient has already borne children she may notice an unusual degree of abdominal enlargement and excessive fetal movements. In late pregnancy she may have discomfort and shortness of breath because of the large size of the uterus. The patient is more likely to become anaemic. Apart from the fact that there is a greater increase in plasma volume than in a single pregnancy, there is a double fetal demand for iron. As well as iron-deficiency anaemia, megaloblastic anaemia is more common with twins. It is important to ensure that the patient has an adequate diet and supplements of iron and folic acid. Oedema of the legs is common and any tendency to haemorrhoids or varicose veins of the legs is accentuated.

On examination the uterus is found to be larger than expected from the duration of gestation. Polyhydramnios may occur with twins, adding to the size and confusing the diagnosis. The diagnosis is simple if two fetal heads can be felt. Both backs and both breeches may be identified, and an unusual number of small parts. The diagnosis is more certain if fetal heart sounds are heard in two separate areas, and sometimes the rates will differ. If heart movements are detected with the ultrasound apparatus in two separate areas or directions the diagnosis of twins is almost certain.

By ultrasound scan in early pregnancy two separate gestation sacs can be identified from about the seventh week or sooner. From about the 12th week separate fetal bodies can be detected and from about the 14th week two heads can be distinguished. If routine scanning of all women is carried out at 16 weeks twins should rarely be missed.

If antenatal supervision is poor the diagnosis of twins is sometimes missed until after the birth of the first twin. The high position of the fundus, abdominal palpation of the second fetus and discovery of a second bag of membranes and fetal parts on vaginal examination will make the diagnosis clear. The risk to the mother and to the fetuses is increased because of the following complications:

Complications of pregnancy

Preterm labour

This is the most important factor in causing the increased perinatal mortality, which may reach 15 per cent. Not only may labour begin before term, but the rate of growth of a twin after the 28th week is slower than that of a single fetus. The reduced rate of growth begins when the total weight of the twins is in the region of 3500 g. The median duration of non-induced twin pregnancy is 37 weeks. About 20 per cent of twin pregnancies do not reach the 36th week.

Pregnancy-induced hypertension

Pregnancy-induced hypertension, including eclampsia, occurs at least three times more frequently than in single pregnancies, and this increases both the maternal and fetal risk.

Anaemia

Because of the increased fetal demand for iron and folic acid maternal anaemia is common in twin pregnancies unless adequate dietary supplements are given.

Polyhydramnios

There will obviously be more fluid in two sacs, but over and above this one sac may contain an abnormally large amount of fluid.

Congenital malformations

Congenital malformations occur about twice as often in twin than in singleton pregnancies.

Complications of labour

Malpresentations

Malpresentations are common with twins. In about 45 per cent of cases both twins present by the head (Fig. 3.11); in about 35 per cent one fetus presents by the head and the other by the breech (Fig. 3.12); in about 10 per cent both present by the breech and in about 10 per cent a transverse lie is associated with a cephalic presentation or a breech. It is very rare for both fetuses to lie

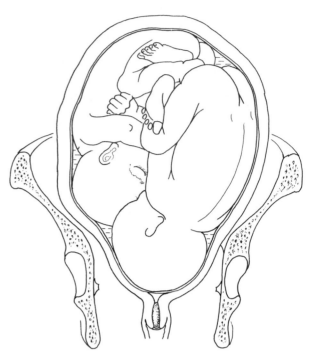

Fig. 3.11   Twin pregnancy. Both presenting by the vertex. Fetuses lying alongside one another. Both heads could probably be felt, one at the brim and the other above it in the iliac fossa. One back and an unusual number of small fetal parts would be recognized and possibly two breeches in the fundus

transversely. Malpresentations increase both the maternal and the fetal risk.

Postpartum haemorrhage

The risk of haemorrhage after delivery is increased because of the large size of the placental site. In the past a general anaesthetic was frequently given to deal with complications of labour and this caused uterine relaxation; with epidural anaesthesia this risk is reduced. If the mother is anaemic at the start of labour any acute blood loss may be serious.

Contrary to earlier teaching, the overdistended uterus usually contracts well during labour, and the duration of labour is not increased.

Cord prolapse

This may occur in association with malpresentation, especially with the second twin at the time when its membranes rupture.

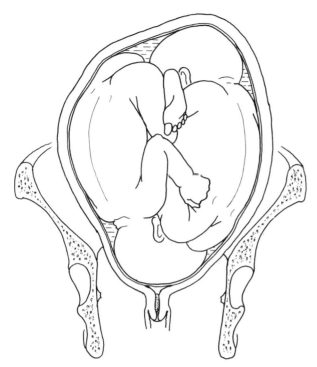

Fig. 3.12 Twin pregnancy. First presenting by the vertex, second by the breech. Fetuses lying alongside one another. This offers the easiest diagnosis; one head would be felt at the brim and one at the fundus; two backs with the small parts in the groove between would be palpable and two poins of maximal intensity of fetal heart sounds would be made out, one on the right and below the umbilicus and the other on the left and above

Locked twins

This very rare complication may prevent spontaneous delivery (*see* p. 140).

Community fetal circulations

On rare occasions the circulation of twins may communicate by anastomoses in the placenta. This may give rise to unequal growth or death of one of both fetuses in pregnancy or in labour.

Management of twin pregnancy

The antenatal care of a patient with a twin pregnancy should be intensified so that the complications listed above can be detected early. The patient is seen more often than usual from midpregnancy onwards. It is important that she should

have adequate rest. The practice of admitting patients with twins to hospital from the 30th to the 35th week is now less common, but it may be advisable if the home conditions are poor. It is by no means certain that rest will prevent premature labour, but it may increase the placental blood flow and so improve fetal growth. There is no convincing evidence that the prophylactic use of tocolytic drugs or cervical suture will reduce the incidence of preterm labour in twin pregnancy. In addition many patients are uncomfortable when carrying twins and need more rest on that account.

Some obstetricians recommend that labour should be induced at the 38th week to avoid the theoretical risk of placental insufficiency, but there is little evidence of any advantage in this. Induction may, however, be indicated for hypertension or growth retardation of one or both fetuses.

Management of twin labour

All preparations should have been made for the resuscitation and special care of babies of low birth weight. Because this can only be effectively done in hospital, and because other complications of labour may occur, all cases of twin labour should be in hospital units.

The first stage

The first stage of labour is managed in the ordinary way; labour is not often prolonged. Epidural analgesia is very suitable for these cases and an intravenous glucose drip should also be set up. The former will allow any necessary operative intervention without delay and the latter will permit an oxytocic infusion to be started at any time. Because of the changing relationships of the fetuses it may be difficult to hear both fetal hearts, but an effort must be made to locate them. Provided that one can be heard at a normal rate no interference should be contemplated for fetal distress, but caesarean section might be performed for prolonged delay in the first stage which did not respond to a careful trial of oxytocin and, rarely, in cases in which both twins were lying transversely or the twins were conjoined.

The second stage

The second stage is also managed in the usual way unless some complication arises. As in other cases the indications for delivery with the forceps or vacuum extractor, or for breech extraction, are undue delay, fetal distress or maternal distress. Unless the perineum is very lax an episiotomy should be performed routinely for the protection of a small baby's head, under local anaesthesia if an epidural injection has not been given.

It is after the birth of the first twin that any problems usually arise, and it is the second twin who is mainly at risk. It may have to be delivered without delay and an anaesthetist must be ready in the labour ward during all twin deliveries. The advantages of epidural analgesia have already been pointed out. A doctor who is able to carry out fetal resuscitation should be available in addition to the obstetrician conducting the delivery.

Usually both twins are delivered before the placentae, but rarely with binovular twins the placenta of the first twin will come away before delivery of the second fetus.

Immediately after the delivery of the first twin the abdomen is palpated to determine the lie of the second fetus. If it is oblique or transverse external version is performed to bring one pole of the fetus over the cervix. It does not matter if this is the breech or the head; if extraction of the second twin should become necessary this is often easier by bringing down the legs of a breech than by application of forceps or the vacuum extractor to a very high head.

The fetal heart rate is monitored continuously, preferably by ultrasound, for if the fetus is distressed immediate delivery is required. Distress may occur because the volume of the uterine cavity is reduced after delivery of the first twin, and there may be separation of the placenta on which the second twin depends. It may also be caused by prolapse of the cord, and a vaginal examination to exclude this should always be performed when the second sac of membranes ruptures.

Uterine contractions are often in abeyance for a few minutes after delivery of the first twin. When they start again delivery of the second twin is usually rapid as the birth canal has already been fully dilated. Delivery is conducted in the ordinary way, whether the head or the breech comes first.

If the uterine contractions do not return within about 5 minutes after the delivery of the first twin, Syntocinon (2 units in 500 ml) is added to the glucose solution in the intravenous drip (which should already be in place) and the second sac of membranes is ruptured. In the past it was custom-ary to wait some time before rupturing the second sac, unless fetal distress occurred. During this interval the cervix sometimes partly closed down, and experience has proved that fewer babies are lost after immediate rupture of the membranes of the second sac, which is usually followed by rapid delivery of the second twin.

If the second twin shows signs of distress or its cord prolapses it must be delivered reasonably quickly. The head may be found presenting but lying high above the pelvic brim, and application of forceps at that level can be difficult. If forceps delivery is attempted the head should be pressed down as far as possible by abdominal pressure from an assistant, or vacuum extraction may be performed. Internal version and breech extraction is another possibility which should seldom be necessary, but if the breech already presents it is comparatively easy to bring down a leg (or both legs) and extract the baby.

Locked twins

This is a very rare complication of twin delivery. If there is unexplained delay in the second stage or difficulty in extracting a first breech it should be considered, and the possibility of conjoined twins should not be forgotten. The diagnosis is made by examination under anaesthesia. General anaesthesia will be necessary if an epidural injection has not already been given.

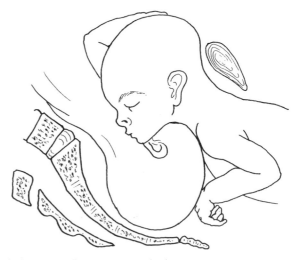

Fig. 3.13 Aftercoming head of the first twin locked with the forthcoming head of the second twin

Locking may occur when the first twin presents as a breech and the second as a vertex. The aftercoming head of the first twin is caught above the chin of the second twin (Fig. 3.13) and if disengagement is not quickly achieved the first twin dies. Caesarean section and delivery of the second twin from above is probably the easiest course, but alternatively under deep general anaesthesia with fluothane the neck of the dead fetus is divided from below and its head pushed up into the uterus to free the head of the second twin. The decapitated head of the first is delivered later with forceps.

Delay can also occur if both heads are in collision at the brim, with the head of the second twin pressed against the neck of the second. Disengagement may be possible, but otherwise caesarean section is performed.

Third stage of labour

There is an increased risk of postpartum haemorrhage because of the large size of the placental site, which may encroach on the lower segment where the contraction of the muscle is relatively ineffective in closing blood sinuses. A prophylactic injection of Syntocinon or ergometrine should be given with the birth of the second twin and the placenta delivered in the usual way. If haemorrhage occurs it is treated as described on page 230.

Caesarean section

Elective caesarean section has a place in twin delivery if the pregnancy is complicated by severe hypertension, or if the patient is older or has a bad previous obstetric history. It may also be considered in cases of preterm labour before 34 weeks if the leading twin presents by the breech.

Triplets and higher multiple births

The increasing use of gonadotrophins and assisted reproduction techniques in infertility has resulted in an increased incidence of triplets and higher multiple births. The exact diagnosis is only likely to be made by ultrasound or radiological examination. All the fetal hazards already described are accentuated, and some of the babies are likely to be very small. The perinatal mortality is high and delivery of triplets or higher multiples is generally best managed by caesarean section. Obviously special arrangements for the provision of adequate expert paediatric help must be made. The impact on neonatal units may be considerable, to say nothing of the difficulties of parenthood.

FETAL LOSS IN EARLY PREGNANCY: ABORTION

Vaginal bleeding in early pregnancy is always a cause for concern. It may occur in cases of abortion or ectopic pregnancy, or with a cervical lesion such as a polyp or carcinoma. On many occasions no certain cause of early bleeding may be found. In such cases the possibility that there has been chorionic separation remains and placental function must be monitored carefully in the later weeks of pregnancy.

FETAL LOSS IN EARLY PREGNANCY

Failure of the pregnancy due to miscarriage is unlikely once the second trimester has been reached, but 10–15 per cent of all pregnancies diagnosed after six weeks amenorrhoea end in spontaneous miscarriage in the first trimester (Fig. 3.14).

The miscarriage rate is higher in women having their first pregnancy. The reasons for this are unclear, but women who have had an uneventful pregnancy and the birth of a normal live baby are much less likely to miscarry. In approximately 1 per cent of women, pregnancy failure is due to ectopic pregnancy and the incidence of the condition is influenced by pelvic infection, tubal surgery and whether there has been difficulty in achieving conception (subfertility or infertility). Vaginal bleeding and lower abdominal pain are the most common symptoms in early pregnancy failure.

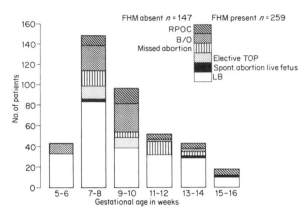

Fig. 3.14 Pregnancy outcome and the detection of fetal life in 406 women with intrauterine pregnancy complaining of vaginal bleeding in relation to the gestational age. RPOC, retained products of conception; B/O, blighted ovum; TOP, termination of pregnancy; LB, live birth; FHM, fetal heart movements

IN WOMEN WITH VAGINAL BLEEDING

Vaginal bleeding occurs commonly in the first trimester, in possibly a quarter of all pregnant women. If painless, the clinical diagnosis is usually threatened miscarriage; the risk of miscarriage increases with advancing maternal age and decreases with advancing gestational age. If fetal life is confirmed on ultrasound by the detection of the embryonic heart beat 95–98 per cent of cases will develop pregnancies which progress beyond 20 weeks gestation.

Half of the women presenting with vaginal bleeding in early pregnancy have a live fetus, indicating that miscarriage is unlikely, one quarter turn out not to be pregnant and the remainder miscarry, many with a blighted ovum. It is particularly important to note that, in spite of the absence of pain, some of these women have an ectopic pregnancy – a life-threatening condition.

IN WOMEN WITH ABDOMINAL PAIN AND VAGINAL BLEEDING

In women who complain of vaginal bleeding and lower abdominal pain the likelihood of ectopic pregnancy is much greater, occurring in up to one in four women with these symptoms. The diagnosis of pregnancy may be difficult to confirm, but women who suspect pregnancy when complaining of lower abdominal pain and bleeding must have the diagnosis of an ectopic conclusively made or rejected, because of the dangers of rupture and internal haemorrhage.

ABORTION

The terms abortion and miscarriage are synonymous and denote the expulsion of the conceptus before the end of the 28th week of pregnancy. There is no sharp demarcation between late abortion and early premature labour; the division is merely of descriptive convenience. It was formerly thought that a fetus born before the 28th week would not survive, and in Britain any such birth is only notifiable if the child is born alive, whereas all deliveries, live or dead, after that time must be notified. Today, with modern paediatric care, many less mature fetuses survive, and the legal convention of viability needs revision.

The obstetrician must understand the diagnosis and treatment of abortion, as it is a common complication of pregnancy, but many of the cases are treated in gynaecological wards rather than obstetric units. A fuller description of the condition and of the law relating to termination of pregnancy will be found in *Gynaecology by Ten Teachers.*

Clinical observation suggests that 10 to 15 per cent of pregnancies end in early abortion, but the loss of very early embryos is certainly greater than this. The most common time for clinically evident abortion to occur is between 7 and 13 weeks.

Causes of abortion

Despite a long list of aetiological factors, the cause of a particular abortion is often uncertain. The known causes include:

Malformation of the zygote

A common cause of abortion is an abnormality of the fetus or chorion which is severe enough to cause fetal death. About 70 per cent of these are caused by chromosomal abnormalities, for which either parent may be responsible, although they mostly arise from spontaneous, unexplained mutation in the zygote itself. Other chromosome disorders which are compatible with life (e.g. Down's syndrome) are also associated with an above average abortion rate. Most abortions of this type are not recurrent, so the prognosis in later pregnancies is good unless several abortions of identical pattern have already occurred.

When there is vaginal bleeding in early pregnancy ultrasound scanning may reveal an empty chorionic sac containing no fetus at all, or one in which the fetal echo is much too small for the dates. This is a blind ovum, in which abortion is bound to happen. Sometimes layers of blood clot collect round the sac as it collapses (*carneous mole*).

Immunological rejection of the fetus

Many investigations of the immune response of the mother to her fetus are now in progress. It has been suggested that the mother is stimulated by antigens in the trophoblast to produce blocking antibodies which inhibit the cell-mediated rejection process. If a couple share more HLA antigens than usual the trophoblast may fail to stimulate the production of maternal blocking antibodies and the pregnancy is rejected (i.e. aborted). Trials to assess the value of injecting donor lymphocytes to stimulate the production of blocking antibodies are currently being carried out.

General disease of the mother

Pregnancy will often continue in spite of maternal disease, but any maternal illness may cause abortion if it is sufficiently severe, especially acute fevers. Maternal infection may involve the fetus, particularly rubella and syphilis, but rarely also malaria, brucellosis, toxoplasmosis, cytomegalic inclusion disease, vaccinia and listeriosis.

Abortion occurs in a few cases of *rubella*, but more often the infected fetus is born alive but with congenital abnormalities. (*Syphilis* does not cause early abortion and it is an uncommon cause of late abortion in the UK; it is more likely to cause intrauterine death after the 28th week.)

The abortion rate is above average in *diabetes* if the disease is not adequately controlled.

Intrauterine death may occur with *hypertension* and *renal disease*, sometimes before the 28th week.

Severe *malnutrition* will cause abortion, but it has to be of a degree which is unlikely to be seen in Britain. Although deficiency of vitamin E will cause abortion in experimental animals there is no evidence that it causes abortion in women, and this substance is always present in adequate amounts in the diet.

Uterine abnormalities

The incidence of abortion is increased if the uterus is double or septate, but in many such cases pregnancy is uneventful.

Retroversion of the uterus is not a cause of miscarriage, except in rare instances in which incarceration of the uterus occurs and is left untreated.

A fibromyoma which is closely related to the cavity and the uterus may cause abortion, but other fibromyomata will not do so.

Lacerations of the cervix involving the internal os may result in abortion in the middle trimester, or in premature labour. Very rarely the cervical weakness is of congenital origin; usually it is the result of obstetric laceration or of over-vigorous surgical dilatation of the cervix. During pregnancy the unsupported membranes bulge through the cervix and rupture; miscarriage follows.

Hormonal insufficiency

It has been claimed that insufficient production of progesterone by the corpus luteum before the placenta is fully formed will lead to inadequate development of the decidua and abortion. The evidence for this is weak (p. 146).

Both thyroid deficiency and hyperthyroidism may be contributory factors in abortion.

Other causes

Other causes of abortion which are unlikely to be encountered in the obstetric unit include irradiation of the uterus; drugs including quinine, ergot and prostaglandins; accidental or operative trauma to the uterus or the insertion of foreign bodies.

Pathological anatomy

In the first trimester of pregnancy the attachment of the chorion to the decidua is so delicate that separation may follow strong uterine contractions produced by any cause. The resulting haemorrhage into the choriodecidual space leads to further separation. In other cases fetal death precedes uterine contractions, which may occur some days later. The decidua basalis remains in the uterus, and in the majority of cases the embryo, with its membranes and most of the decidua capsularis, is expelled. In some cases the gestation sac is retained in the uterus for days or weeks as a missed abortion, layers of blood clot collect around it to form a carneous mole (*see* p. 146).

By the 12th week the placenta is a definite structure, and after this time the process of abortion is similar to that of labour. Bleeding and painful contractions are followed by dilatation of the cervix, rupture of the membranes and expulsion of the fetus and placenta. If all the conceptus is expelled (complete abortion) normal uterine involution follows, but frequently part of the placenta is retained with some blood clot (incomplete abortion). Rarely the uterine contractions mould the retained contents into a polypoid mass, described as a *placental polyp*.

Clinical varieties of abortion

The following terms are used to describe varieties of abortion:

threatened
inevitable
complete
incomplete
septic
missed
recurrent.

Threatened abortion

In these cases haemorrhage occurs without dilatation of the cervix and with very little or no pain. The clinical distinction from inevitable abortion is based on the relatively slight degree of bleeding and the absence of cervical dilatation. If the bleeding is heavy, or increases, the prognosis is bad, but the abortion should not be regarded as inevitable until the cervix begins to dilate. There may be repeated short episodes of bleeding without the abortion becoming inevitable, and if a slight red loss is followed for some days by old brown altered blood this may have little significance.

The patient is put to bed immediately, and, provided an ultrasound scan confirms that pregnancy is progressing, rests until some days after all red loss has ceased. A gentle vaginal examination and the passage of a speculum will exclude any other unsuspected cause for the bleeding, such as a cervical polyp for example, and may also reveal any dilatation of the cervix.

There is no specific treatment and the essential task is to establish that the abortion is only threatened and is not becoming inevitable. Ultrasound examination will determine the size of the fetus and show if the fetal heart is beating. In normal pregnancy a gestation sac of about 8 mm diameter can be identified by the sixth week, and during the eighth week the fetal crown–rump length increases from 15 to 21 mm. Repeated scanning is without risk to the fetus and can establish continuing growth. By the 14th week the crown–rump length averages 90 mm; thereafter growth can be monitored by measuring the biparietal diameter of the fetal head. If ultrasound shows an empty pregnancy sac it is probable that there is serious chromosomal abnormality and abortion will eventually occur. Attempts to conserve such a pregnancy are of no value. Ultrasound will also help in the differential diagnosis; if the abortion becomes inevitable dilatation of the cervix and descent of the gestation sac into the cervical canal may be seen.

Serum progesterone levels can be measured, and decreasing levels may indicate that the attachment or the survival of the embryo is precarious, but the value of administrating progesterone is doubtful.

If the pregnancy continues the mother may be anxious about the possibility that the fetus is abnormal; she can truthfully be told that this is very unlikely, especially if the ultrasound scan is normal.

Inevitable abortion

The process is now irreversible. There is more bleeding and rhythmical and painful uterine contractions cause cervical dilatation.

The uterus usually expels its contents unaided. All examinations are carried out with careful aseptic technique. Analgesics such as pethidine may be required. If haemorrhage becomes severe or the abortion is not quickly completed the uterus should be evacuated under anaesthesia with a suction curette.

In all cases of inevitable abortion anti-D gammaglobulin 100 micrograms is injected intramuscularly unless the patient is known to be rhesus positive.

Complete abortion

When all the uterine contents have been expelled spontaneously there is cessation of pain, scanty blood loss and a firmly contracted uterus. If careful inspection of the products of conception confirms complete expulsion, or if an ultrasound scan shows an empty uterine cavity, no further treatment is required. Many women who have a complete abortion do not require hospital admission.

Incomplete abortion

This term means that part of the products of conception, usually chorionic or placental tissue, is retained. Bleeding continues and may be severe. There is a danger of shock and of sepsis. If blood loss is heavy or continues for more than a few days after an abortion it must be assumed that there are retained products, particularly if the uterus is still found to be enlarged and the cervix is open. The products can be seen on ultrasound scanning. The chief dangers are haemorrhage and sepsis, and they continue until the uterine cavity is empty.

Severe bleeding associated with shock may necessitate blood transfusion by a mobile emergency unit before the patient is moved from home to hospital. Intramuscular ergometrine, 500 micrograms, is given immediately and any placental debris in the cervical canal is removed, under direct vision, using a speculum and ring forceps. The foot of the bed is raised and transfusion is continued until the blood pressure reaches a level safe enough for transfer of the patient to hospital. There the uterus is evacuated under anaesthesia with the suction curette or ring forceps. A postoperative prophylactic antibiotic such as ampicillin is given.

In some cases of incomplete abortion the bleeding is not severe but it continues intermittently for several weeks and the uterus remains enlarged. Surgical evacuation of the uterus is then essential, with histological examination of the products. Some of these cases are due to a placental polyp. (*see* p. 144).

Septic abortion

Infection may occur during spontaneous abortion but it more often occurs after induced abortion. Blood clot and necrotic debris in the uterus form an excellent culture medium. Infection may spread rapidly to surrounding structures, causing pelvic or generalized peritonitis, pelvic cellulitis and salpingitis, sometimes with septicaemia. There is fever and a raised pulse rate, and there may be lower abdominal pain. Permanent blockage of the fallopian tubes may occur as the end-result of salpingitis.

The most common infecting organisms in cases of septic abortion in Britain now are *Staphylococcus aureus*, coliform bacteria, *Bacteriodes* organisms and *Clostridium welchii*, and of these the most dangerous arc the Gram-negative and anaerobic organisms which produce endotoxic shock. The potentially lethal cases of infection with the β-haemolytic streptoccus group A are, fortunately, seldom seen.

The patient must be admitted to hospital and isolated from other obstetric and surgical patients. High vaginal swabs and blood specimens are sent for bacteriological culture, while treatment is started with wide-spectrum antibiotics. There is much debate about the best choice; one that has been recommended is cephradine, 250–500 mg every six hours together with metronidazole 500 mg. Both of these can be given intravenously if the patient is vomiting. When the bacteriological report is received the antibiotic treatment is modified according to the sensitivities of the organisms discovered.

Anaemia may occur from haemolysis as well as from haemorrhage, and the haemoglobin level must be determined. Blood transfusion may be necessary.

The uterus must be emptied, but if the bleeding is not too serious evacuation is best postponed until 24 hours after the start of antibiotic treatment. In cases with serious bleeding it cannot be deferred. In most cases evacuation is performed under anaesthesia with a suction curette or ring forceps. In cases of more than 14 weeks gestation in which a dead fetus is retained its expulsion may be achieved by oxytocin infusion and vaginal insertion of prostaglandins.

Some patients are gravely ill, especially if anaerobic infection has occurred, with high swinging fever, anaemia and sometimes haemolytic jaundice. Endotoxic shock may be superimposed on hypovolaemic shock, with circulatory failure due to peripheral vasodilation caused by endotoxins released from coliform organisms which have invaded the bloodstream. Before surgical intervention massive doses of intravenous penicillin and metronidazole are given. Both are usually given by mouth, but in severely ill patients the intravenous route may be preferable. Intravenous hydrocortisone is sometimes helpful if restoration of the blood volume does not quickly restore the blood pressure. The urinary output must be carefully watched, since oliguria may indicate renal cortical or tubular necrosis (*see* p. 79).

Missed abortion

This occurs when the embryo dies or fails to develop, and the gestation sac is retained in the uterus for weeks or months. Haemorrhage occurs into the choriodecidual space and extends around the gestation sac. The amnion remains intact and becomes surrounded by hillocks of blood clot with a fleshy appearance, hence the term *carneous mole*. Mild symptoms like those of threatened abortion are followed by absence of the usual signs of progress of the pregnancy. The uterine size remains stationary and the cervix is often tightly closed. Urinary gonadotrophin pregnancy tests remain equivocal for weeks, but repeated ultrasound scans will show no growth of the fetal crown–rump measurement and absence of fetal heart movements.

All missed abortions would eventually be expelled spontaneously, but there may be a delay of weeks or months and many patients become distressed once the diagnosis is made, so that active treatment is often chosen. In a few late cases there is a risk of hypofibrinogenaemia after retention of a dead fetus for some weeks, probably caused by thromboplastins from the chorionic tissue entering the maternal circulation.

Successful evacuation of the uterus is usually achieved in late cases with a combination of intravaginal prostaglandins and an intravenous Syntocinon infusion. In early cases the uterus may be emptied surgically with a suction curette after dilating the cervix.

Recurrent abortion

By convention this term refers to any case in which there have been three or more consecutive spontaneous abortions. Unless each successive abortion has occurred at about the same time and in similar fashion it should not be assumed that there is an underlying and recurrent cause. Repeated miscarriages can occur by unlucky chance from different causes each time.

Early repeated abortion has been attributed to progesterone deficiency. But estimations of serum progesterone have shown no consistent abnormality, nor have controlled clinical studies shown any significant improvement from treatment with progestogens in these cases. Advocates of this treatment give twice-weekly intramuscular injections of 17-α-hydroxyprogesterone hexanoate (Proluton Depot) 250 mg. Other progestogens are contraindicated because they are partly androgenic and may have a virilizing effect on a female fetus. An alternative treatment is to support the corpus luteum with chorionic gonadotrophin 10 000 units intramuscularly twice-weekly.

Repeated midtrimester abortions may result from incompetence of the internal os of the cervix, which is usually caused by previous obstetric trauma, injudicious surgical dilatation, cone biopsy or cervical amputation. In the non-pregnant state this condition may be diagnosed by a hysterogram or finding that a dilator 1 cm in diameter can be easily passed. During pregnancy it is suspected from a history of repeated, almost painless, abortions after the 16th week, or sometimes by observing the membranes bulging through the partly dilated cervix.

Recurrent abortion is treated by insertion of a purse-string suture of non-absorbable material in the thickness of the wall of the cervix at the level of the internal os before the 16th week (Shirodkhar operation). This is removed shortly before term.

While there have been some adverse reports about the need for or success of this operation, the criticism may perhaps be directed at the choice of patients rather than at the procedure itself.

When a definite cause for habitual abortion cannot be established simple general advice is given. Any defect of general health is rectified if possible. Coitus is discouraged at the time of the previous abortion, and the patient may be admitted to hospital for rest in bed, especially at the time at which previous abortions occurred. In all cases the patient will need constant encouragement and support.

Trials are taking place to assess the value of injecting the partner's lymphocytes into the mother in the hope of stimulating her to produce blocking antibodies which prevent cell-mediated rejection of the pregnancy.

ECTOPIC PREGNANCY

An ectopic or extrauterine pregnancy occurs when the fertilized ovum embeds in some site other than the uterine decidua. Nearly all ectopic implantations are in the fallopian tube, but very rarely the cervix, the ovary or the peritoneal cavity is the site of implantation. In Britain the incidence of ectopic pregnancy is about 1 case to 150 mature intrauterine pregnancies, but much higher incidences are found in countries where pelvic infection is common, e.g. 1 in 28 in the West Indies.

Most of the cases are treated in gynaecological wards, and a fuller account of the condition is given in *Gynaecology by Ten Teachers*.

Aetiology

Fertilization of the ovum normally occurs in the ampulla of the fallopian tube, and the ovum takes about five days to reach the uterine cavity where it implants at the blastocyst stage in the prepared secretory endometrium.

Delay or arrest in transit along the tube may be caused by a number of factors. Previous salpingitis may have destroyed part of the ciliated epithelium, or formed pockets of epithelial folds within the lumen; peritoneal adhesions may kink or compress the outside of the tube. Rarely a congenital diverticulum or abnormal length of the tube may be causative factors. There is a higher incidence of ectopic pregnancy in women using an intrauterine contraceptive device, possibly caused by interference with normal tubal peristalsis or by ascending infection. Previous tubal surgery is also an important cause and patients who have had such surgery should be warned of the risks of tubal pregnancy.

Pathological anatomy

The ampulla is the commonest site of implantation of the fertilized ovum. In less than a quarter of the cases the embryo is lodged in the isthmus; the other sites are very rare. The process of embedding is similar to that in an intrauterine pregnancy but, because the tube has no decidua, after the epithelium is penetrated by the trophoblast the embryo burrows directly into the thin muscular wall, where it grows and distends the tube (Fig. 3.15).

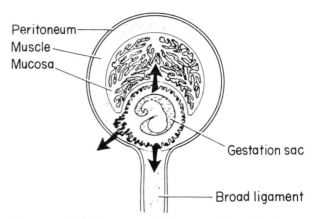

Fig. 3.15 Tubal pregnancy. Diagram to show that the embryo becomes embedded in the muscular wall of the tube. The gestation sac may then rupture into the lumen of the tube, through the wall of the tube and into the peritoneal cavity, or between the layers of the broad ligament. Of these, the last is the least common

Tubal blood vessels are eroded with resulting haemorrhage around the embryo which then bursts either into the lumen of the tube (*intratubal rupture*) or through the wall (*extratubal rupture*) into the peritoneal cavity or occasionally between the layers of the broad ligament.

The uterus also hypertrophies and the endometrium undergoes normal decidual changes. After death of the embryo the decidua is shed either in fragments or as a decidual cast, with some external bleeding.

Clinical course and management

Symptoms most commonly arise after one menstrual period is missed, although they may occasionally begin before this. However, it is rare for ectopic pregnancy to advance beyond eight weeks without the occurrence of pain or bleeding, a point which is sometimes helpful in differentiating between a uterine abortion and an ectopic pregnancy.

The dominant feature is low abdominal pain. This often originates on the side of the ectopic implantation and can be acute and severe. This is followed by slight irregular bleeding from the uterus. Profuse intraperitoneal haemorrhage and severe pain may result in sudden shock and collapse of the patient, which may be fatal unless immediate transfusion and laparotomy are undertaken.

A tubal pregnancy may terminate in the following ways:

Tubal mole

Bleeding around the embryo results in embryonic death, the embryo is retained in the tube surrounded by clot (Fig. 3.16). The patient complains of pelvic pain, sometimes unilateral, and slight dark vaginal blood loss. On bimanual examination a very tender swelling is palpable beside a bulky uterus. The diagnosis from salpingitis or torsion of a small ovarian cyst may be difficult. An immunological test for pregnancy is often positive for a time. Ultrasound scan and laparoscopy may be helpful, but if there is a pelvic mass exploratory laparotomy is usually performed, and the damaged tube is removed.

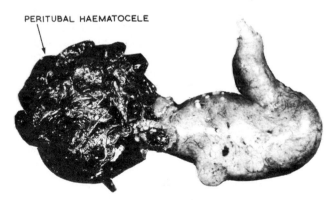

PERITUBAL HAEMATOCELE

Fig. 3.16 Tubal mole, with bleeding through the ostium of the tube

Tubal abortion

As the name implies, this occurs when separation of an ampullary ectopic gestation is followed by its expulsion through the ostium of the tube into the peritoneal cavity. Blood escapes from the tube to collect in the rectovaginal pouch as a *pelvic haematocele*. This blood becomes walled off by adhesions, producing a tender cystic swelling behind the uterus. With a large haematocele the cervix is pushed forwards and upwards, and occasionally retention of urine may occur. Later on, when absorption of the blood has begun, an untreated haematocele may have a lumpy and uneven consistence. There is often slight fever.

Surgical removal of the damaged tube and the haematocele is required.

Tubal rupture

This usually follows implantation in the isthmus of the tube. In this narrow part of the tube early rupture occurs into the peritoneal cavity. The patient rapidly develops signs of severe intraperitoneal bleeding, with pain, fainting or collapse, pallor, rapid pulse and low blood pressure and signs of an acute abdomen. The whole lower abdomen is extremely tender and there may be some distention. Shifting dullness can sometimes be demonstrated. When the patient lies down the blood tracks up to reach the diaphragm and causes referred shoulder-tip pain. On pelvic examination there is exquisite tenderness, but no mass will be felt as the ruptured tube is now empty.

Immediate blood transfusion is required, followed without delay by laparotomy to clamp the bleeding points and remove the damaged tube and the blood clot.

In rare instances the rupture occurs downwards between the layers of the broad ligament to form an *intraligamentous haematoma*. The management is similar to that of a tubal mole, since the differential diagnosis may be impossible before laparotomy.

Secondary abdominal pregnancy

Intraperitoneal rupture, as described above, is occasionally accompanied by relatively little bleeding. On very rare occasions the embryo may then be partially extruded into the peritoneal cavity and may continue to grow, developing partial placental attachment to surrounding structures. If the amnion remains intact the pregnancy may progress. Towards the end of the pregnancy the patient may experience a mock labour which is followed by death of the fetus and thrombosis of vessels going to the placental site. This very rare condition is known as *secondary abdominal pregnancy*. Ultimately mummification of the fetus occurs with subsequent calcification, forming a *lithopaedion*. If infection does not occur this may be retained for many years in the abdominal cavity, only to be discovered if the patient presents with intestinal obstruction or an abdominal mass. In modern practice the diagnosis of intra-abdominal pregnancy is usually made by ultrasound. It may be suspected because the fetus is felt very easily through the abdominal wall, the lie is oblique and there is a soft mass, the uterus, occupying the pelvic cavity. With careful observation in hospital the pregnancy can sometimes be maintained until the fetus is viable. Because of the relatively inefficient placenta, a reflection of the poor blood flow to the abnormal site, retarded growth and fetal death are likely at about 32 weeks. Delivery by laparotomy is needed to avoid this.

There is a risk of severe haemorrhage if the placenta is separated from its attachment to other structures. It is best to leave the placenta *in situ* and to close the abdomen, allowing spontaneous absorption to occur.

Interstitial (cornual) pregnancy

The site of implantation is in the part of the tube which lies in the uterine wall. The pregnancy may continue until about the 12th week, but sooner or later there is extensive rupture of the uterine cornu with very free bleeding from the vascular myometrium. This will necessitate enucleation of the gestation sac and wedge resection of the cornu, or even hysterectomy if there is uncontrollable bleeding.

Ovarian pregnancy

This is exceedingly rare and clinically indistinguishable from a ruptured tubal pregnancy. The diagnosis can only be proved by careful histological examination of the gestation sac and ovary after removal.

Rupture of a pregnant rudimentary horn

Rupture of a pregnant rudimentary horn of a bicornuate uterus is not strictly an extrauterine pregnancy, but it is a serious accident with intraperitoneal bleeding. This occurs later than rupture of a tubal pregnancy, often at about the 14th week. The diagnosis is usually made at laparotomy, when the horn is removed.

Cervical pregnancy

Very rarely the embryo implants in the cervical canal. Because of the restriction in its growth the pregnancy seldom progresses beyond the sixth week. There is free bleeding and there may be pain from uterine contractions. Evacuation of the pregnancy by curettage does not always stop the bleeding because there is little contractile muscle in the cervix, and deep sutures may have to be inserted to arrest the haemorrhage.

OTHER CAUSES OF HAEMORRHAGE DURING EARLY PREGNANCY

Bleeding may come from lesions of the cervix:

Cervical erosion

Cervical erosion is very common during pregnancy, when the high level of oestrogens causes proliferation of the columnar epithelium of the cervical canal so that this extends outwards on the vaginal aspect of the cervix, forming a velvety red area, with well-defined edges, around the external os. Such erosions very occasionally cause a slight blood-stained discharge, but with any bleeding the possibility of malignancy must be considered. If there is any doubt, a biopsy should be done, but in most cases as long as a cervical smear is examined and found to be normal, no treatment is required during pregnancy, and most erosions resolve after delivery.

Cervical adenomatous polypi

These may be found during pregnancy as small, soft, red tumours, attached by a stalk to the cervix near the external os. If they are not causing more than a slight blood-stained discharge, and a smear arouses no suspicion of malignant disease, they may be left alone during pregnancy; otherwise they are easily removed for biopsy.

Carcinoma of the cervix

See page 67.

4

NORMAL LABOUR

THE CAUSE OF THE ONSET OF LABOUR

The uterus contracts strongly to expel any foreign body or solid tumour from its cavity. In discussing the cause of the onset of labour the problem is not to discover why the uterus starts to contract at term, but to find out why it usually remains quiescent during pregnancy. The uterus clearly has the power of expelling its contents before term, as in miscarriage, premature labour and when labour is induced before term.

It has been suggested that progesterone inhibits the uterine muscle during pregnancy. In rabbits the onset of labour can be postponed by giving large doses of progesterone, but this is not the case in women. Nor has it been shown that the blood concentration of progesterone falls significantly before term.

It has also been suggested that the rising levels of oestrogen during pregnancy sensitize the uterine muscle, so that it eventually responds more easily to stimuli or to oxytocin. There is no increase in secretion of oxytocin at term and labour starts normally in hypophysectomized animals. A prostaglandin pessary (PGE_2) placed in the vaginal vault near term induces labour.

There is some evidence that the fetal adrenal gland plays a part in initiating labour. Anencephalic fetuses may have defective adrenal cortices and with some of these fetuses pregnancy is greatly prolonged unless labour is induced artificially.

The possible part played by prostaglandins in the onset of labour has yet to be fully investigated. It has been shown that mechanical stimulation of the cervix by the insertion of a finger and separation of the membranes leads to local secretion of prostaglandins. Prostaglandins are present in the decidua and membranes of late pregnancy. It is possible that premature labour may be caused by increased prostaglandin production following rupture of the membranes or ascending infection. A prostaglandin pessary placed in the vaginal vault near term can induce labour.

During normal pregnancy the growth of the uterus keeps pace with that of its contents and the limit of stretch is probably not reached even at term; the intrauterine pressure does not rise. However, in cases of polyhydramnios or twins, premature labour is common, so that in abnormal cases over-stretching of the uterus may play some part in the onset of labour.

Quite apart from the natural mechanism of onset, in some instances labour may be started artificially by rupture of the membranes, by oxytocin infusions or by the local or systemic administration of prostaglandins.

Labour follows intrauterine death of the fetus, but there is usually an interval of several days or even weeks before its onset.

During normal pregnancy the uterus contracts intermittently, but these contractions are not strong enough to overcome the resistance of the normal cervix. However, if the internal os of the cervix is damaged or incompetent even these weak contractions may dilate the cervix and labour will follow.

THE UTERINE SEGMENTS

In describing the phenomena of labour the uterus may be divided into two functional segments.

The upper part of the uterus (known as the *upper segment*) contracts strongly, and with each successive contraction the smooth muscle fibres comprising it become shorter and thicker. This powerful segment draws the weaker, thinner and more passive lower part of the uterus up over its contents, and in so doing 'takes up' and then dilates the cervix.

The *lower segment*, consisting of the lower part of the body of the uterus and the cervix, can contract (as is evident if ergometrine is given) but is relatively passive as compared to the upper segment.

The upper and lower segments are not fully formed until the end of the first stage of labour when they can be clearly seen and the transition between them is quite abrupt (Fig. 4.1). In the non-pregnant uterus and during early pregnancy it is not possible to define the limits of the eventual lower segment, but at the end of pregnancy the lower segment is recognizable; in front it corresponds fairly well with the lower limit of firm peritoneal attachment to the uterus. Below this point the uterovesical peritoneum is loosely attached.

During labour, as the cervix dilates and the lower segment is drawn up, its shape changes from a hemisphere to a cylinder. If there is obstruction to delivery the retraction of the upper segment is even more pronounced, and the junction between the two segments forms a distinct ring known as the *retraction ring of Bandl*. In extreme cases this may be palpable and visible per abdomen.

In labour the lower uterine segment, cervix, vagina, pelvic floor and vulval outlet are dilated until there is one continuous birth canal. The forces which bring about this dilatation and expel the fetus are supplied by the contraction and retraction of the muscle of the upper uterine segment, with assistance in the second stage from

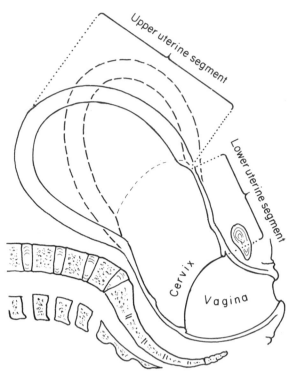

Fig. 4.1 The thick upper segment and the thin lower segment of the uterus at the end of the first stage of labour. The dotted lines indicate the position assumed by the uterus during a contraction

the abdominal muscles, including the diaphragm.

The muscle fibres of the upper segment of the uterus not only contract but also retract. When contracting the fibres become shorter and thicker. When the active contraction passes off the fibres lengthen again, but not to their original length. If contraction was followed by complete relaxation no progress would be made. In retraction some of the shortening of the fibres is maintained. Each successive contraction starts at the point where its predecessor ended, so that the uterine cavity becomes progressively smaller with each contraction. Retraction is a property which, though not peculiar to uterine muscle, is more marked in the uterus than any other organ. Later in labour when the placenta is expelled, retraction enables the uterine walls to come together so that there is hardly more than a potential cavity.

THE STAGES OF LABOUR

Labour is divided into three stages:

the *first stage*, or stage of dilatation, lasts from the onset of true labour until the cervix is fully dilated

the *second stage*, or stage of expulsion of the fetus, lasts from full dilatation of the cervix until the fetus is born

the *third stage* lasts from the birth of the child until the placenta and membranes are delivered and the uterus has retracted firmly to compress the uterine blood sinuses.

Premonitory symptoms

In most primigravidae the presenting part sinks into the pelvis during the last three or four weeks of pregnancy, and in lay terms this is spoken of as 'lightening' because the descent of the fundus of the uterus, together with the reduction in the amount of liquor in late pregnancy, reduces the upper abdominal distension, making the patient more comfortable.

In many multiparae the presenting part does not engage in the pelvis until labour begins. Not infrequently, multiparae experience uterine contractions which are strong enough to be painful, some days, or even weeks, before real labour starts. Such 'false pains' differ from labour pains only in that they are less regular and are ineffective in dilating the cervix.

Symptoms and signs of the onset of labour

These are:

painful uterine contractions
the show
rupture of the membranes
shortening and dilatation of the cervix.

The contractions

The uterus contracts irregularly and painlessly throughout pregnancy (Braxton Hicks contractions). Labour is recognized by the changes in the contractions when they become regular and painful enough to distract the patient from her usual activities and cause the cervix to be taken up and dilated. The uterus can be felt to harden during each contraction, which begins gradually, works up to a period of maximum intensity and then dies away, the whole lasting about 45 seconds.

At the onset of labour the interval between contractions may be variable and can be as long as 20 minutes. However, it is quite common for the interval between contractions to be as short as five minutes right from the onset.

Contractions are often preceded by backache and tend to increase in frequency and duration, gradually becoming more painful. By the end of the first stage of labour the contractions may come every two or three minutes and may last as long as a minute.

The contractions are not within the control of the patient's will and occur even when she is unconscious, although they may be lessened in frequency or temporarily abolished by emotional disturbance or by distension of the bladder. They may be increased in strength and frequency by such stimuli as a purgative or enema, stretching of the cervix or pelvic floor by the presenting part, by prostaglandins or by injection of oxytocin.

The pain of labour has the same character as that of spasmodic dysmenorrhoea and probably has the same cause – ischaemia of the uterine muscle from compression of the blood vessels in the wall of the uterus. It is analogous to the myocardial pain which occurs when the blood flow in the coronary arteries is restricted. The fact that the contractions are intermittent and not continuous is of great importance to both the fetus and the mother. During a contraction the circulation through the uterine wall is stopped, and if the uterus contracted continuously the fetus would die from lack of oxygen. The intervals between the pains allow the placental circulation to be re-established and give the mother time to recover from the fatiguing effect of the contraction. The uterus is a very large muscle and contractions use up a lot of the patient's energy; if continued too long this would produce maternal exhaustion.

Electrical records of the pattern of uterine contractions show that in normal labour each contraction wave starts near one or other uterine cornu. The contraction spreads as a wave in the myometrium, taking 10 to 30 seconds to spread over the whole uterus. As each point is reached by the wave, contraction starts and takes about another 30 seconds to reach its peak.

The upper part of the uterus contracts more strongly than the lower part, and the duration of the contraction is longer in the upper than in the lower segment. This dominance of the upper segment leads to the stretching and thinning of the lower segment and to dilatation of the cervix.

If the wave pattern is abnormal, with the lower part of the uterus contracting first or as strongly as the upper part, no progress in labour will be made. Sometimes the wave spreads erratically in the myometrium and the contractions are unco-ordinated (*see* p. 180).

The duration and strength of each contraction are relevant both to their efficiency and to the pain felt by the patient. The resting tone between contractions in early labour is about 1.33 kPa (10 mmHg); the intrauterine pressure at which a contraction can be felt by the hand of an observer is about 2.66 kPa (20 mmHg); and the pressure at which the patient feels pain is about 3.325 kPa (25 mmHg). Efficient first stage contractions reach 6.65 kPa (50 mmHg), and they may reach 9.975 kPa (75 mmHg) in the second stage. The pain threshold of patients varies, and may vary in one woman during the course of labour. It is the anxious worried patient, a long time in labour, who may feel pain at a pressure as low as 1.995 kPa (15 mmHg).

The show

This is a mucous discharge from the cervix, mixed with a little blood. As the internal os is drawn, or taken, up (Fig. 4.2) the membranes are separated

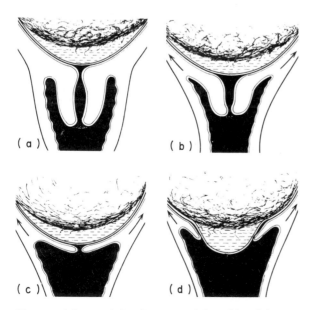

Fig. 4.2 The cervix is taken up and then dilated during pregnancy

from the lower uterine segment, and a variable amount of oozing of blood results.

Rupture of the membranes

The membranes may rupture at any time during labour, although this usually occurs towards the end of the first stage. When the membranes rupture spontaneously near term it is probable that labour will begin within a short time, although in a few instances the onset is still delayed. Early rupture of the membranes is more likely to occur if the presenting part is not engaged or if there is a malpresentation, but it also occurs in many normal cases.

Shortening and dilatation of the cervix

At the beginning of labour the cervix of a nulliparous woman is usually a thick-walled canal, of at least 2 cm in length. However, in other cases the cervix may be found to be shortened (or taken up) and partly dilated in the later weeks of pregnancy.

When labour begins the contraction and retraction of the upper uterine segment stretches the lower segment and the upper part of the cervix; the lower part of the cervical canal remains at first unaltered. As the internal os is pulled open, the cervix is dilated from above downwards, becoming shorter, until no projection into the vagina is felt, but only a more-or-less thick rim at the external os, the whole cervix being taken up and its cavity made one with that of the body of the uterus. Without true shortening of the cervix it is unwise to diagnose that a primigravida is in labour (*see* Fig. 4.2).

In women who have delivered children the external os will often admit a finger before labour has begun, and the finger-tip can somtimes be passed through the internal os. Very often the cervix has been taken up. In this case the projection of a small bag of membranes (Fig. 4.2(d)) during a contraction will show that labour has begun.

THE FIRST STAGE OF LABOUR

The contractions of the uterus dilate the cervix. The dilatation of the internal os causes separation of the chorion from the decidua closest to it. Thus a small bag of membranes is formed and is forced into the internal os by the intrauterine pressure. At the beginning of each contraction a little more liquor is forced into the bag of membranes, the head then comes down like a ball valve and separates the liquor amnii which is above it from that in the bag, called respectively the hind and forewaters. The bag of membranes may remain intact until nearly the end of the first stage, but even if the membranes rupture early the cervix will normally still become dilated as it is drawn up over the presenting part by the retraction of the upper segment.

During the first stage the fetus does not move downwards to any great degree. When a certain amount of liquor has left the uterus after the membranes have ruptured a new form of pressure comes into play, namely the *fetal axis pressure*. The upper pole of the fetus, normally the breech, is pressed on by the fundus of the uterus, while the lower pole is pressed down onto the lower segment and cervix. When the membranes rupture early the fetal axis pressure will operate at an early stage, and in modern practice the membranes are often deliberately ruptured during labour because this is believed to encourage more efficient uterine action and shorten labour.

The normal first stage should not exceed 12 hours in a primigravida, and should be even shorter in a multipara. During the early part of the first stage the pains may not be very severe, but towards the end of this stage they are often very distressing. They recur frequently, and as progress in dilatation of the cervix is not apparent to the patient she is under the mistaken impression that they are not effective. Vomiting is not uncommon at this time. This is often the most painful part of labour.

In the past much has been written about the disadvantage of early rupture of the membranes, but today it is agreed that in normal vertex presentations early rupture is of no consequence. As long as the bag of membranes is intact, the intrauterine pressure is distributed equally over all parts of the fetus. This is still true in a normal case after the membranes have ruptured except for the small part of the fetus which is related to the cervix, because the well-fitting presenting part prevents much liquor from draining away. If, however, there is a malpresentation or disproportion, early rupture of the membranes may be followed by loss of nearly all the liquor and the uterus becomes closely applied to the fetus. If labour is prolonged the placenta and cord may be unduly compressed by the retraction of the uterus, fetal hypoxia ensues, and in extreme circumstances the fetus may die.

If the membranes remain unruptured when the cervix is fully dilated the onset of the expulsive stage may be delayed, the cervix not receiving the pressure of the head which should stimulate the uterus to increased activity. If the membranes remain intact after full dilatation they should be ruptured with toothed forceps or a sterile plastic amnihook during a contraction.

THE SECOND STAGE OF LABOUR

There may be very little descent of the fetus during the first stage. However, in the second stage the resistance offered by the lower uterine segment and the cervix has been overcome and the presenting part can be pushed down onto the pelvic floor. The resistance of the pelvic floor then has to be overcome by the uterine contractions, aided by the action of the voluntary muscles of the abdominal wall and the diaphragm.

The normal second stage should not last much more than an hour in a primigravida, and may be very much shorter in a multipara. The pain felt during the second stage is often less than that at the end of the first stage, partly because cervical dilatation is now complete. The patient realizes that some progress is being made and that she can help herself. As the head passes through the pelvis she may complain of cramp in the legs from pressure on the sacral nerves and, especially in first labours, there is sharp discomfort during the stretching of the vulval outlet.

In the second stage the character of the pains is different from that in the first stage. As the contraction comes on the patient takes a deep breath, then holds her breath and bears down with all the force of her abdominal muscles. During the height of the pain there may be expiratory groans. These expulsive efforts are partly voluntary but largely reflex.

During a contraction the fetal heart rate is often slowed, but it regains its normal rate as soon as the contraction has passed. Such transient bradycardia is of little significance, but if bradycardia is prolonged after each contraction this is a sign of fetal distress.

With each contraction the presenting part is forced down onto the pelvic floor. During the intervals between the contractions, however, the pelvic floor at first pushes the presenting part up again. Retraction now plays an important part, so that the progress made by each contraction is not completely lost during the succeeding interval. Eventually, after being pushed down many times by the contractions and slipping back in the intervals between them, a time comes when the presenting part is stationary at the end of a contraction. After this, with each contraction and expulsive effort the head slowly moves down in a forwards direction, becoming more visible. In a primigravida the head may be visible for some time at the vulva before it can emerge. When the widest diameter of the head distends the vulva it is said to be crowned.

As the head passes through the vulva of a primigravida the stretching pain may be very severe, and will probably cause the patient to cry out, and so to cease from bearing down. To some extent this saves the perineum from damage, as it is likely to be torn if the patient bears down hard while the head is passing through the vulval orifice. It is at this stage that episiotomy may be necessary.

The body of the child is generally born by the next contraction if not by the contraction which expelled the head, and is followed by a gush of liquor.

The caput succedaneum

That part of the head which is most in advance is free from pressure during labour, while the rest of the head is pressed upon by the cervix and lower segment. As a result of venous congestion serum is exuded and an oedematous swelling forms on the scalp, superficial to the periosteum of the cranial bones and not limited by them. This is known as the caput succedaneum. After delivery, over a few hours or days, it gradually disappears.

If some other part presents, e.g. the face or breech, a comparable oedematous swelling will be formed over the part most in advance.

Moulding

The change in the shape of the head during labour is called moulding.

The bones of the base of the skull are incompressible, and are joined to each other in such a way that movement is not possible between them. The bones of the vault of the skull *are* compressible, and the sutures allow some movement between the individual bones. The parietal bones and the tabular portions of the occipital and frontal bones can be shaped by pressure, and when forcibly compressed the parietal bones can override the occipital and frontal bones, and one parietal bone can override its fellow. By moulding and overlap the biparietal diameter can be reduced by as much as 1 cm, but excessive moulding may result in intracranial damage.

THE THIRD STAGE OF LABOUR

At the end of the second stage of labour the uterus contracts down to follow the body of the fetus as it is being born. As the cavity of the uterus becomes smaller the area of the placental site is diminished so that the placenta is shorn off the spongy layer of the decidua basalis. Further uterine contractions now expel the placenta from the upper segment into the lower segment and vaginal vault. This process, whereby the placenta leaves the upper segment and occupies the lower segment and vagina, is referred to as *separation* of the placenta.

Immediately after the birth of the child the normal uterus is quiescent for a few minutes. Uterine contractions then begin again, but are not usually painful. When the placenta has separated it presses on the pelvic floor, causing the woman to have an involuntary desire to bear down. The placenta is expelled from the vagina, followed by the membranes and any retroplacental blood clot. There is generally an escape of less than 200 ml of blood as the placenta is delivered. If the uterus does not retract well there is further bleeding, but in the great majority of cases the strong retraction of the uterine muscle compresses the uterine sinuses so effectively that there is little further loss. The uterus can then be felt as a hard round ball about 10 cm in diameter, with the top of the uterus just below the level of the umbilicus.

There are two ways in which the placenta may pass through the vulva. In the Schultz method the placenta presents by its centre, which comes out first dragging the membranes behind it.

In the Matthews Duncan method the placenta presents by an edge and slips out of the vulva sideways. It is erroneous to suppose that the way in which the placenta leaves the vagina necessarily implies that that was the way in which it separated from the upper into the lower segment.

Normally the third stage lasts 10 to 20 minutes;

with modern active management this can be shorter (*see* p. 167).

DURATION OF LABOUR

Labour in primiparae usually lasts eight to 12 hours, the precise time of onset is often uncertain; in multiparae four to eight hours is usual. The first stage in primiparae usually lasts seven to 11 hours, the cervix taking much longer to dilate than in multiparae. In the second stage the perineum and vaginal orifice also offer greater resistance in primiparae. In some multiparae labour may last only two or three hours and the child may be born with only two or three contractions after full dilatation of the cervix.

When labour is very rapid it is referred to as being precipitate. Once a patient has had a precipitate labour subsequent deliveries tend to be of the same type.

THE MECHANISM OF NORMAL LABOUR

The following terms are used to describe the position of the fetus in relation to the uterus and maternal pelvis.

Lie

This means the relation which the long axis of the fetus bears to the uterus. The lie may be longitudinal, oblique or transverse.

Presentation

The presenting part of the fetus is that part which is in or over the pelvic brim and in relation to the cervix. When the head occupies the lower segment of the uterus the presentation is termed *cephalic*. If the head is flexed on the spine the *vertex* presents.

If the head is fully extended on the spine there is a *face presentation*, and if it is partly extended a *brow presentation*.

If the breech occupies the lower segment the presentation is termed *podalic*.

If the fetus lies obliquely the shoulder generally lies over the cervix and this is called a *shoulder presentation*.

Any presentation other than a vertex presentation is described as a malpresentation.

Position

Position describes the relationship which some selected part (the denominator) of the fetus bears to the maternal pelvis. The denominator varies according to the presentation being described. With a vertex presentation the denominator is the occiput, while with a face presentation it is the chin (mentum) and with a breech presentation, the sacrum.

It is conventional to describe four positions for each presentation. For example with a vertex presentation the occiput could be related to:

the left iliopectineal eminence – left occipito-anterior position (LOA) (Fig. 4.3)
the right iliopectineal eminence – right occipito-anterior position (ROA)
the right sacroiliac joint – right occipitoposterior position (ROP) (Fig. 4.4)
the left sacroiliac joint – left occipitoposterior position (LOP).

However, the occiput most commonly lies in the transverse diameter of the pelvic brim, and the terms left occipitotransverse position (LOT) and right occipitotransverse position (ROT) are useful.

Attitude (flexion or extension)

This term refers to the relation of the different parts of the fetus to one another. Normally the head, back and limbs of the fetus are flexed. In some abnormal presentations, which will be described in later chapters, the head or limbs may be extended.

In 96 per cent of cases at term the fetus lies longitudinally, with the head presenting. The reason for this is that the fetus adapts itself by its movements to the shape of the uterus. In the early months of pregnancy the liquor amnii is compara-

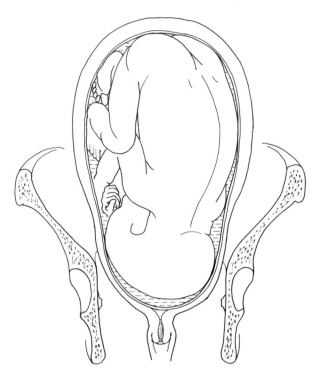

Fig. 4.3 Left occipitoanterior position

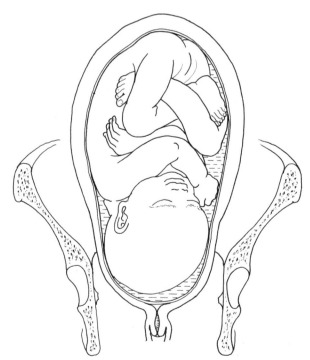

Fig. 4.4 Right occipitoposterior position

tively more abundant, and the fetus can float freely; but as pregnancy advances the fetus rapidly increases in size and the volume of liquor becomes comparatively less, so that the fetus is constrained to fit the shape of the uterus. When the attitude is one of complete flexion the buttocks, together with the adjacent parts of the thighs and the feet, constitute a mass which is larger than the head. The cavity of the uterus at term is pear-shaped, with the wider end uppermost; therefore the fetus fits into it best when the breech lies in the upper part of the uterus and the head in the lower part.

If the head cannot readily enter the brim of the pelvis a malpresentation may occur, for instance when the pelvic brim is severely contracted, or when a low-lying placenta or a pelvic tumour reduces the available space in the lower segment.

If the tone of the uterine and abdominal muscles is poor, as may be the case in a woman who has had many children, the factors which normally constrain the fetus to lie longitudinally are absent, and there may be a transverse or oblique lie. If the fetus is dead it may lie abnormally because it does not move and lacks muscular tone.

MECHANISM OF LABOUR WITH VERTEX PRESENTATIONS

The term 'mechanism' refers to the series of changes in position and attitude which the fetus undergoes during its passage through the birth canal. These should be studied with the help of a fetal model and a pelvis, as well as by observation of patients in labour.

The head is more or less oval, and fits fairly tightly into the birth canal through which it is pushed. The largest diameter of the pelvis is transverse at the inlet and anteroposterior at the outlet. The head, which normally enters the brim in the transverse or one of the oblique diameters, undergoes rotation and also some change in its attitude as it passes through the pelvic cavity. If the head and pelvis are both of normal size the mechanism of labour is determined by the soft parts rather than the bony pelvis.

Although four oblique positions of the occiput are conventionally described, in most cases the fetal head enters the brim in the transverse diameter. In less than 15 per cent of cases the occiput lies in relation to one of the sacroiliac joints at the onset of labour; it is never in direct relation to the promontory of the sacrum.

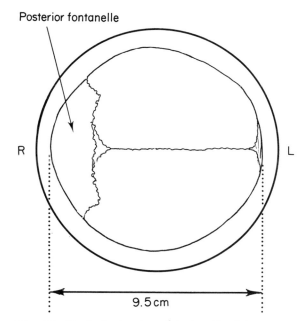

Posterior fontanelle

R   L

9.5 cm

Fig. 4.5 Vaginal palpation of the head in right occipitolateral position. The circle represents the pelvic cavity with a diameter of 12 cm. The head is well-flexed and only the sutures around the posterior fontanelle are felt

The degree of flexion or extension of the head is a most important factor in determining the mechanism of labour and therefore its outcome (Fig. 4.5).

MECHANISM WITH THE OCCIPUT IN THE TRANSVERSE OR ANTERIOR POSITION

For convenience of description the mechanism will be described for the LOT or LOA positions. (For the ROT or ROA positions the same description applies, but with substitution of 'right' for 'left' throughout.)

While the head is descending it makes five movements:

flexion
internal rotation
extension
restitution
external rotation.

Flexion

The head is often well flexed before labour starts, but if flexion is incomplete when labour starts it

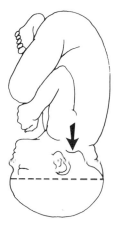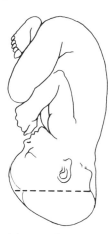

Fig. 4.6 Flexion of the head during labour. The arrow shows the direction of fetal axis pressure and the dotted line indicates the reduction in diameter of the flexed head

becomes complete as the uterine contractions drive the head down into the lower uterine segment. This is because:

any ovoid body being pressed through a tube tends to adapt its long diameter to the long axis of the tube

of the so-called head lever (Fig. 4.6).

The occipitospinal joint is nearer to the occiput than to the sinciput (forehead), so the head can be regarded as a lever with a long anterior and a short posterior arm. When the breech is pressed on by the uterine fundus the fetus is subjected to axial pressure and the lever comes into play. The long anterior arm meets with more resistance than the short posterior arm and the head flexes.

Flexion has the advantage of bringing the shortest suboccipitobregmatic diameter of the head into engagement, when the posterior fontanelle of the skull will be at a lower level than the anterior fontanelle.

Internal rotation

In the second stage of labour the forces propel the fetus progressively down the birth canal. When the head meets the resistance of the pelvic floor the occiput rotates forward from the LOT or LOA position to lie under the subpubic arch, with the sagittal suture in the anteroposterior diameter of the pelvic outlet (Fig. 4.7). This internal rotation of the head occurs because with a well-flexed head

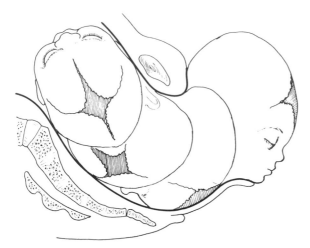

Fig. 4.7 Descent and flexion of the head followed by internal rotation and ending in birth of the head by extension

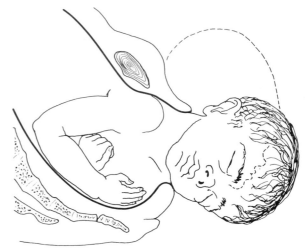

Fig. 4.8 External rotation of the head after delivery as the anterior shoulder rotates forward to pass under the subpubic arch

the occiput is leading and meets the sloping gutter of the levatores ani muscles which, by their shape, direct it anteriorly.

Extension

Further advance of the head leads to its passage through the vulva by a process of extension. Once the occiput has escaped from under the symphysis pubis the head extends, with the nape of the neck pressed firmly against the pubic arch. This extension of the head causes the anterior part to stretch the perineum gradually, until the moment of crowning when the greatest diameter slips through the vulva. Further extension allows the forehead, face and chin successively to escape over the perineum (Fig. 4.7).

Restitution

As the head descends with its suboccipitofrontal diameter in the transverse or right oblique diameter of the pelvis the shoulders enter the pelvic brim in the anteroposterior or the left oblique diameter. When internal rotation of the head takes place the head is twisted a little on the shoulders. As soon as it is completely born it resumes its natural position with regard to the shoulders, the occiput turning towards the mother's left thigh. This movement, which sometimes occurs almost with a jerk, is called restitution, because by it the

neck becomes untwisted and the head is restored to its natural relation to the shoulders.

External rotation

As the shoulders descend the right and anterior shoulder is lower and meets the resistance of the pelvic floor before the left shoulder. The right shoulder rotates to the space in front, as did the occiput, and the shoulders now occupy the anteroposterior diameter of the pelvis. As they rotate, the head, which has already been born, rotates with them and may make a further movement towards the mother's left thigh. The head now lies with the face to the right and the occiput to the left (Fig. 4.8).

Delivery of the body

The shoulders then emerge, the right one escaping under the pubic arch, while the left slides over the perineum. The rest of the body is usually born without any difficulty as its diameters are less than those of the head or the shoulders. The arms are usually folded on the chest, with the hands under the chin.

MECHANISM WITH THE OCCIPUT IN THE POSTERIOR POSITION

The ROP position is more common than the LOP

position, and will be described. (For the LOP position the same description applies but with the interchange of 'left' for 'right' throughout.)

The mechanism in the occipitoposterior positions depends on whether the head is well flexed or incompletely flexed.

The well-flexed head

If the head is well flexed the occiput is in advance when the head meets the resistance of the pelvic floor. The occiput slides down the gutter formed by the levator muscles, undergoing long rotation through three-eighths of a circle, to reach the free space under the pubic arch.

When the occiput lies behind and to the right (ROP) it rotates along the right side of the pelvis to reach the front, the shoulders rotating with the head from the left oblique diameter into the anteroposterior diameter. From this point the mechanism is the same as that of the ROA position, with birth of the head by extension.

Delay, which occurs in some cases of occipitoposterior position, is not because of this additional long rotation. If the head is fully flexed, as it must be for long rotation to occur, there is no delay in the labour and no difficulty. The cause of delay, if it occurs, is incomplete flexion, so that normal long rotation does not occur.

The incompletely-flexed head

When the occiput occupies the posterior part of one of the oblique diameters of the pelvis the biparietal diameter lies in the sacrocotyloid region of the pelvic brim. (This is the bay to one side of the promontory.) When the head is pushed down into the pelvis in this position the biparietal diameter is hindered in descending if the pelvis is small or the head is large, and so the forepart of the head descends more easily than the occiput and the head enters the pelvis incompletely flexed (Fig. 4.9).

If the head is incompletely flexed the larger occipitofrontal diameter of the head, which measures 11.5 cm, has to pass through the pelvis instead of the suboccipitobregmatic diameter, which measures 9.5 cm. It is this, and the fact that sometimes neither the occiput or the sinciput is sufficiently in advance of the other to influence rotation, that explains why some cases of occipitoposterior positions cause difficult and prolonged

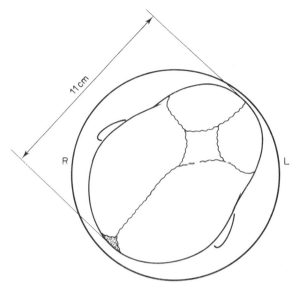

Fig. 4.9 Vaginal palpation of the head in the right occipitoposterior position. The circle represents the pelvic cavity with a diameter of 12 cm. The head is poorly flexed, so that the anterior fontanelle presents. Moulding is seen

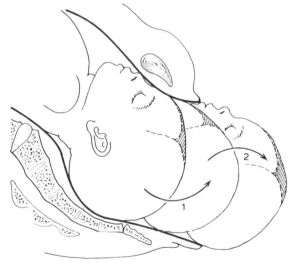

Fig. 4.10 Delivery of the head in the face-to-pubes position. 1, shows the head being born by flexion, this is followed by extension, shown in 2

labour. However, in some cases in which long rotation of the occiput does not occur spontaneously delivery takes place by an alternative mechanism, as follows.

If the head is incompletely flexed with an occipitoposterior position the forehead is as low as the occiput, and being at the anterior end of the oblique diameter of the pelvis it meets the resistance of the pelvic floor before the occiput. The forehead rotates to the front to the free space under the pubic arch, turning through one-eighth of a circle while the occiput rotates backwards into the hollow of the sacrum. The head may now be born with the face towards the posterior surface of the symphysis pubis. The root of the nose is pressed against the bone, and the head flexes about this fixed point. The vertex is born by *flexion* and followed by the occiput. As soon as the occiput is born the head extends, the face and chin emerging from under the pubic arch. The vulval orifice is stretched by the occipitofrontal instead of the suboccipitofrontal diameter, with a difference in size of 2 cm, and a severe perineal tear may result (Fig. 4.10).

DEEP TRANSVERSE ARREST OF THE HEAD

In some cases the head becomes arrested with its long axis in the transverse diameter of the pelvis, the degree of extension being such that neither the occiput nor the forehead is sufficiently in advance

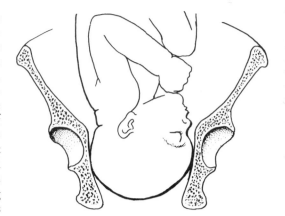

Fig. 4.11   Deep transverse arrest of the head

to influence rotation (Fig. 4.11).

This is described as deep transverse arrest of the head and calls for assistance (*see* p. 186). Some of these cases are the result of incomplete forward rotation from an occipitoposterior position. Others, perhaps the majority, are the result of the descent of a head which originally lay in the occipitotransverse position and which has failed to rotate anteriorly.

MANAGEMENT OF NORMAL LABOUR

In Britain today the majority of women are confined in hospital simply because obstetric emergencies such as fetal distress or postpartum haemorrhage may suddenly arise in apparently normal cases. The expertise and facilities to deal with an emergency are immediately available in hospital whereas there is inevitable delay if the crisis occurs in the patient's home, a delay which may be the deciding factor between life and death for the woman or her baby. Many women have the impression that childbirth is an entirely physiological event without risk, but this is not so in a proportion of cases. As a compromise for those who prefer home delivery many hospitals arrange for delivery in hospital and early discharge home after 24 or 48 hours, provided that there is a domiciliary midwife and a doctor willing to be responsible when the women returns home. Some units have facilities for a woman to be looked after by her own midwife and general practitioner while she is in hospital and some have rooms which are furnished like ordinary bedrooms in order to make the woman feel more at home. The presence of the child's father, or of a close relative, is welcomed throughout labour. Should an emergency arise in such a 'birthing room' the patient can be transferred to the main part of the hospital immediately.

Modern management of labour is carried out by a team consisting of obstetrician, senior registrar or registrar, senior house officer, midwife and obstetric nurse.

The role of the midwife is of the utmost importance. At present a midwife is the senior person present in at least 70 per cent of normal deliveries. Midwives are normally responsible for the care of women in labour, observing the progress of labour and the condition of the mother and her fetus, alleviating pain, preventing infection and supervising safe delivery. They look for abnormalities in labour and procure medical assistance when necessary, being ready to take emergency measures (e.g. urgent breech delivery or manual removal of the placenta) in the absence of medical help.

No labour is certainly normal until the third stage is safely concluded. Danger, especially to the fetus, can arise suddenly and unexpectedly, and to secure the greatest safety of the mother and baby, labour is best managed by intensive care techniques. There is no reason why modern methods of monitoring during labour should be psychologically harmful or interfere with normal labour; indeed there is some evidence that they may prevent unnecessary intervention. If their purpose is explained to the patient they should be reassuring to her.

Although the dangers of infection have been much reduced by the use of antibiotics, it is still very important to minimize the risk of introducing infection into the genital tract during labour. Full sterile precautions must be taken by those delivering the patient. Vaginal examinations should be limited as far as possible.

The first stage of labour is proceeding normally if the cervix is progressively dilating and the fetal condition is satisfactory. The second stage is normal when there is progressive descent of the head and the fetus is in good condition. These statements may seem very obvious, but they are the basis on which most of the observations made during labour rest.

Because of the increased risk to mother and fetus during prolonged labour, labours are no longer permitted to continue for great lengths of time. Delay in the first stage is overcome by active management, and delay in the second stage by the use of forceps or the vacuum extractor.

MANAGEMENT OF THE FIRST STAGE

On admission, the woman's antenatal record is reviewed to discover whether there have been any abnormalities during her pregnancy. In a few instances there will have been no antenatal care; in such circumstances a complete history must be taken. In every case the woman's general condition is assessed, her pulse rate and blood pressure are recorded, and her urine is tested for protein and sugar. By abdominal examination the presentation

and position of the fetus, and the relation of the presenting part to the brim of the pelvis, are determined. Abdominal examination will also show the frequency and strength of the uterine contractions. The fetal heart rate is counted for a full minute and any abnormality of rate or rhythm is noted. A vaginal examination will show the degree of dilatation of the cervix, whether the membranes are intact or ruptured and the level and position of the presenting part.

Much of the apprehension from which many women suffer during labour may be removed by adequate explanation beforehand. The best time to give this is in antenatal classes to which the woman may go with her partner. She will find it a great comfort to hear what labour entails in her partner's presence, knowing that he will be at her side all through the confinement. If it is explained to them that the first stage of labour may last up to ten hours, during which it will be difficult for her to appreciate that there is much progress, it will be much easier to reassure her at the time that all is well. She should, however, always be kept informed about dilatation of the cervix and of the condition of her baby. If it is decided that the best way of checking the fetal heart is with a monitoring device its purpose must be explained. The reason for any intervention must also be discussed fully with the woman and her partner. If there is free communication between attendants and patient there will almost always be full cooperation. At no time in labour should the woman be left alone. The partner should be with her all the time, and the midwife as much as possible.

It is unnecessary to give an enema or to clip or shave the vulval hair. These practices are of no particular benefit and are generally disliked. A warm bath or shower, however, is both hygenic and pleasant.

If the head is engaged there is no need for the woman to remain in bed during early labour. If she is up and about the weight of the liquor and the fetus helps to dilate the cervix and pressure on the lower segment stimulates the uterus to contract. If the presenting part is not engaged the woman is kept in bed to diminish the likelihood of prolapse of the cord when the membranes rupture.

Discomfort during the early part of the first stage may not be severe, although in primiparae it may cause distress. Towards the end of the first stage the pains become more severe. If epidural analgesia (*see* p. 173) is not employed, drugs such as pethidine 100 mg intramuscularly may be given when labour is established if the woman is distressed, but a woman who has been appropriately prepared for labour should be allowed to decide for herself whether, and when, she wants any analgesia. The knowledge that help is available gives her confidence and she may prefer to defer its use for a time. As pethidine sometimes causes nausea, metoclopramide (Maxolon) 10 mg may also be injected intramuscularly. Some women obtain relief by means of transcutaneous electrical nerve stimulation (TENS) but the method is not universally available.

There may be a frequent desire to pass urine during the first stage. When the head is deep in the pelvis the woman may be unable to pass urine and the bladder rises up into the abdomen where it can be seen and felt as a suprapubic swelling. A soft catheter should be passed, as a full bladder has an inhibiting effect on the uterine contractions.

During labour there is delay in the emptying time of the stomach, and food or fluids may remain there for several hours. If a general anaesthetic has to be given for any reason there is a risk of vomit being inhaled and the acid contents of the stomach may cause bronchiolar spasm (Mendelson's syndrome). Alkali given by mouth may reduce the severity of this complication, but it is better to withhold solid food during labour, and if fluid or glucose is required for dehydration or ketosis this should be given intravenously.

Dextrose solutions given intravenously during labour must be properly controlled. There have been instances of injudicious administration of large volumes of fluid containing no sodium, resulting in maternal and fetal hyponatraemia. If large volumes of intravenous fluid are given for any reason during labour, physiologically balanced infusions such as Hartmann's solution must be employed. Modern drip counters allow strict control of the volume of fluid used.

Large volumes of water are retained during pregnancy, chiefly in the maternal extracellular compartment (p. 29) and unless there has been excessive vomiting significant dehydration or ketosis are unlikely in a labour lasting less than 24 hours.

Towards the end of the first stage, if epidural analgesia is not used, administration of nitrous oxide and oxygen may be started with the onset of each contraction (*see* p. 174).

Partogram

Once labour has become established, or the membranes have ruptured, all events during labour are noted on a partogram – a most useful graphical record of the course of labour. Routine observations of the mother's pulse rate and blood pressure, with an assessment of the strength of the uterine contractions are entered on it. Records of the findings at successive vaginal examinations are plotted on a graph, showing the dilatation of the cervix in centimetres against the time in hours. The curve obtained is compared with an average curve for normal primigravidae or multigravidae as may be appropriate in any given population. If the patient's progress is normal her curve will correspond with the normal curve, or lie to the left of it.

Friedman, who introduced the idea of the partogram, has described two phases of labour:

> the *latent phase*, from the onset of labour until the cervix is about 3 cm dilated, which may last three to seven hours in a primigravida
> the *active phase*, during which dilatation from 3 to 10 cm is more rapid, taking three to seven hours, so that the slope of the partogram curve will be steeper in this phase (Fig. 4.12).

If labour is not progressing normally in the active phase, dilatation of the cervix will become slower or may cease and the patient's partogram will be to the right of the normal curve. A vaginal examination should be made every three or four hours, and if there is delay the membranes should be ruptured and uterine action augmented by administration of an oxytocic infusion if there is no progress after the membranes are ruptured (*see* p. 177).

All this information about the strength and frequency of the uterine contractions, the dilatation of the cervix and (later in labour) descent of the head, and the state of the mother and fetus can be shown on the partogram. Drugs that are given should also be recorded (Fig. 4.13).

Fetal monitoring

The other important observations which must be made during labour relate to the fetus. If simple clinical observations are all that are possible these must be made and recorded regularly. The fetal heart rate is counted with a stethoscope at half-hourly intervals in early labour and at 10 minute intervals in the active phase of labour. The normal

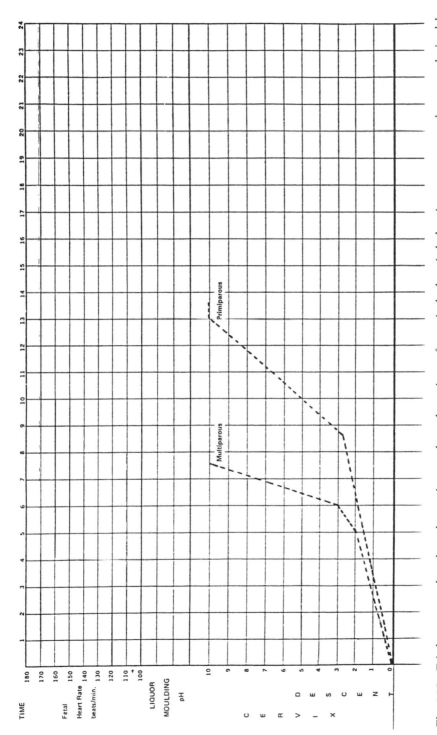

Fig. 4.12 Friedman curves based on observations made on the patients of a particular hospital, showing average normal progress during labour in that population. The time of admission will vary from patient to patient, and therefore the starting point of the observations will also vary. In general, the active phase of labour begins when the cervix is about 3 cm dilated. For practical use in the labour ward it is possible to prepare a series of stencils which can be superimposed on the partogram according to the parity of the patient and the degree of dilatation when she is first seen

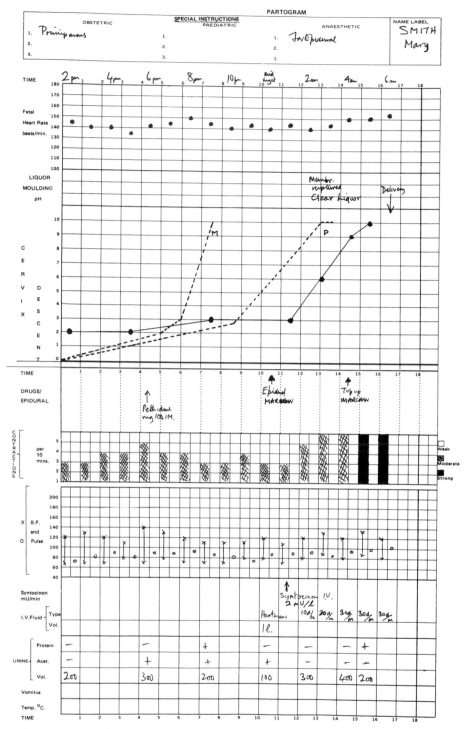

Fig. 4.13 Example of a partogram. Only the middle section is shown. At (a) there is a chart of the fetal heart rate and at (b) there is a chart of the maternal blood pressure and pulse rate. In the illustrative case shown there was a prolonged latent phase. The membranes were artificially ruptured with little effect on the contractions. With intravenous oxytocin (2 units/500 ml) at 10 and then 20 drops per minute the uterine contractions improved and the active phase soon followed. At the point marked M, meconium was seen in the liquor and there were some decelerations in the fetal heart rate, but a fetal blood sample showed a pH of 7.3 and labour was allowed to continue, ending in an easy forceps delivery. (The partogram shown is part of that devised by Mr J Studd and used at King's College Hospital)

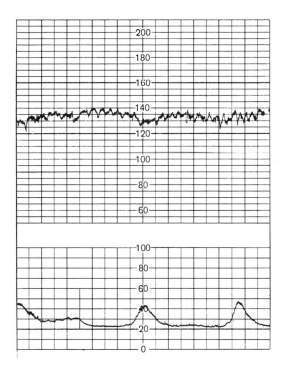

Fig. 4.14 Fetal heart rate, normal trace. The lower trace records the uterine contractions

rate is between 120 and 160 beats per minute and there is no change of rate, or only a very transient slowing, with the uterine contractions. For signs of fetal distress *see* page 216.

Most hospitals now employ fetal monitoring during labour. The uterine contractions can be recorded with a strain gauge strapped to the mother's abdomen, and the fetal heart can be monitored with an ultrasonic device attached in the same way (Fig. 4.14). The ultrasound record of the fetal heart rate is not always satisfactory, although this simple method can be tried first. After the membranes have ruptured and the cervix has started to dilate a more reliable record can be obtained by attaching a clip to the fetal scalp (through the cervix) from which a lead passes to a machine which calculates the heart rate continuously by measuring the intervals between R waves in the fetal electrocardiographic cycles. In normal labour the basal heart rate between contractions is between 120 and 160 beats per minute, with a continuous slight 'beat-to-beat' variation of the order of five beats per minute. In normal labour the heart rate may slow with each uterine

contraction, but the slowing is neither profound nor prolonged. Prolonged deceleration or loss of beat-to-beat variations may be sinister signs. Details of these and other abnormalities which may be observed in the trace are discussed on page 218.

Where resources are limited monitoring may only be possible for high-risk cases and those in whom clinical signs suggesting fetal distress appear, but to secure the best possible surveillance of the fetus the ideal would be to monitor every labour, because half the instances of hypoxia during labour occur without evident preceding high risk factors. However, some women object to the routine use of monitoring. They dislike any apparent interference in a normal labour and the limitation of free movement caused by the electrical leads to the recording machine; they may also fear fetal injury from the scalp electrode. Restriction of mobility may in future be overcome with apparatus that sends radio signals to the recording machine, so that leads are not required, but this is, at present, very expensive. Particularly in high risk cases, the patient's cooperation can usually be obtained if the purpose and advantage of monitoring is explained.

If the monitor or clinical observations suggest that there may be fetal distress a sample of fetal blood is taken from the fetal scalp to determine its pH and thus, indirectly, whether there is fetal hypoxia or not (*see* p. 220).

These rather technical methods of checking that all is well with the mother and baby must never be allowed to take the place of close contact between doctors, midwives and the patient, and clinical assessment of well-being must not be omitted or disregarded.

Active management of labour

Most obstetricians believe that by abandoning the historical teaching of masterly inactivity, and with the help of modern technology, they can ensure that childbirth is a safer and happier experience for the mother and her baby. In the first stage of labour this includes effective analgesia (including epidural block); monitoring the fetal heart with a ratemeter and the uterine contractions with a tocograph; recording cervical dilatation on a partogram to make sure that progress is being made and the occasional use of an oxytocic drip. Provided that the woman understands the reasons for these measures she will usually accept them in the knowledge that they are undertaken for her benefit and for that of her baby. It is stressed that they are to be used selectively, not routinely, and in particular that it is only necessary to accelerate labour with an oxytocic drip if progress is abnormally slow.

MANAGEMENT OF THE SECOND STAGE

During the second stage the woman should be on her bed and the midwife or doctor should stay with her.

Early in the second stage it does not matter what position the woman adopts, but if she is well propped up in the lithotomy position with her head upright and her hands behind her knees she will be in a comfortable position to push effectively, with some assistance from gravity. Occasionally, because of supine hypotension, slowing or other changes in the fetal heart rate occur with the patient in the dorsal position (*see* p. 219). If such changes occur the patient is turned onto her side.

As each uterine contraction pushes the head down onto the pelvic floor the expulsive reflex comes into play and the woman will generally take a deep breath, hold it, and strain down. In a first labour the woman needs to be encouraged to relax the muscles of the pelvic floor at the time of the contraction. The progress of the descent of the head can be judged by watching the perineum. At first there is a slight general bulge as the patient strains. When the head stretches the perineum the anus will begin to open, and soon after this the caput will be seen at the vulva at the height of each contraction. Between contractions the elastic tone of the perineal muscles will push the head back into the cavity of the pelvis. The perineal body and vulval outlet become more and more stretched until eventually the head is low enough to pass forwards under the subpubic arch. When the head no longer recedes between contractions this indicates that it has passed through the pelvic floor and that delivery is imminent.

When the head begins to appear at the vulva it must be decided whether the woman is to be delivered on her back or on her side. If little help is available the left lateral position is probably better, and it may be easier to control the birth of the head in this position. When assistance is available most women are delivered in the dorsal position, as described above.

Different positions may be adopted in the second stage according to individual preference. There has been a recent tendency for a minority of women to ask to give birth in such positions as on all fours, squatting, kneeling or standing upright, claiming that such positions make delivery easier. Birthing chairs have been tried in some hospitals, and usually given up. In Russia babies have been delivered under water in large tanks. There is little evidence that delivery in any of these positions is more rapid or comfortable, and they have the disadvantage that they make proper observation of the fetal heart rate and control of analgesia very difficult, and care of the perineum hardly possible. However, the right of every woman to deliver her baby in the manner she wishes must be considered sympathetically.

If delivery is left entirely to nature laceration of the perineum often occurs during birth of the head. By the time that the head begins to appear at the vulva some form of analgesia is usually desirable. An epidural or pudendal block or local infiltration may be used (*see* p. 174) but alternatively inhalation of a mixture of nitrous oxide and oxygen is often effective.

At this stage the accoucheur must control the head to prevent its being born suddenly, and it must be kept flexed until the largest diameter has passed the vulval outlet. Once the head is crowned the woman should be discouraged from bearing down by telling her to take rapid shallow breaths. The head may now be delivered carefully by pressure through the perineum onto the fore part of the head by means of a finger and thumb placed on either side of the anus, pushing the head forwards slowly before it is allowed to extend and complete its delivery and controlling the rate of escape with the other hand (*see* Fig. 4.15).

If extension of the head begins before the biparietal diameter has passed through the vulval orifice a larger diameter than the suboccipitofrontal will distend the vulva and a tear may result. Even if the head has become crowned gradually, perineal rupture may occur if the head is then expelled suddenly and rapidly; it is important that the head should be born slowly and in an interval between pains.

Episiotomy, or incision of the perineal body, is necessary in some cases (*see* p. 277) and a clean incision is always preferable to an irregular laceration, or even to a grossly overstretched perineal body. Because of adverse lay propaganda against episiotomy it is important to explain to the woman

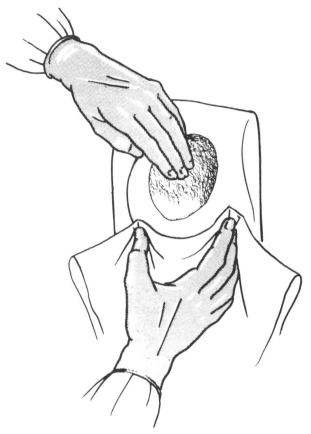

Fig. 4.15 Care of the perineum. The left hand is preventing sudden expulsion of the head, while the fingers and thumb of the right hand are gently helping the head forwards by pressure on each side of the anus

beforehand that it is sometimes necessary, and to assure her that it will not be performed as a mere routine.

Directly the head is born a finger is inserted to feel whether a loop of cord is round the neck. Such a loop should be slipped over the head; if this cannot be done the cord is clamped with two pairs of artery forceps and divided between them.

The shoulders usually follow with the contraction following the birth of the head, the anterior shoulder being delivered before the posterior. Even if the head has been born without perineal laceration the shoulders can cause damage unless they are carefully delivered.

If the shoulders do not descend after the birth of the head the mother should be exhorted to bear down. If the shoulders still do not move and the baby's head is becoming cyanosed birth must be

assisted. If the shoulders have not rotated into the anteroposterior diameter of the pelvis they must be rotated by digital pressure. If there is still delay attempts must then be made to bring the anterior shoulder under the subpubic arch by bending the neck laterally (towards the anus). Once the anterior shoulder has passed the symphysis pubis the posterior shoulder can usually be delivered after pulling the head forwards. As little force as possible should be used, for fear of injury to the brachial plexus. An assistant can help by pressing on the fundus of the uterus at the same time.

In cases of extreme difficulty a finger may be passed up to the anterior axilla of the fetus and the shoulder pulled down; or else a hand may be passed behind the posterior shoulder into the hollow of the sacrum and the posterior arm brought down over the perineum by flexing it at the shoulder and elbow. This makes more room and the anterior shoulder is then easily delivered.

After delivery of the shoulders the rest of the body quickly follows. As soon as the child is delivered it is held with its head downwards so that any liquor or mucus in the mouth can run out. The mouth and pharynx are sucked clear with a mucus extractor. A healthy baby breathes and cries very soon after it is born; if it fails to do so it is treated as described on page 295.

In a normal case the cord should not be clamped until the child has cried vigorously and pulsation in the cord has ceased. If it is clamped immediately the baby is deprived of about 50 ml of blood which would be drawn out of the placenta by the expansion of the lungs. It is best to keep the baby at the same level as the placenta or a little below it. If the baby is held high above the placenta (which may be done inadvertently at caesarean section) blood may run back into the placenta with the risk of hypovolaemia or subsequent anaemia in the baby. For this reason the fashionable practice of placing the baby on the mother's abdomen 'skin to skin' immediately after birth is of doubtful wisdom, and the unwrapped baby may also suffer heat loss. Once the baby is breathing normally and the cord has been divided it should be wrapped up and handed to the mother to hold, cuddle and enjoy.

At first the cord is divided between two artery forceps placed about 15 cm from the umbilicus. Later a plastic Hollister crushing clamp is placed on the cord 1 to 2 cm from the umbilicus and the cord is cut again 1 cm beyond the clamp. When this is done the cut end of the cord is examined to make sure that both umbilical arteries are present (*see* p. 171).

If spontaneous respiration is not established soon after birth resuscitation is the immediate priority and the baby is taken to the resuscitation table directly after the cord is divided.

MANAGEMENT OF THE THIRD STAGE

In a normal delivery, if oxytocic drugs are not injected, the uterus will generally remain quiescent for a few minutes after the delivery of the baby. Regular contractions then begin again. These detach the placenta and push it down into the lower uterine segment and vagina (Fig. 4.16). The mother will become aware of its presence on the pelvic floor, and by straining expel it through the vagina.

The following signs indicate that the placenta has separated and been expelled from the upper uterine segment:

the cord moves down. It may be difficult to be sure of this, and in case of doubt the fundus of the uterus may be gently pressed upward by a hand placed just above the pubis. If the placenta is still in the upper segment the cord will be drawn up with the uterus

the uterus rises up because it is now perched on the lower segment which contains the placenta, and when it contracts the empty upper segment feels hard, round and movable from side to side

there is often a small gush of blood when the placenta leaves the uterus

the placenta can be felt with a finger inserted into the vagina.

The third stage of labour is a natural process which can be managed by simple observation and without interference unless bleeding or delay occurs, but even with such conservative management postpartum haemorrhage sometimes occurs if the uterus relaxes. However, nearly all obstetricians now advocate an alternative and more active method of management of the third stage because this has been found to be safer.

Active management of the third stage

After 1935 ergometrine became available as an effective and non-toxic oxytocic agent. It was at first used for the treatment of postpartum haemorrhage after the uterus had been emptied but it was soon found that by giving it at the time of birth, or immediately afterwards, the number of cases of excessive bleeding (defined as a loss of more than 500 ml) was reduced. Ergometrine causes a prolonged contraction of the uterus without periods of relaxation, and while the uterus is contracting there is not likely to be any bleeding. It is therefore a most valuable drug given in a dose of 500 micrograms by intramuscular or intravenous injection in cases of excessive blood loss.

However, ergometrine may cause nausea and vomiting and there is usually a significant rise in

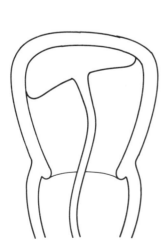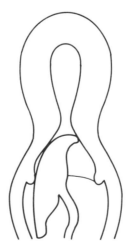

Fig. 4.16   Signs of descent of the placenta. After separation the contracted upper segment is at a higher level and feels more rounded

blood pressure. Because of these disadvantages there is a tendency for obstetricians to prefer Syntocinon, 5 units, for routine management of the third stage of labour. Syntocinon is given by intramuscular or intravenous injection with delivery of the anterior shoulder in a primigravida or while the head is crowning in a multipara. With this method the third stage of labour is shortened and blood loss is reduced. As soon as the signs of separation are present, showing that the placenta is in the lower uterine segment and vagina, the placenta is delivered by the Brandt-Andrews' method, as described below.

By injecting an oxytocic drug before the placenta has separated there is a small risk that the placenta may be grasped by the contracting upper segment and become retained, with a slight increase in the number of cases in which manual removal of the placenta becomes necessary. But this disadvantage is small compared with the advantage of reduction in incidence of postpartum haemorrhage.

Syntometrine is a preparation containing 500 micrograms of ergometrine and 5 units of Syntocinon per ml. It can be given as an alternative to Syntocinon alone or ergometrine, but as it has the disadvantages of ergometrine it is not preferred to Syntocinon alone.

Brandt-Andrews' method of delivering the placenta

With the patient lying on her back the obstetrician places his left hand over the anterior surface of the uterus just above the symphysis pubis, at the presumed level of the junction of the upper and lower segments. An artery forceps is placed on the umbilical cord, which is held just taut but without strong traction with the right hand (Fig. 4.17). The uterus is pushed gently upwards with the left hand and if this can be done satisfactorily it means that the placenta is below the level of the lifting hand and is in the lower segment or vagina. Lifting is now discontinued and, with the uterus contracted, pressure is made with the same (left) hand in a downward direction while the cord is still held taut until the placenta is seen at the introitus. After the placenta has been expelled the uterus is lifted out of the pelvis, as this is thought to diminish the tendency to haemorrhage. It will be noted that the principle of the method is not cord traction but rather elevation of the uterus, which helps to

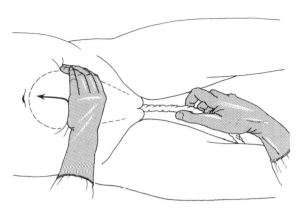

Fig. 4.17 Brandt–Andrews method of delivery of the placenta

prevent acute inversion of the uterus (*see* p. 224) as a complication.

The membranes generally slip out after the placenta. However, if they do not come away with gentle traction on the placenta they should be held with artery forceps and gently pulled, when they will usually be extracted.

Examination of the placenta, membranes and cord

These must always be examined carefully as soon as possible. The maternal surface of the placenta will be seen to be divided into cotyledons, but these should all fit together when the maternal surface is made concave. If any part is missing a gap will be seen.

The membranes should form a complete bag except for the hole through which the fetus passed. The amnion and chorion can be separately examined after peeling the amnion off the chorion. An important but rare abnormality is that in which blood vessels run off the edge of the placenta to a small detached island of placental tissue called a *succenturiate lobe* (*see* p. 72). If this has come away with the main placenta and membranes it will be plainly seen, but if it is retained there will be a hole in the chorion corresponding to it, to which the vessels pass.

The cut end of the cord should be examined. A rare abnormality is absence of one umbilical artery. This is important as it may be associated with other congenital abnormalities.

If a piece of placenta is retained it is almost certain to cause postpartum haemorrhage, therefore it should be removed as soon as the diagnosis is made. In cases of doubt an ultrasound scan will show whether the uterus is empty. However, if a piece of membrane is retained within the uterus, be it large or small, it will not cause any complications and will come away in two or three days; uterine exploration is not necessary.

Examination of the perineum

After the placenta is delivered the vulval outlet must be examined carefully for lacerations after separating the labia, with the woman on her back. Any tear other than a minute one must be sutured immediately.

THE RELIEF OF PAIN IN LABOUR

The obstetrician James Young Simpson was the first person to use chloroform for the relief of pain in labour in 1847. Dr John Snow administered chloroform to Queen Victoria during the births of her two youngest children, and 'chloroform à la Reine' became popular for analgesia during normal labour.

The amount of pain experienced during labour appears to vary enormously from patient to patient. A few women find that labour is almost painless, but the majority have pain that they describe as severe. Some will manage with minimal doses of analgesic drugs while others demand much more.

During the first stage of labour pain is felt with each uterine contraction. The pressure in the uterus between contractions is of the order of 1.33 kPa (10 mmHg). During a first stage contraction the pressure is about 6.65 kPa (50 mmHg). Most patients do not feel pain until the pressure reaches 3.325 kPa (25 mmHg); the beginning of the contraction can be felt with the hand or recorded with a tocograph before the patient feels pain. The pain is believed to be caused by ischaemia of the myometrium, which occurs when the blood flow is arrested or impeded by the contraction.

The nerve pathway for the pain of uterine contractions is the hypogastric plexus and then the preaortic plexus, entering the cord as high as the 11th and 12th dorsal segments via the posterior nerve roots.

Pain is also caused by dilatation of the cervix, and this is severe at the end of the first stage. Sensory impulses from the cervix probably enter the cord via the sacral roots; pain towards the end of the first stage is often referred to the sacral region.

The upper vagina distends easily and this does not seem to cause much pain, but during the second stage, when the head is stretching the vulval orifice, severe pain is felt which is different from that of uterine contraction. Pain impulses from the vulva and perineum are carried by the pudendal nerves, and to a small extent by the ilioinguinal, genitofemoral and posterior femoral cutaneous nerves.

During the antenatal period patients should be told about the stages of labour in simple terms, avoiding technical words and the jargon of the labour ward. It is particularly important to explain that the first stage of labour is long compared to the second, and that during the first stage the cervix is being opened up, and that there will be no sensation of progress or descent of the baby. In a normal second stage the patient will be encouraged by feeling the descent of the baby and the realization that the end of labour is not far away. The severity of pain may not be altered by explanation, but fear of the unknown and fear that the labour is not progressing normally can greatly add to mental distress.

There are those who believe that if the patient is tense and anxious this will impede the progress of labour, and that if she is relaxed labour will be both quicker and less painful. While it is agreed that a tense pelvic floor might delay delivery, there is nothing to show that dilatation of the cervix will be affected by the patient's state of mind. However, it is probable that the patient who relaxes completely and rests between pains is conserving her energy, and will be able to make stronger voluntary efforts in the second stage. Moreover, labour will be a less unpleasant experience for her.

Various courses of antenatal exercises have been recommended. If they give the patient confidence they are useful and helpful, although there is little or no scientific evidence that they have any other effect on the course of labour. It is wrong to tell women that if only they follow some pattern of exercises or relaxation that they will have little pain and that labour will be quick and normal; when this sometimes proves to be untrue disappointment may turn into anxiety and recrimination.

Patients should be told about the various means of relieving pain, and that these will be available on demand. Secure in the knowledge that help is available many women will not ask for any analgesic until the first stage is well advanced. Drugs should never be given in a routine fashion, but always with respect for the patient's wishes and need. During antenatal instruction classes the patients should visit the labour ward and if possible meet the staff who will look after them there, and be given a demonstration of such equipment as the gas and oxygen machine.

During labour women should never be allowed to feel that they have been left alone and deserted. A sensible and affectionate partner can give much support and comfort, provided that he has also been given a little instruction and told what to expect. The knowledge that a trusted doctor or midwife is present or immediately available will make labour more tolerable.

THE IDEAL ANALGESIC

An ideal analgesic for labour will not harm or endanger the mother or the fetus. In particular it should not:

interfere with uterine action
lead to more operative intervention
depress the respiratory centre of the newborn infant.

In addition to its analgesic effect it should be:

easy to administer
foolproof
predictable and constant in its effects.

ANALGESIA IN THE FIRST STAGE OF LABOUR

Three methods are in common use during the first stage:

drugs which are given by intramuscular injection. This method is simple and convenient. Oral administration of drugs during labour is unsatisfactory because absorption is unreliable

an anaesthetic agent which is inhaled. This method is not suitable for use over long periods, and is therefore only used in the latter part of the first stage; it is more appropriate for the second stage

an epidural or caudal block. This gives complete relief of pain, but requires skill in injection, and has a few hazards.

ANALGESIC DRUGS

Over the years many drugs have been used, but *pethidine* is now in almost universal use. It is a synthetic drug which is less effective than morphine in relieving pain, but has less of a depressant effect on the respiratory centre of the newborn infant. However, it is untrue to say that it has no depressant effect, and it should not be given if delivery is expected within two hours. The usual dose is 100–150 mg intramuscularly and 50–100 mg can be repeated after two hours. In an average labour the total dose should not exceed 400 mg. Pethidine sometimes has an emetic effect, this can be counteracted with metoclopramide (Maxolon) 10 mg intramuscularly.

Morphine sulphate 15 mg, sometimes combined with hyoscine 0.4 mg, is seldom used today for normal labour because of its effect on the infant's respiratory centre, but in cases in which the fetus is dead or grossly abnormal (e.g. anencephalic) such drugs will give good pain relief.

Respiratory depression in the newborn from pethidine or morphine can be counteracted by injecting naloxone (Narcan neonatal) into the umbilical vein. The preparation contains 20 micrograms/ml, and the dose is 5 micrograms/kg.

INHALATION ANALGESIA

See p. 174.

EPIDURAL BLOCK

This is usually started in the first stage, and it may be continued throughout labour. It is preferable to spinal anaesthesia during pregnancy, because the latter causes vasomotor paralysis of the lower part of the body, and if this is combined with interference with the venous return by the large uterus sudden and severe hypotension may occur.

The anaesthetic is injected into the epidural space through a Tuohy needle which is usually inserted between the 1st and 2nd lumbar spines. Lignocaine (Xylocaine) 1 per cent is used if rapid analgesia is required. Marcain 0.5 per cent has more prolonged action but takes longer to produce analgesia. A polythene catheter is threaded through the needle and left in the epidural space so that further injections of the anaesthetic can be given as required. The injection calls for some skill and experience of the method, and whoever gives it must maintain continuous supervision and be prepared to deal with immediate complications such as hypotension or temporary respiratory paralysis from accidental inthrathecal injection. Long-term neurological sequelae such as weakness or paraesthesia of the legs or bladder disturbances are very rare.

In some hospitals epidural anaesthesia is provided for more than half of the patients in normal labour, but a 24 hour service makes heavy demands on anaesthetic staff. With epidural analgesia the incidence of low forceps delivery will be increased because voluntary expulsive efforts are often ineffective, but apart from this there are no adverse fetal effects. Because it is not affected by the analgesic drug used, the fetus is usually born in the most favourable condition, breathing and crying as soon as the head is out. Uterine tone is good, and the risk of postpartum haemorrhage is reduced.

Epidural anaesthesia is excellent for cases of prolonged labour from inco-ordinate uterine action, for vaginal operative procedures such as rotation and forceps delivery of a head in the occipitoposterior position, for breech delivery, for severe cases of hypertension and for caesarean section.

CAUDAL BLOCK

This is an alternative method of introducing an extradural block. A malleable needle is inserted through the sacral hiatus into the sacral canal and a catheter may be left in the extradural space to continue the injection. The lumbar route is now generally preferred.

TRANSCUTANEOUS ELECTRICAL NERVE STIMULATION (TENS)

This is a self-administered method for relieving pain based on the gate control theory of pain. It supposes that excitation of large myelinated afferent nerve fibres reduces the pain impulses conducted by small myelinated and non-myelinated fibres. Part of the analgesic effect may be due to the production of endogenous opioids. A battery-powered stimulator is connected by wires to electrodes placed on either side of the spine in the dermatome corresponding to the pain. It is a harmless method which gives a measure of relief from pain in the first stage of labour in about half of the patients who try it.

ANALGESIA FOR THE NORMAL SECOND STAGE OF LABOUR

Two methods are in common use:

intermittent inhalation of anaesthetic mixtures
epidural or nerve block.

INTERMITTENT INHALATION METHODS

Nitrous oxide mixtures

Nitrous oxide and oxygen can be given as the patient requires it with the Entonox machine. This has gas cylinders containing a mixture of nitrous oxide and oxygen in equal proportions. The cylinders must not be kept below room temperature, because at lower temperatures the gases separate out. Self-administration depends on the patient fitting the mask accurately to her nose and mouth, and closing the valve with her finger. She should take a deep breath as soon as the pain starts and continue breathing throughout the contraction.

EPIDURAL OR NERVE BLOCK

These methods have many advantages. They do not affect the baby's respiratory centre, nor the uterine action. Except for epidural analgesia, the services of an anaesthetist are not required. In comparison with general anaesthesia they are much safer during labour because the risk of the unprepared patient inhaling vomit is avoided. Furthermore many woman like to be fully conscious during delivery. Methods in general use include:

Epidural block

This has been described above.

Pudendal block

This simple method can be used for normal delivery, including repair of an episiotomy or perineal tear, for forceps delivery or vacuum extraction, for breech and twin delivery. The pudendal nerve is derived from the 2nd, 3rd and 4th sacral nerves. These roots unite above the level of the ischial spine. The nerve passes out of the greater sciatic foramen posteriorly to the ischial spine and re-enters the pelvis through the lesser sciatic foramen. It then enters the pudendal canal where the vessels lie lateral to the nerve. The nerve divides into:

 the inferior haemorrhoidal nerve, giving branches to the anal sphincter and the skin around the anus
 the perineal branch, supplying the perineal muscles and the skin of the perineum and labia majora
 the dorsal nerve of the clitoris, supplying the clitoris and labia minora.

Fibres from the posterior femoral cutaneous nerve and from the ilioinguinal nerve also reach the perineum.

Lignocaine hydrochloride 1 per cent is used throughout (without adrenaline). The total amount injected should not exceed 50 ml. A skin weal is raised half-way between the anus and the ischial tuberosity. The index finger of the left hand is inserted in the vagina and the left ischial spine is located. A 20 cm 20 gauge needle is passed through the weal and directed towards the ischial spine with the guidance of the vaginal finger (Fig. 4.18). The needle is directed just posteriorly to the inferior tip of the spine. The plunger of the syringe is withdrawn to make sure that the needle is not in a vein and about 5 ml of lignocaine solution is injected. The needle is inserted a further centimetre and, after testing for intravasation by withdrawing the plunger again, another 5 ml of lignocaine is injected. The process is repeated on the right side.

Some prefer to insert the needle through the vaginal wall rather than the perineal skin.

Pudendal block is usually combined with local infiltration of the vulva, a weal being raised at the fourchette and lignocaine injected here and on each side, extending well forward in both labia majora. If the local infiltration is carried out before the pudendal block it will reduce the discomfort of the manipulations required for the block.

Perineal infiltration

If an episiotomy is required in advanced labour with the presenting part well down, direct infiltration of the line of incision with 10 ml of lignocaine 1 per cent is employed.

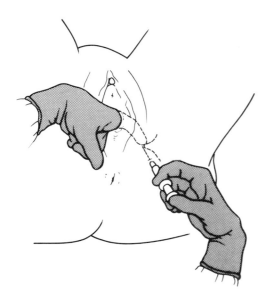

Fig. 4.18 Pudendal block. The index finger of the left hand helps to direct the needle to the correct position

ANAESTHESIA FOR OPERATIVE DELIVERY

Numerous anaesthetic techniques are available for operative deliveries. For vaginal delivery, an epidural or pudendal block is used whenever possible, but sometimes general anaesthesia is unavoidable. For lower segment caesarean section some abdominal relaxation is required and general anaesthesia (including the use of a relaxant, *see* p. 291) is often employed. Many caesarean operations are performed under epidural block, when the woman can be awake and given her baby to hold soon after its delivery. Section can also be performed under regional infiltration of the abdominal wall. Whatever method is used, morphine and allied drugs which may depress the respiratory centre of the newborn infant should not be given for premedication.

THE DANGER OF GENERAL ANAESTHESIA IN OBSTETRICS

The Reports on Confidential Enquiries into Maternal Deaths in England and Wales show that a number of fatalities occur every year from complications of general anaesthesia. Most of these are caused by inhalation of vomit when solid particles obstruct the bronchioles, or by acid secretion causing intense bronchial spasm (Mendelson's syndrome). It is extremely dangerous to give a general anaesthetic if the head of the obstetric bed cannot be lowered immediately should vomiting occur, and without proper suction apparatus ready.

Although the responsibility for the technical details of general anaesthesia during labour does not fall to the obstetrician, it must never be forgotten that any patient in labour may unexpectedly need an anaesthetic. Solid food should never be given to women in labour, because during labour there is gastric stasis and the stomach may contain food which has been taken many hours before. In cases of abnormal labour in which treatment under general anaesthesia is a possibility, cimetidine 200 mg may be given 8-hourly by mouth. The passage of a gastric tube is sometimes prudent before an emergency anaesthetic; 15 ml of 0.3 M solution of sodium citrate, or an H_2 receptor blocker such as ranitidine 150 mg is more commonly given by mouth before induction of anaesthesia. A most useful preventative measure against inhalation of vomitus during induction of anaesthesia is cricoid pressure. As the patient is falling asleep and the relaxant that is commonly used is taking effect, an assistant pushes the cricoid cartilage back against the cervical vertebrae so as to compress the oesophagus and prevent regurgitation into the pharynx until the cuffed endotracheal tube is passed and inflated.

Should vomiting occur the head of the patient must be lowered at once and turned on one side so that vomit can flow out of the mouth. The pharynx is immediately cleared with suction apparatus. If inhalation has occurred the patient must be carefully observed afterwards lest there should be collapse of the lungs. If Mendelson's syndrome develops 500 mg of hydrocortisone is given intravenously and oxygen used as required. Further injections of hydrocortisone 250 mg 6-hourly may be required, and prophylactic antibiotics are given.

An administrative problem is that emergency obstetric anaesthesia is often required at inconvenient hours, or when senior anaesthetists are already engaged with other work. In large obstetric units provision of anaesthetic cover at all times for the labour ward is a necessity, not only for the comfort but for the safety of the patients.

THE USE OF OXYTOCIC DRUGS

OXYTOCIN (SYNTOCINON)

In 1906, Dale found that extracts of posterior pituitary gland had an oxytocic action. These extracts were first used in obstetrics by Blair Bell three years later. They contained:

antidiuretic hormone (vasopressin)
oxytocin.

Nowadays the unwanted antidiuretic effect of vasopressin has been eliminated by using a synthetic preparation of oxytocin – Syntocinon.

Oxytocin is an octapeptide. It causes contraction of the myometrium and also of the myoepithelial cells of the breast.

The response of the myometrium to oxytocin (Syntocinon) is relatively slight until late pregnancy when, in response to physiological doses, strong but rhythmical contractions occur (unlike the prolonged spasm produced by ergometrine). However, abnormally large doses of Syntocinon will cause sustained contraction, which can arrest the placental blood flow and cause fetal hypoxia or even death. There have been a number of cases of uterine rupture after administration of Syntocinon. This is not so much a condemnation of the drug as of the mode of administration. If the treatment is properly supervised so as to produce contractions which are no stronger than those of normal labour the risk of rupture is no more than in spontaneous labour. Clearly there is some risk of rupture if the patient has a caesarean scar, when even more careful supervision is required.

An increase in neonatal hyperbilirubinaemia has

been reported after the use of Syntocinon to induce labour. The reason for this is uncertain, but it is possible that oxytocin causes osmotic swelling of erythrocytes, reducing their plasticity so that they are more easily haemolysed.

Oxytocin is destroyed in the gastrointestinal tract and Syntocinon is therefore administered by intravenous infusion. The dose is measured in units based on a standard preparation.

CLINICAL USES OF OXYTOCIN

To induce labour

Syntocinon is most effective as term is approached or passed, but it has some effect even in cases of missed abortion or hydatidiform mole (for which high concentrations can be used) (*see* p. 70).

To augment slow labour

A Syntocinon infusion may be used to accelerate labour if there is delay from inadequate uterine action (*see* below) but care must be taken to exclude mechanical obstruction as a cause of the delay (*see* p. 208).

In the third stage of labour

Syntocinon may be used for the preventative treatment of postpartum haemorrhage, given intramuscularly as an injection of 5 or 10 units, or by intravenous infusion at a level of 100 mU/min.

During therapeutic abortion

Syntocinon is sometimes used to enhance uterine contractions during therapeutic abortion induced with prostaglandins.

METHOD OF ADMINISTRATION FOR INDUCTION OR AUGMENTATION OF LABOUR

Any patient receiving intravenous Syntocinon must be under continuous supervision, ideally by means of a cardiotograph, which records simultaneously the fetal heart rate and uterine contractions.

Infusion pumps regulate the flow of solution better than gravity drips. By adding 10 units of Syntocinon to 500 ml of isotonic saline, one drop

of the infusion will contain approximately 1 mU of Syntocinon (assuming 20 drops/ml of infusion).

The starting dose is 2 mU/min, increasing at intervals of 15 min according to the strength and frequency of the uterine contractions to a maximum of 32 mU/min. This may be achieved by manual control, or if an intrauterine pressure catheter (IUPC) has been inserted, by a monitor which has an automated feedback mechanism. Once contractions are occurring regularly the rate of infusion can often be decreased, but the infusion should be kept running until the third stage of labour is complete. If at any time there is evidence of fetal distress or hypertonic uterine contractions the infusion is stopped immediately.

ERGOMETRINE

In the Middle Ages epidemics of ergotism (St Anthony's fire – with gangrene of the limbs and toxic effects on the central nervous system) used to occur after eating rye which had been infected by a fungus, *Claviceps purpurea*. It was found that an infusion of infected rye would expedite labour. Various vasoconstrictors such as ergotamine and ergotoxin were extracted from crude ergot, but it was not until 1932 that Chassar Moir and Dudley separated ergometrine, the substance which is responsible for the strong action of ergot on the uterus.

Ergometrine has an almost specific action on the myometrium, but it also has general vasoconstrictor action, which may cause a rapid rise in blood pressure in patients who are already hypertensive. It may also induce nausea and vomiting. Ergometrine maleate may be injected intravenously, intramuscularly or given by mouth. After intravenous injection of 500 micrograms a strong uterine contraction occurs within 40 seconds, and persists for 30 minutes. After intramuscular injection the time before the uterus contracts is about six minutes, and even if hyalase is added to the injection the time will be four minutes. Therefore if ergometrine is to be used for postpartum haemorrhage it should be given intravenously, or by direct injection through the anterior abdominal wall into the uterus if peripheral vasoconstriction has rendered the intravenous route difficult. As an alternative for preventing postpartum haemorrhage a mixture of Syntocinon 5 units and ergometrine 500 micrograms (Syntometrine) may be given intramuscularly. The Syntocinon will act in about two minutes, its action will be followed and maintained by that of the ergometrine.

If the uterus remains flaccid after one dose of 500 micrograms of ergometrine a second, similar dose may be given. No more than two doses should be given, as occasional cases of severe peripheral vasoconstriction have been reported. If oxytocic action is still inadequate a Syntocinon infusion can be used.

The risk of causing a rise of blood pressure, particularly in a patient who is already hypertensive, has been mentioned. Because of this Syntocinon alone is now often preferred for active management of the third stage of labour, and ergometrine is only used if haemorrhage occurs. It has also been suggested that ergometrine should be withheld in cases of cardiac disease, but there is little evidence of any risk.

Ergometrine should never be given to expedite the delivery of a living child, as the uterine spasm which it produces will stop the placental blood flow, and there is also a risk of uterine rupture.

Ergometrine is used in the treatment of abortion and at caesarean section. It is also sometimes used in puerperium if the loss is unduly heavy, but it is futile to give it with the hope of increasing the rate of uterine involution; it causes contraction, not involution.

5

ABNORMAL LABOUR

PROLONGED LABOUR

When obstetricians speak of prolonged labour they invariably mean prolongation of its first stage, a condition which occurs most commonly in primiparae. Prolongation of the second stage of labour is referred to as delay and is dealt with in Chapter 8, which details those procedures that can hasten delivery of the infant through a fully dilated cervix. The physiology of the first stage of labour and the proper management of normal labour have been described in Chapter 4.

Progress in labour is judged by:

dilatation of the cervix, measured from 0–10 cm
descent of the fetal head, measured in fifths of the fetal head palpable per abdomen or in centimetres above or below the ischial spines on vaginal examination.

Additional assessments made during the first stage of labour are:

the condition of the mother, i.e. her pulse rate, temperature, blood pressure, urine output, urinary protein and ketones and psychological state
the condition of the fetus as judged by such methods as auscultation of the fetal heart rate at regular intervals and looking for meconium in the amniotic fluid; or by more modern means such as cardiotocography and measurement of fetal scalp blood pH
the size of caput and the extent of moulding, the presence of either or both indicating a tight fit between the fetal head and the maternal pelvis.

THE PARTOGRAM

In all but the most rapid labours progress is usually charted on a partogram (see Chapter 4, p. 164). That portion of the partogram which plots cervical dilation (cm) against time (h) is called the cervimetric graph (or cervicogram) and is the focus of attention in the recognition and classification of prolonged labour. The cervicogram is usually started when labour becomes established (sometimes a difficult diagnosis) or at the time when an amniotomy is done as part of the surgical induction of labour.

The first stage of labour is divided into the latent and active phases. The latent phase is the time spent achieving 3 cm cervical dilatation, and can take six hours. The active phase is from 3 to 10 cm dilatation and, at just under 1 cm dilatation per hour, also takes about six hours, making a total of about 12 hours for the acceptable normal duration of the first stage of labour in a primipara; multiparae do not take this long.

Types of prolonged labour

When the first stage of labour exceeds the time limits given above the patient's cervimetric graph moves to lie to the right of the accepted norm (*see* Fig. 5.1) and labour is prolonged. Three types of prolonged labour are recognized:

prolonged latent phase, lasting for more than six hours

primary dysfunctional labour, when uterine activity is either inert or incoordinate from the start of the active phase

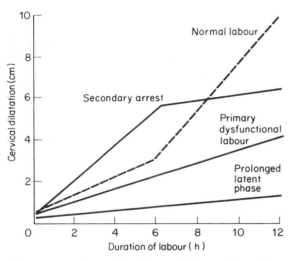

Fig. 5.1 Cervicographs of normal labour (dotted line) and the three types of prolonged labour. *See* table 5.1 for information about fetal and maternal outcome in each group

secondary arrest, when the rate of cervical dilatation, which is normal at first, slows down.

The characteristic cervimetric graphs for each of these three types of prolonged labour are shown in Figure 5.1 and data about the outcome of normal labour and the three types of prolonged labour are given in Table 5.1.

Prolongation of the first stage of labour occurs in about one in three primiparae and in about one in eight multiparae. In both types of patient prolonged labour is associated with a much higher (10- to 16-fold) caesarean section rate and a roughly four-fold increase of low five minute Apgar scores (6 or less) over those that are found in patients whose pattern of labour is normal (*see* Chapter 9, p. 296 for a detailed discussion of Apgar scores). It is small wonder that prolonged labour is regarded as a high risk condition requiring the best hospital facilities and specialist skills.

The causes of prolonged labour

Cephalopelvic disproportion (see p. 205)

This diagnosis is made whenever the presenting fetal head seems to be too big for the birth canal that it has to pass through; it is by far the most important cause of prolonged labour.

The causes of cephalopelvic disproportion are:

Fetal
malpositions (*see* Chapter 4)
malformation (e.g. hydrocephaly)
macrosomia or a large baby.

Table 5.1 Incidence and outcome of various types of labour in primiparae and multiparae who go into labour spontaneously (from Cardozo LD, Gibb DMF, Studd JWW *et al. British Journal of Obstetrics and Gynaecology*: **89**, 33–38 and 708–711

	Cervimetric pattern	Incidence (%)	Caesarean section rate in each group (%)	Apgar scores of 6 or less at 5 min (%)
Primipara (n=684)	Normal	63.9	1.6	2.6
	Prolonged latent phase	3.5	16.7	8.3
	Primary dysfunctional labour	26.3	20.0	5.5
	Secondary arrest	6.3	27.9	–
Multipara (n=847)	Normal	88.4	0.5	2.4
	Prolonged latent phase	1.4	8.3	8.3
	Primary dysfunctional labour	8.1	8.8	4.3
	Secondary arrest	2.1	5.9	–

Maternal
  contracted pelvis.
A combination of A and B.

Abnormalities

Abnormalities which can cause prolonged labour in the absence of cephalopelvic disproportion are:

  Fetal malpresentation (brow, shoulder, face or breech – *see* p. 186)
  Maternal abnormalities
    pelvic tumour
    stenosis or scarring of the cervix
    septae or stenosis of the vagina
    primary uterine dysfunction (i.e. uterine dysfunction or inertia which is not secondary to disproportion).

The investigation of prolonged labour

The first thing that must be considered before making a diagnosis of prolonged labour is the possibility that there has been uncertainty about timing the onset of labour. Next it is important to assess and examine the patient in order to identify the cause and to determine the condition of mother and baby. To do this it is necessary to take a history, assess the contractions, review cardiotocographic recordings and also to make general, abdominal and vaginal examinations.

The treatment of prolonged labour

There are two alternative courses of action:

  to allow the labour to continue in the hope of a vaginal delivery
  to undertake an operative delivery.

A prolonged labour should never be allowed to degenerate into an obstructed labour – the potentially disastrous outcome of which is described on page 209.

Allowing the labour to continue

In the absence of fetal distress, maternal distress or severe cephalopelvic disproportion the labour may be allowed to continue in the hope of achieving a vaginal delivery. If the labour is allowed to continue it is important to ensure:

  adequate analgesia (often the only way of achieving this is by an epidural block)
  good maternal fluid balance with treatment of dehydration by adequate volumes of normal saline or dextrose/saline given intravenously
  rupture of membranes if they are still intact
  good uterine activity, which often means augmentation of labour with a Syntocinon infusion.

Syntocinon infusions for augmenting labour are usually started at a dose of 2 mu/min and the dose is gradually increased until optimum uterine activity is obtained (but not beyond 32 mu/min). In these circumstances it is important to assess uterine contractions or activity with care and accuracy. The best method available is an intrauterine transducer, particularly if it can be linked to a monitor which automatically measures and prints out uterine activity above the resting baseline in kPas (kiloPascalseconds), a normal value being about 1500 kPas/15 min.

In the absence of such sophisticated equipment fluid-filled intrauterine catheter systems or external sensors which give qualitative recordings of uterine activity are available. In the units where there is no monitoring equipment, the timing and assessment of the strength of uterine contractions by hand becomes one of the functions of the birth attendant, who must keep a careful record, preferably on a partogram.

If prolonged labour is being managed conservatively it is vital to establish good communications with the patient and her partner, relatives or friends, who are invariably anxious and impatient. Detailed and careful explanations of the rationale and the nature of all aspects of management should be offered. Doctors and midwives supervising such patients should recognize this responsibility and when they go off duty they should take care to introduce the patient to the new team to whom the responsibility is being transferred.

Operative delivery

In the presence of fetal distress, maternal distress, evidence of arrest of cervical dilatation despite good contractions or frank cephalopelvic disproportion the baby will have to be delivered; the usual method is by caesarean section. In rare circumstances it might be possible to achieve a ventouse extraction (*see* p. 286) before full dilatation of the cervix but this should only be attempted if there is no caput or moulding, the head is well down in a roomy pelvis, there is no fetal distress and the sole reason for prolongation of labour seems to be ineffective uterine activity.

In Third World countries, where there is poor access to hospitals, there may be a reluctance to do caesarean sections because of possible rupture of the uterine scar in subsequent pregnancies and labour. Under these circumstances prolonged labour due to frank cephalopelvic disproportion may, in rare and carefully selected instances, be treated by symphysiotomy. However, this procedure should only be undertaken by trained experts and should only be attempted when there are good uterine contractions, when the leading part of the moulded head is deep in the pelvis and when the cervix is more than 5 cm dilated. The immediate complication of symphysiotomy is damage to the urethra and bladder; long-term problems are instability of the symphyseal joint with a painful waddling gait and stress incontinence of urine.

FETAL MALPOSITION AND MALPRESENTATION

OCCIPITOPOSTERIOR POSITIONS OF THE VERTEX

The mechanism of labour in occipitoposterior positions of the vertex has already been described in Chapter 4 (pp. 160–162). In most cases in which the occiput lies posteriorly at the onset of labour normal vaginal delivery occurs. With good flexion of the head, the occiput (being the first part of the head to meet the pelvic floor) usually undergoes long rotation forward through three-eighths of a circle and is thus directed to the space below the pubic arch. In about 20 per cent of the cases this does not occur and the malposition persists. A short backward rotation of one-eighth of a circle may then take place which results in the occiput being directed to lie in the hollow of the sacrum. This may occur because the head is poorly flexed, so that the first part of the fetal head to meet the pelvic floor is the sinciput, and this part of the head then rotates forward. In patients who have epidural anaesthesia, the musculature of the pelvic floor loses some of its resistance. This lack of resistance may increase the incidence of failure to rotate when a vertex in the occipitoposterior position meets the pelvic floor.

The direction of rotation of the fetal skull may also be influenced by the shape of the cavity and outlet of the pelvis. In the android type of pelvis (p. 202) there is narrowing of the pelvic cavity from side to side, and the size of the cavity tends to diminish in the lower straits. The pubic arch is narrower and the ischial spines project more into the birth canal. There therefore tends to be less room in the anterior part of the pelvis and a posterior position of the occiput may persist even with good flexion of the head.

With an occipitoposterior position the head is pushed downwards and forwards against the back of the symphysis pubis rather than directly downwards onto the cervix. Thus some of the effectiveness of the uterine contractions is lost, cervical dilatation tends to be slow and labour is prolonged. The cervix may be compressed between the head and the pubis, so that progressive oedema of the anterior lip of the cervix occurs.

Diagnosis

Diagnosis during pregnancy is of no importance except that the occipitoposterior position must be recognized as a cause of non-engagement of the head before the onset of labour. During labour a lack of flexion of the head may be suspected if there is early rupture of the membranes.

Abdominal examination

During the intervals between uterine contractions slight flattening of the lower abdomen may be observed, and the limbs, being in front, are easily felt. It may be difficult to define the back or to hear the fetal heart. This should be listened for well to the side of the abdomen and towards the mother's back, but it may sometimes be best heard in the midline when the sounds are heard through the anterior chest wall of the fetus. The head usually descends through the pelvic brim as labour proceeds, but descent may be slow because with poor flexion a wider diameter presents.

Vaginal examination

Early in labour it may be difficult to reach the presenting part and the membranes may rupture early. When the head has entered the pelvic cavity the most striking feature is the ease with which the anterior fontanelle can be felt behind the pubis. The anterior fontanelle is more easily felt because the head is less well flexed, and also because it lies well forward when the head is in the occipitoposterior position. An attempt should be made to assess the degree of flexion of the head, as the well-flexed head is more likely to rotate. If only the anterior fontanelle can be felt the head is poorly flexed; it is less poorly flexed if both the anterior and posterior fontanelles can be felt; it is well flexed if only the posterior fontanelle is felt (Fig. 5.2).

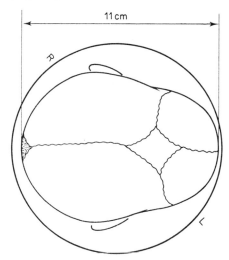

Fig. 5.2 Vaginal palpation of the head in the right occipitoposterior position. The circle represents the pelvic cavity with a diameter of 12 cm. The head is poorly flexed, so that the anterior fontanelle is easily felt

Although the diagnosis should be made early in labour, it frequently happens that the position is unrecognized until there is delay in the second stage of labour. Diagnosis by vaginal examination may then be difficult owing to the formation of a caput succedaneum over the presenting part. Before forceps delivery, when it is essential to have accurate knowledge of the direction of the occiput, the fingers may be passed higher to feel the sutures above the caput and the free margin of an ear, which will point to the occiput.

The course of labour in occipitoposterior positions

In about 70 per cent of cases spontaneous rotation of the occiput to the anterior position occurs, and in about another 10 per cent of cases the occiput undergoes short rotation so that delivery in the occipitoposterior position (face-to-pubes) can occur. In the remainder assisted rotation will be required.

During labour the uterine contractions may be ineffective because the poorly-flexed head fails to press down upon the cervix and provide the reflex stimulation of the lower segment that is produced by the more pointed vertex with full flexion. A long first stage is likely to be followed by a long second stage because the woman is tired and the uterus may be less capable of further strong contractions.

Moulding of the head

When the fetal head descends through the birth

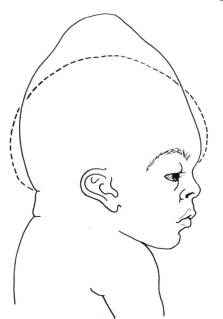

Fig. 5.3 Moulding of the head and formation of caput succedameum is persistent occipitoposterior position

canal and flexion of the head is poor the skull will be compressed in the occipitofrontal diameter (Fig. 5.3). If the alteration in shape is extreme the structures of the skull may not adapt well to the relatively sudden change. Great compression along the occipitofrontal diameter causes tension in the posterior vertical part of the falx cerebri. This elevates the tentorium cerebelli, which may ultimately tear at its free margin. The upward dislocation of the tentorium may result in rupture of the great cerebral vein (vein of Galen) or a tributary of it, and fetal damage or death from intracranial haemorrhage.

Management of the first stage of labour

The first stage is managed as in a normal case. Nothing can be done to correct the malposition or to influence the rotation of the head at this stage.

The frequency, duration and strength of the uterine contractions, the dilatation of the cervix and the fetal heart rate are observed in the ordinary way and recorded on a partogram. A continuous epidural block will not only give pain relief but will allow time for spontaneous rotation of the occiput into the anterior position. If progressive cervical dilatation does not occur augmentation of the uterine action with a Syntocinon drip by the method described on page 181 may be tried. If this does not result in better progress in a few hours caesarean section is performed. Caesarean section will also be required if fetal distress occurs.

Management of the second stage of labour

A mistaken diagnosis of full dilatation of the cervix is not uncommon in these cases, when the patient complains of rectal discomfort and a desire to bear down. Vaginal examination is essential to establish that the second stage has been reached. The degree of flexion of the head and its position are determined by palpation of the fontanelles. Continued deflexion, a large caput succedaneum or marked over-riding of the skull bones suggest that spontaneous rotation may not occur.

In most cases, provided that the uterine contractions are strong and the patient is able to make good expulsive efforts the occiput rotates forward and normal delivery takes place. In other cases the baby may be delivered face-to-pubes without any difficulty, although there is a greater risk of a perineal tear.

The indications for interference in these cases are:

> failure of the presenting part to descend
> fetal distress
> maternal distress.

It is desirable for the head to be in the occipitoanterior position, because it presents a smaller and more favourable diameter and therefore the first step in assisting delivery is rotation of the fetal head. This can be performed:

> manually
> with Kielland's forceps
> with the vacuum extractor during traction if the cup is applied to the occipital part of the vertex.

Manual rotation

Unless an epidural anaesthetic has already been given, a pudendal block or general anaesthesia will be required. After careful diagnostic examination the head is rotated with the hand in the appropriate direction. Thus, if the fetus is in the right occipitoposterior position the head is rotated so that the occiput travels round the right wall of the pelvis until it is directly anterior; the opposite direction of rotation is followed for a left occipitoposterior position. The shoulder girdle of the fetus should be rotated at the same time as the fetal head. If this is not done the head will tend to slip back after rotation into an oblique or transverse diameter of the pelvis. Rotation of the shoulder girdle may be achieved by pressure through the abdominal wall with an external hand (Fig. 5.4).

It is undesirable to displace the head upwards and this should be avoided, as it will make subsequent application of the forceps more difficult. It is often possible to achieve rotation with the half hand. Rotation is effected by tangential pressure on the side of the head with the fingers only, without grasping the head with fingers and thumb. After rotation to the occipitoanterior position has been achieved the fingers are kept in place to hold the head in position until the obstetric forceps are applied to complete the delivery.

Difficulties arise if the forceps are applied to the head in any position other than with the sagittal suture in the anteroposterior diameter of the pelvis. If this position is not achieved the forceps will not lock properly and the handles will not lie

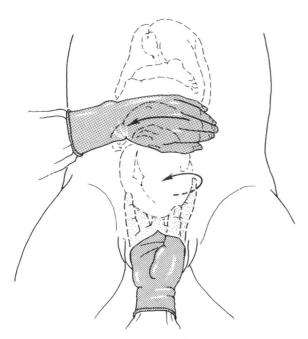

Fig. 5.4 Manual rotation of the fetus in the occipitoposterior position. The right hand passes between the pelvic wall and the fetal head and is about to rotate the head. The left hand placed on the abdomen will assist this rotation by pressure on the shoulder

together. Squeezing the handles will only compress the head and may cause fetal injury, and when traction is applied the blades may slip off and also cause maternal injury.

Kielland's forceps

This instrument is of relatively light construction and is designed so that it can be used for rotation of the fetal head, in addition to traction. The pelvic curve of the shank has been eliminated and the lock allows one shank to slide upwards or downwards on the other (*see* Fig. 8.14) Without a pelvic curve the circle described by the blades during rotation is a small one, thus avoiding damage to maternal tissues, bladder and rectum. In experienced hands the instrument is safe and most satisfactory, but it is potentially dangerous in the hands of anyone not trained in its use. The technique of application of Kielland's forceps differs from that for ordinary forceps in that the instrument is applied with reference to the fetal head in whatever position it lies, and not in relation to the pelvis. These forceps are used before traction is applied to

rotate the head until the occiput lies anteriorly. Details of the method of use are given on page 284. If the instrument is incorrectly used damage to both maternal tissues and the fetal head may occur.

Vacuum extraction

If the extractor is applied as near to the occipital end of the vertex as possible, and traction is applied, forward rotation of the head often occurs. For the method of application *see* page 286.

Arrest at the pelvic outlet

If it is found that arrest has occurred when the head is so low in the pelvic cavity that with each contraction of the uterus the fetal scalp is easily visible it is probable that further progress is being prevented by the muscles of the pelvic floor. To reach this level the head will already have undergone a considerable degree of moulding into the shape described for the persistent posterior position of the occiput (p. 183). It may be found easier to perform an episiotomy and assist the delivery of the baby in the unrotated occipitoposterior position. The large occipitofrontal diameter, albeit shortened by moulding, will have to pass through the pelvic floor and therefore the episiotomy should be adequate. Traction with the obstetric forceps must be careful and only moderate force should be used. The instrument was not designed to fit the head in this position and may slip off. However, only moderate traction is necessary to complete the delivery of a fetal head which is arrested by the perineal muscles at this low level. The vacuum extractor can be used instead of the forceps.

Trial of forceps with an occipitoposterior position

If the baby seems unduly large, if two-fifths of the head are still abdominally palpable, if there is marked caput or moulding, if the ischial spines are unduly prominent, if there is any suggestion of outlet contraction (a rare condition) or if the head is not visible at the height of a second stage contraction, there could be difficulty in rotating and delivering a head in the occipitoposterior position. Under these circumstances it is appropriate to conduct a *trial of forceps*. This means embarking on a forceps delivery with everything prepared for caesarean section and with the patient under general or effective epidural anaesthesia. Should there be any difficulty in applying the blades, or if it appears that too much force is needed to extract the baby's head, it is then easy and perfectly proper to abandon the attempt at operative vaginal delivery and to resort to caesarean section without delay and without undue risk to mother or baby.

Failed forceps is the term used to describe an unsuccessful attempt to deliver the baby which has been made in the absence of preparations for a possible caesarean section. It is a situation which should never arise.

DEEP TRANSVERSE ARREST OF THE HEAD

This term denotes arrest in labour when the fetal head has descended to the level of the ischial spines and the sagittal suture lies in the transverse diameter of the pelvis. The occiput is on one side of the pelvis and the sinciput on the other; the head is badly flexed. The condition is only diagnosed during the second stage of labour. If the head is firmly fixed in the transverse position obstructed labour will occur.

The occiput may have been obliquely posterior at the onset of labour and only partly rotated forward, or it may have descended from an initial transverse position.

In an android pelvis the anterior surface of the sacrum may be flattened and the ischial spines may be prominent because the side walls of the pelvis are convergent. The head fails to descend to the pelvic floor, where rotation of the head normally occurs.

Diagnosis

Because the progress of labour has ceased the diagnosis rests on vaginal examination made during the second stage of labour. The head will be found to be arrested at the level of the ischial spines, with the sagittal suture lying in the transverse diameter of the pelvis. Both fontanelles are usually palpable.

Management

The head must be rotated so that the occiput is brought to the front and then, and only then, is traction applied. Rotation may be done manually

or with Kielland's forceps. Exactly the same procedure is followed, and exactly the same precautions are taken as have already been described for rotation of the head from occipitoposterior position.

FACE PRESENTATION

Face presentation, in which the head is fully extended, occurs about once in 300 labours (Fig. 5.5)

Causes

The most common type of case is one in which a normal fetus actively holds its head extended; even after delivery the infant may keep its head in an attitude of exaggerated extension for some days. In spite of this the head can be flexed on to the chest, showing that there is no spinal or muscular abnormality.

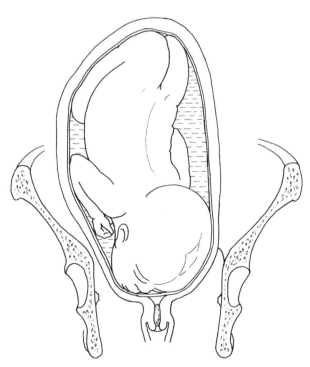

Fig. 5.5   Face presentation, right mentoposterior position. The face from the chin to the bregma presents, the submentobregmatic diameter occupying the right oblique diameter of the pelvic inlet. The back faces forwards and to the left, but is extended instead of flexed as in a vertex presentation, so that the breech is more prominent and is more easily palpated

In anencephaly the abnormal head of the fetus is set on the shoulders with the face directed upwards, and the face may present in labour. With congenital tumours of the neck the head may also be extended.

Rarely, with a contracted pelvis, the biparietal diameter of the head is too large to enter the brim of the pelvis, the occiput is held up and the sinciput descends, so that the head becomes extended.

Mechanisms

The chin is the denominator and four positions are conventionally described, analogous to the corresponding positions of the vertex from which they may be said to arise:

right mentoposterior
left mentoposterior
left mentoanterior
right mentoanterior.

The mentoanterior positions are relatively more frequent (Fig. 5.6).

In a mentoanterior position the head engages and descends with increasing extension, so that the submentobregmatic diameter (9.5 cm) comes through the cervix. When the chin reaches the pelvic floor it undergoes internal rotation through

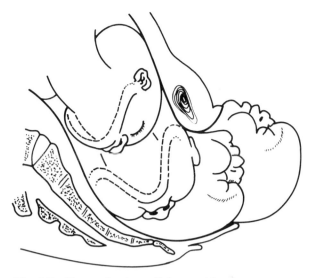

Fig. 5.7 The mechanism of labour with a face presentation. The head descends with increasing extension. The chin reaches the pelvic floor and undergoes forward rotation. The head is born by flexion

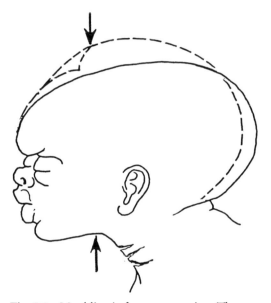

Fig. 5.8 Moulding in face presentation. The arrows indicate the direction of the pressure which shortens the diameter between the submentovertical and submentobregmatic diameters. The splitting of the skin in the front of the neck and the swelling of the face are also shown

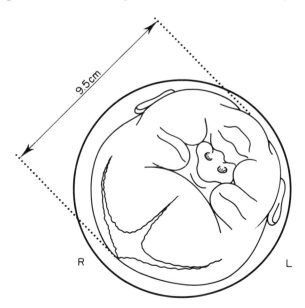

Fig. 5.6 Vaginal examination in the left mentoanterior position. The circle represents the pelvic cavity with a diameter of 12 cm

one-eighth of a circle and the submental region comes to lie under the subpubic arch. The head is then born by a movement of flexion. Restitution occurs and is followed by external rotation as in vertex presentations.

In a mentoposterior position a similar mechanism occurs, except that the chin has to undergo internal rotation through three-eighths of a circle (Fig. 5.7).

Backwards short rotation of the chin sometimes occurs, but a fetus in such a persistent mentoposterior position cannot be delivered unless it is very small. This is because the head is already fully extended and so further extension to deliver the head is impossible. The head and thorax become impacted in the pelvis and obstructed labour occurs unless assistance is given.

Moulding

In a face presentation the submentovertical diameter of the head is compressed, causing elongation of the occipitofrontal diameter (Fig. 5.8). This shape of the head is called dolichocephaly.

Diagnosis

Abdominal examination

With a mentoposterior position the cephalic prominence is very easily felt; it appears to overlap the symphysis and is felt on the same side as the back, from which it is separated by a deep sulcus. It may be difficult to locate and hear the fetal heart sounds.

With a mentoanterior position the cephalic prominence is again felt on the same side as the back but, being posterior, it is difficult to feel and may be confused with the prominent chest. The fetal heart is easily heard over the chest, and small parts may be felt on the same side.

Vaginal examination

As the face fits less well than the vertex the membranes may rupture early. When the presenting part has engaged in the brim and can be felt, the supraorbital ridges, the bridge of the nose and the alveolar margins within the mouth are recognized. If the face is oedematous it can be mistaken for the breech.

Prognosis

Many face presentations are delivered naturally without difficulty. Face presentations are less favourable than vertex presentations because the face is a less efficient dilator of the cervix, and because spontaneous rotation of the mentoposterior positions occurs late in the second stage of labour. The emerging diameter, the submentovertical (11 cm), is larger than that with a normal vertex presentation.

Management of labour and delivery

The patient is kept in bed during the first stage and a vaginal examination is made as soon as the membranes rupture to exclude prolapse of the cord. An epidural block or infiltration of the perineum with local anaesthetic and an episiotomy are advisable in primigravidae if there is any delay when the cervix becomes fully dilated and the face reaches the pelvic floor. With a mentoanterior position spontaneous delivery is to be expected. If there is delay in the second stage from inadequate expulsive forces an experienced operator will have no difficulty in applying the forceps.

With a mentoposterior position time should be allowed for spontaneous rotation, which will only occur late in the second stage. If spontaneous rotation does not occur manual rotation of the head to the mentoanterior position is attempted under epidural block or general anaesthesia, after rotation delivery is completed with the forceps. The expert may prefer to use Kielland's forceps, with which the chin is rotated forwards while traction is applied. When undertaking rotation and delivery for a mentoposterior position the obstetrician should conduct the delivery as a trial of forceps. Vacuum extraction is obviously totally contraindicated with a face presentation.

Caesarean section becomes necessary when there is some complication, such as a contracted pelvis, prolapse of the cord, when the presenting part fails to descend or when there is difficulty with rotation.

The face is always somewhat swollen and discoloured after a face delivery, and the parents should be warned that it may be temporarily unsightly, but that complete recovery is to be expected.

BROW PRESENTATION

The causes of a primary brow presentation (Fig. 5.9) include those of a face presentation, but often

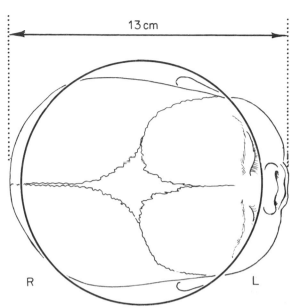

Fig. 5.10 Vaginal examination with brow presentation. The circle represents the pelvic cavity with a diameter of 12 cm. The mentovertical diameter of 13 cm is too large to permit engagement of the head

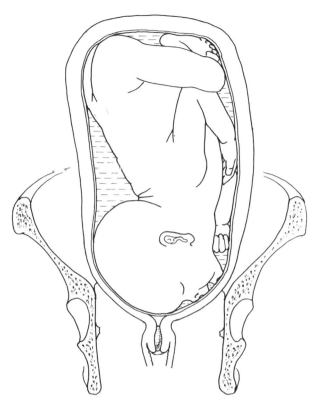

Fig. 5.9 Brow presentation. The head is above the brim and not engaged. The mentovertical diameter of the head is trying to engage in the transverse diameter at the brim

the reason for partial extension of the head is not evident.

Extension of the head before labour may be termed primary, and extension during labour secondary.

Two types of secondary extension occur, one at the level of the pelvic brim and the other at a lower level in the pelvis. If the pelvic brim is contracted, descent of the wide biparietal diameter of the head may be impossible and the narrower anterior part of the head may descend a little into the pelvis, so that the head becomes partially extended.

Similarly, in some cases of occipitoposterior position, the wider occipital end of the head may be held up in the sacral bay of the pelvis, while the sinciput descends and extension of the head occurs in the cavity of the pelvis. This can only occur with a small fetus.

A persistent brow presentation is fortunately rare. If a head of normal size lies with its longest diameter of 13 cm across the brim of a normal

pelvis it cannot engage (Fig. 5.10). If this occurred in a fetus of average size obstructed labour would result. However, when the fetal head is small in proportion to the pelvis it may be driven down into the pelvic cavity and be born as brow presentation.

With a brow presentation the head becomes very much moulded, with compression of the mentovertical diameter and lengthening of the occipitofrontal diameter.

Diagnosis

In cases in which extension of the head occurs early in labour the diagnosis may be difficult. On abdominal examination the head is above the brim, with some overlap, and the cephalic prominence is on the same side as the back. This malpresentation should always be suspected when non-engagement of the head is noted, particularly after the membranes rupture in a patient who has had previous easy deliveries.

As a rule the membranes rupture early in labour, and there is some risk of prolapse of the cord. On vaginal examination, except in the case of extension of a head lying in the occipitoposterior posi-

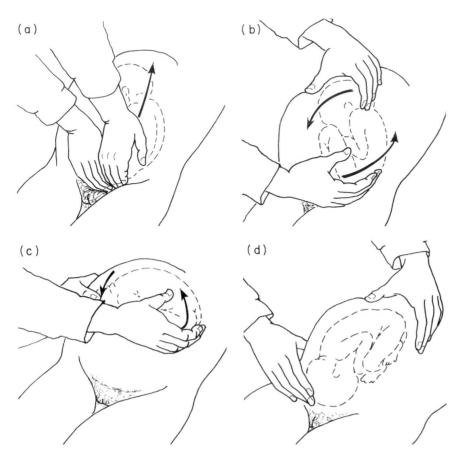

Fig. 5.15   External cephalic version. (a) the breech is disengaged from the pelvic inlet; (b) version is usually performed in the direction which increases flexion of the fetus and makes it do a forward somersault; (c) on completion of version the head is often not engaged for a time. The fetal heart rate should be checked after the external version has been completed

flexion (Fig. 5.15). Only if the long axis of the fetus can be brought across the long axis of the uterus will version succeed. Steady pressure is more likely to be effective than jerky movements. After any attempt at version, successful or otherwise, the fetal heart rate should be counted. Immediately after version the head is often high and not engaged, and this should not be taken as evidence of disproportion.

If, by 36 weeks, version had not been successful it used to be common practice to attempt version under anaesthesia with the hope of relaxing the abdominal muscles and the uterus. The only anaesthetic agents now in common use that will relax the uterus (as distinct from the abdominal muscles) are ether, cyclopropane and fluothane (Halothane). The last carries some risk of hepatic necrosis. Anaesthesia for version has the great disadvantage that increased force is liable to be used on the uncomplaining patient, with a risk of placental separation or premature labour. The vast majority of obstetricians do not now use anaesthesia for version.

Planning the method of delivery

If a breech presentation persists every effort should be made to prove that the pelvis is normal in shape and size, this should be done in all patients, regardless of parity. The history of previous confinements and clinical examination of the bony pelvis are of importance. Most (but not all) obstetricians recommend a lateral X-ray of the pelvis. Those against lateral X-ray pelvimetry cite the danger of irradiating the fetus and the inaccuracy of measurements on X-rays as evidenced by the frequent disparity between the predicted and actual outcome of labour in cases of suspected cephalopelvic disproportion.

An attempt should also be made to assess the size of the baby. Clinical assessment should not be overlooked but the best predictions of fetal weight are made from ultrasound measurements of fetal abdominal and head circumference. Any baby whose estimated birthweight is over 4 kg is best delivered by caesarean section if it is presenting by the breech. The same is true in any circumstances where there is reason to believe that the shape and/or size of the pelvis are abnormal; breech birth is very dangerous in the presence of even slight disparity between the size of the baby and the size of the pelvis.

The role of induction of labour

It was once argued that, ideally, breech delivery should occur at around 38 weeks, a time when the fetus is mature, smaller than it would be at 40 weeks and supported by an optimally functioning placenta. The view that this would constitute a good indication for inducing labour at 38 weeks no longer stands. Indeed, many believe that vaginal delivery should only be contemplated if labour is of spontaneous onset, caesarean section being preferable to induction of labour, whatever the indication.

The place of caesarean section in breech delivery

Before discussing the management of vaginal breech delivery it must be asked whether, in view of the fetal risk, caesarean section should not always be preferred. The maternal risk is increased by section, yet in Britain at least 30 per cent of women with breech presentations are delivered by caesarean section, and the percentage is increasing.

With vaginal breech delivery it is possible that fetal death may occur, but even if the fetus is born alive there is some risk of it being injured. Many women know this and request delivery by caesarean section. Many obstetricians agree with them, and also point out that even if labour is allowed to begin, many cases will end in section for delay or fetal distress.

Even if this view is not wholly accepted, it is generally agreed that any additional complication during pregnancy or labour, or anything untoward in the patient's history, is an indication for section. It would be advised for any primigravida over 35 years of age, and for any woman who has previously been infertile or has had stillbirths. It is now also a generally held (but unproved) view that caesarean section is preferable to vaginal delivery with babies whose gestational age is less than 34 weeks, the very preterm baby being unduly susceptible to intracranial bleeding caused by trauma or asphyxia.

Pelvic contraction, even if it is only slight, is an indication for section. An android pelvis is particularly unfavourable. Section would be performed in cases associated with placenta praevia, and in cases of prolapse of the cord before full dilatation of the cervix.

Management of vaginal breech delivery

The conduct of the first stage of labour is exactly as described for a vertex presentation. Early rupture of the membranes may occur as the presenting part, particularly of a flexed breech, may not fit the brim well. As soon as the membranes rupture a vaginal examination should be made to exclude prolapse of the umbilical cord. Throughout this stage of labour a watch is kept, as always, for failure to progress or any evidence of maternal or fetal distress and any of these complications are best treated by caesarean section.

In the second stage a vaginal examination must always be made to confirm full dilatation before the patient is allowed to bear down. Spontaneous descent of the breech onto the pelvic floor usually occurs, whether the legs are extended or not. When the breech reaches the pelvic floor the patient should be placed in the lithotomy position. So that the intact perineum will provide no obstacle to the delivery of the breech, and to facilitate the ultimate delivery of the head, an episiotomy is performed as a routine as soon as the baby's anus becomes visible at the height of a contraction. Epidural analgesia will provide total pain relief and good relaxation of the pelvic floor, but may interfere with bearing down efforts. As an alternative, pudendal block or local infiltration with lignocaine is necessary for the episiotomy.

In the case of a flexed breech the feet and legs present and as they appear they may be eased out.

If the legs are extended no assistance should be given to the birth, which must be allowed to take place as the result of maternal effort and the force of uterine contractions. First the anterior, and then the posterior buttock is torn by a process of lateral flexion, so that the buttocks appear to climb the maternal perineum. After the buttocks have been born the baby's feet may need to be released by flexing first the anterior and then the posterior leg at the knee.

Arrest of descent of the breech

It is uncommon for the breech to be arrested before it has descended into the pelvic cavity.

Arrest of the breech in midcavity (i.e. at the level of the ischial spines) in the second stage of labour usually means that the fetus is too big for the maternal pelvis and is therefore best delivered by caesarean section, even though the cervix is fully dilated. Before abdominal delivery became as safe as it is today, arrest of the breech in midcavity in the second stage used to be treated by breech extraction. Breech extraction is a procedure which is now only used for expediting the delivery of a second twin and requires good epidural analgesia or general anaesthesia. With the patient in lithotomy the whole hand is inserted into the birth canal and the breech is pushed up to the level of the pelvic brim. A foot (preferably that belonging to the anterior leg) is then grasped (the leg may have to be flexed to bring the foot into reach) and care is taken not to mistake a foot for a hand by feeling for the heel, the big toe (or absence of a thumb) and the malleoli. The foot is brought down and by traction on the leg in the axis of the birth canal the buttocks and the other leg are easily delivered.

If a breech with extended legs gets arrested at the pelvic floor the buttocks may be assisted by gentle digital traction in the anterior groin (Fig. 5.16) and then by traction in the posterior groin as the breech is born. Traction should be made to coincide with uterine contractions and great care must be taken to avoid fracturing the baby's femur by digital pressure during traction.

Delivery of the trunk and head

As soon as the umbilicus is born pulsation of the cord can be observed. Compression of the cord by the side walls of the birth canal may sometimes cause spasm of the umbilical vessels and obliterate

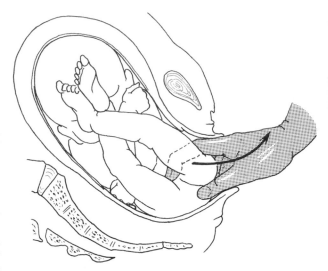

Fig. 5.16 Groin traction during delivery of breech with extended legs after episiotomy

the fetal pulse. Absence of pulsations in the cord during delivery is only an indication for haste if the fetal trunk is pale and limp and the danger of asphyxia seems greater than rapid extraction of the fetus with its risk of intracranial haemorrhage.

A finger should be inserted into the vagina to make certain that the arms are lying folded on the chest. As soon as the body descends so that the inferior angle of the anterior scapula becomes visible at the introitus, the anterior arm can be gently hooked out after which the posterior arm can be released. The baby's body is now allowed to hang down to exert slight traction in the direction of the pelvic axis. As soon as the head has descended onto the pelvic floor and the nape of the neck can be seen below the pubic arch, the baby's legs are held just above the ankles, and by exerting slight traction its body is lifted to the horizontal position. The face will then appear at the vulva and, as the baby can now breathe, the head can be delivered slowly and carefully. Lifting the baby's body upwards before the head has passed completely through the brim will not assist delivery, and may injure the cervical spine. In most units forceps are used routinely for the delivery of the head, as described on p. 197.

Extension of the arms

Easy delivery may not occur if the arms are

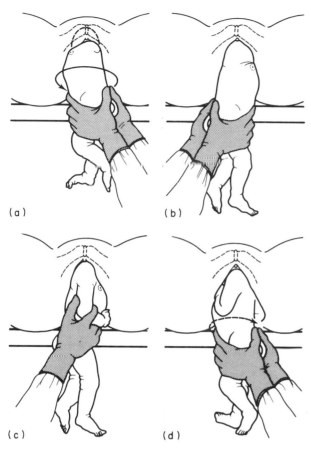

(a)

(b)

(c)

(d)

Fig. 5.17 Løvset's manoeuvre

extended. This should be suspected if descent of the fetus is not continuous after delivery of the thorax, and if the arms cannot be felt in the pelvic cavity. This complication must be dealt with at once by Løvset's manoeuvre. This depends on the fact that the subpubic arch is the shallowest part of the pelvis. By downward traction the anterior shoulder is brought to lie behind the symphysis pubis so that the inferior angle of the scapula can be seen. When this is done the posterior shoulder will lie below the promontory of the sacrum and below the pelvic brim. The pelvic girdle and thighs are than firmly held with both hands and the fetus is turned through 180° with the back upwards, while moderate traction is maintained (Fig. 5.17(a)). By this means the posterior arm is brought to the front and inevitably appears under the pubic arch (Fig. 5.17(b)). The arm may be delivered spontaneously; otherwise it is easily hooked out with a finger (Fig. 5.17(c)). The other

shoulder now lies in the hollow of the sacrum. The fetus, therefore, is again rotated through 180° in the opposite direction, the fetal back again being kept upwards (Fig. 5.17(d)). The remaining arm will appear under the pubic arch and can easily be delivered.

Difficulty with the aftercoming head

After the birth of the shoulders the flexed head normally enters the pelvis in the transverse diameter of the brim. As descent occurs the head undergoes internal rotation so that the occiput comes to lie behind the symphysis pubis. The neck rests under the pubic arch and normally the head is born by a movement of flexion. In most cases the head will enter the pelvis if the fetal trunk is allowed to hang downwards for not more than one minute. Any failure of descent or difficulty in the delivery of the head calls for immediate assistance. The body of the baby having been born, the placental circulation is impaired by retraction of the uterus and pressure on the cord, and respiratory efforts will certainly be made. If the birth is not completed within the next few minutes death from asphyxia is likely. The obstetric forceps must be available for immediate use at every breech delivery whenever the descent of the head is arrested. The body of the baby is lifted upward by an assistant and the blades are applied beneath it. The fingers of the right hand steer the left blade of

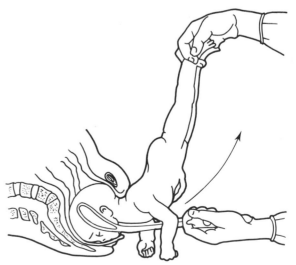

Fig. 5.18 Delivery of the aftercoming head with forceps

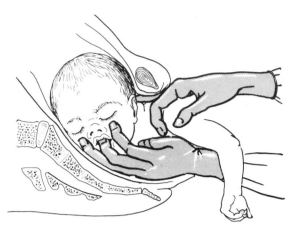

Fig. 5.19 Jaw and shoulder traction applied to a fetus with the head at the level of the pelvic brim. Forceps could not be applied at this level

the forceps to the left side of the pelvis, and then the right blade is applied. Only moderate traction should be required to complete delivery as episiotomy has already been performed (Fig. 5.18).

Very rarely the fetal head cannot be made to enter the pelvic brim. This means that an error of judgement has been made and pelvic contraction has been overlooked (or very rarely that hydrocephalus is present). Apart from the fact that the head may be lying transversely, flexion will almost certainly be poor, and the application of forceps at this level would be difficult and dangerous. The best hope of saving a desperate situation is to pass one hand up in front of the fetal thorax, where one finger presses on the jaw to produce flexion. The other hand is passed along the back until the index and middle fingers can curve over the shoulders to exert traction (Fig. 5.19). The head is drawn down by traction on the shoulders, and if necessary rotated until the neck lies under the pubic arch. Delivery may then be completed with forceps as already described. This sort of traction may cause injury to the cervical spine or to the brachial plexus.

Difficulty at the pelvic outlet may occur if it is contracted, or if the occiput has rotated posteriorly; delivery is achieved with forceps. If the occiput lies posteriorly and cannot be rotated the forceps are applied in front of the baby's body, which is supported by an assistant.

Most of the difficulties encountered in breech delivery can be avoided if:

vaginal delivery is only attempted if the pelvis is capacious, there is no hint of delay in the first stage of labour and the breech readily descends to the pelvic floor in the second stage of labour

full dilatation of the cervix is confirmed before bearing down efforts are encouraged

an episiotomy is performed under adequate analgesia

Løvset's manoeuvre is used if the arms are extended

forceps are used for slow delivery of the after-coming head.

Spontaneous expulsion of the buttocks, rapid and minimally assisted delivery of the trunk and shoulders and slow forceps delivery of the head are the ideal.

TRANSVERSE AND OBLIQUE LIE (SHOULDER PRESENTATION)

The fetus may lie with its long axis transverse or oblique in the uterus, when the point of the shoulder is usually the presenting part (Fig. 5.20). After rupture of the membranes an arm may prolapse. In the absence of antenatal care shoulder presentations occur about once in 500 labours, but

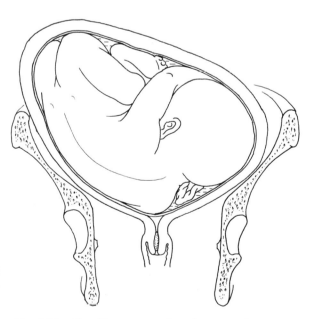

Fig. 5.20 Shoulder presentation, dorsoanterior position. The head is in the left iliac fossa, the back lies anteriorly and obliquely and the breech is on the right above the right iliac fossa

in many cases can be corrected by external version before labour.

Cause

By far the most common cause of an oblique lie is multiparity associated with a lax uterus and abdominal wall. It is not infrequently found on antenatal examination before 36 weeks and it is therefore more common in cases in which labour starts prematurely. An oblique lie may be found with polyhydramnios or multiple pregnancy, and may be caused by anything which prevents engagement of the fetal head, such as contracted pelvis, placenta praevia or a pelvic tumour. If a transverse lie occurs in a primigravida or recurs in successive pregnancies the possibility that it is caused by a uterine malformation (arcuate or subseptate uterus) must be considered.

Positions

The fetus may lie with the head in either iliac fossa, with the back sloping obliquely across the pelvic brim, while the breech usually occupies a somewhat higher position than the head, on the opposite side of the abdomen. Only two positions are described, dorsoanterior and dorsoposterior, the former being the more common.

Diagnosis

On abdominal examination the uterus appears asymmetrical, and is broader than usual with the fundus lower than expected for the duration of pregnancy. On palpation the hard round head is felt in one iliac fossa, with the softer breech on the opposite side. No presenting part is felt over the brim. In the centre of the abdomen the back will be felt in dorsoanterior positions, and small parts in dorsoposterior positions. The fetal heart sounds are usually heard just below the umbilicus (Fig. 5.21).

On vaginal examination at the beginning of labour the presenting part is too high to be felt. During labour the membranes usually rupture early. When the cervix becomes dilated an arm or a loop of cord may prolapse. Diagnosis of a shoulder presentation depends on recognition of the acromion process, scapula and adjacent ribs. A prolapsed arm must be distinguished from a leg; the elbow is sharper than the knee, and absence of a

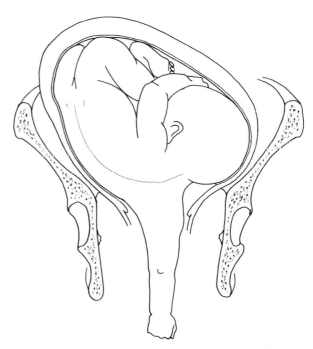

Fig. 5.21 Shoulder presentation with prolapse of the arm. The shoulder and arm, forming the apex of the wedge, are driven into the brim; the head and neck on the side and the trunk on the other form the sides of the wedge

heel and abduction of the thumb will distinguish a hand from a foot.

Course of labour

A fetus lying obliquely cannot be born naturally unless it is macerated or very premature. There is no true mechanism of labour, and an untreated case will end in obstructed labour and fetal death.

Spontaneous rectification to a vertex or more rarely a breech presentation may sometimes occur in early labour, but cannot do so after prolapse of an arm. Spontaneous delivery may rarely occur with a macerated or very premature infant when the body is delivered doubled up (Fig. 5.22).

Prognosis

Neglected or unrecognized shoulder presentations are extremely serious, since all the risks of obstructed labour are present, including rupture of the uterus. Fetal death is usual from interference

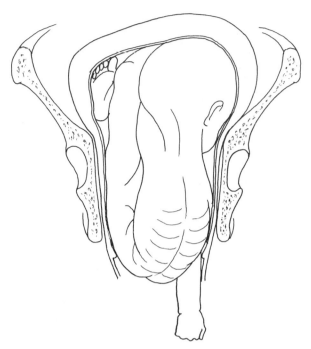

Fig. 5.22 Spontaneous evolution. The body is squeezed past the head by extreme flexion; the ribs distend the perineum, while the breech occupies the sacral hollow

with the placental circulation or prolapse of the cord.

Treatment

During pregnancy

For treatment of an oblique lie before the onset of labour see the section on unstable lie, which follows on this page.

During early labour

If an oblique lie is discovered early in labour it may still be corrected by external version if the membranes are intact. Once the lie has been corrected the membranes should be ruptured and the uterine contractions will usually maintain a longitudinal lie. If an oblique or transverse lie persists in labour caesarean section is performed, being safer than the dangerous operation of internal podalic version, in which a leg of the fetus is pulled down and it is then delivered as a breech.

Late in labour when the shoulder has become impacted

In neglected cases, when the uterus is tonically retracted, any form of version is extremely dangerous, owing to the very great risk of rupturing the thinned out lower uterine segment. If the fetus is alive, which is seldom the case, caesarean section is performed. Even if the fetus is dead caesarean section is probably the safest procedure. In this case a low vertical incision in the uterus is preferable to the usual low transverse incision.

Decapitation is an alternative which was formerly recommended. After division of the neck of the fetus, which can be done with heavy scissors, the trunk can be delivered by traction on the prolapsed arm, and the head is then delivered with forceps.

UNSTABLE LIE

Unstable lie is a self-descriptive term referring to a fetus which frequently changes its axis from transverse to longitudinal to oblique. The condition may be associated with polyhydramnios, placenta praevia, pelvic tumour or contraction but usually occurs in multiparae with a lax uterus and abdominal wall. Gentle external version should be used to correct the malpresentation whenever the patient is examined. Such patients should be warned to come to hospital immediately if they rupture their membranes or have any symptoms suggestive of the onset of labour. Those patients who live at some distance from the hospital should be admitted from 38 weeks onwards to await the spontaneous onset of labour by which time the malpresentation has usually corrected itself.

The place of induction

If it is not practical to await the spontaneous onset of labour or there are obstetric indications for delivering the baby, induction can be contemplated. With an unstable lie it is best, after correcting the fetal lie to longitudinal, to start with a Syntocinon infusion and to delay amniotomy until there are uterine contractions and the presenting part has settled into the pelvic brim. Care should be taken to keep the presenting part in the pelvis when the forewaters are ruptured and to be on the lookout for cord prolapse at that time. Controlled release of liquor is desirable and may be achieved by using a long needle rather than an amniotomy hook to puncture the membranes. Whenever an induction is done with an unstable lie the labour ward staff should be informed so that everything is ready for caesarean section if the cord prolapses or if there is recurrence of the malpresentation during labour.

COMPOUND PRESENTATIONS

Prolapse of a limb with a vertex presentation is known as a compound presentation. Commonly it is a hand which comes down, very rarely a foot. Prolapse of an arm occurs when the head does not fit the brim well. If the head is not low in the pelvic cavity the arm often goes back as the head descends, and active treatment is not required. If the head is lower in the pelvis and its progress is arrested the arm should be replaced under anaesthesia. Delivery is completed with forceps if the cervix is fully dilated.

When a foot presents with the head it may be pushed up under anaesthesia, or it may be better to pull on the foot and push up the head, turning the fetus into a breech presentation. If any difficulties are encountered with the manoeuvres described the baby should be delivered by caesarean section.

FETAL MALFORMATIONS THAT CAUSE DIFFICULTY IN LABOUR

These are mentioned in this chapter to complete the discussion of fetal causes of difficult labour.

HYDROCEPHALY

This may be discovered during pregnancy if the head is noticed to be unduly large, or during the course of investigation of suspected disproportion. The diagnosis is confirmed by ultrasound scan. During labour the wide separation of the cranial bones at the sutures may be recognized on vaginal examination. As the head cannot enter the pelvis a breech presentation may occur.

Obstruction during labour is treated by perforation of the head. It is often sufficient to pass a widebore needle into the head and draw off the cerebrospinal fluid. This may be done through the maternal abdominal wall. It can also be done through the cervix when it is 5 cm dilated. After withdrawal of the fluid the head may collapse sufficiently for spontaneous delivery to occur.

If the fetus presents by the breech the aftercoming head can be collapsed after the trunk has been delivered by passing a metal cannula up through the spinal canal (via a spina bifida if one is present).

If spontaneous delivery does not follow tapping, traction can be applied to the scalp with Morris toothed forceps.

INIENCEPHALY

In this abnormality the head is hyperextended and the tissues over the occiput and sacrum are fused. It is recognized by ultrasound or radiographically. Induction before the 32nd week may avoid the need for caesarean section.

ANENCEPHALY

In some cases of anencephaly difficulty in delivery of the shoulders may occur, because they are often wide and have not been preceded by a head of normal size. There should be no hesitation in dividing the clavicles (cleidotomy) with strong scissors and applying strong traction in the axilla.

CONJOINED TWINS

Conjunction of twins may be suspected during pregnancy if ultrasound or radiological examination shows that the twins constantly maintain the same relative positions, especially if they are facing one another. In other cases the diagnosis is made during twin labour when there is delay and a hand is passed into the uterus to determine the cause. Surprisingly, vaginal delivery has not infrequently been reported when the twins have been small and the junction between them has been fairly pliable, but in most cases caesarean section is unavoidable, and is preferable to embryotomy.

PELVIC ABNORMALITIES AND DISPROPORTION INCLUDING SHOULDER DYSTOCIA

PELVIC ABNORMALITIES

The size of the female pelvis is of primary importance; if it is large enough there will be no difficulty in the passage of an average fetal head through it. The shape of the pelvis is of secondary importance, and only has a bearing on the mechanism of labour and the ease of delivery if the pelvic dimensions are small in relation to those of the head.

Certain terms are used to describe variations in the shape of the pelvis which were discovered by anatomical and radiological studies. Very few pelves fit the criteria exactly, and any pelvis may be a mixture of the types about to be described.

Gynaecoid pelvis

The gynaecoid pelvis conforms to the accepted female type in that the brim is rounded, with the widest transverse diameter slightly behind its centre (Fig. 5.23). The subpubic arch is rounded, with an agle of at least 90 degrees.

Android pelvis

The android pelvis has many of the characteristics of the male pelvis. The brim is heart-shaped, so that the widest transverse diameter is much nearer to the sacrum than it is in the gynaecoid pelvis (Fig. 5.24). The side walls tend to converge, the ischial spines are prominent, the sacrum is straight and the subpubic arch is generally narrow, with an angle of 70 degrees or less. Both the anteroposterior and transverse diameters of the outlet tend to be reduced. This type of pelvis is funnel-shaped, with diameters which decrease from above downwards, and disproportion thus becomes worse as labour proceeds.

Anthropoid pelvis

The anteroposterior diameter of the brim exceeds the transverse diameter (Fig. 5.25). The pelvis tends to be deep and the sacrum often has six segments instead of five; this is known as a high assimilation pelvis. Very often the sacrum and the axis of the pelvic cavity are less curved than in the gynaecoid pelvis and the subpubic arch may be a little narrow, but the sacrosciatic notches are wide and the anteroposterior diameter of the outlet is large, so there is no difficulty.

Platypelloid pelvis

The platypelloid pelvis is described as the simple (non-rachitic) flat pelvis. The brim is elliptical with a wide transverse diameter (Fig. 5.26). The subpubic arch is wide and rounded.

It is emphasized that, except in the case of the android pelvis, these variations in shape have little effect on the normal mechanism of labour unless

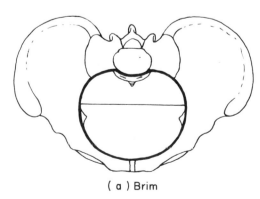

(a) Brim

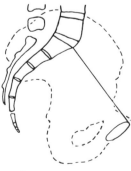

(b) Lateral view

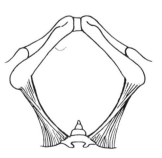

(c)Outlet

Fig. 5.23 The gynaecoid pelvis

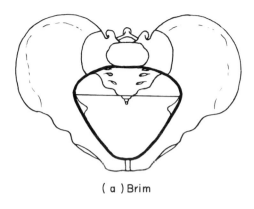
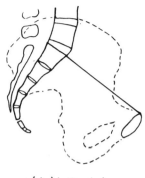
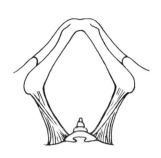

(a) Brim

(b) Lateral view
(the one seen on X-rays)

(c) Outlet

Fig. 5.24 The android pelvis

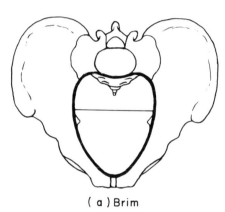
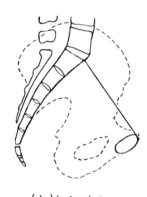
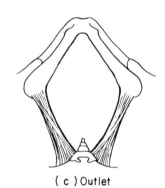

(a) Brim

(b) Lateral view

(c) Outlet

Fig. 5.25 The anthropoid pelvis

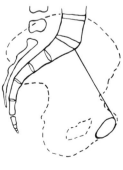
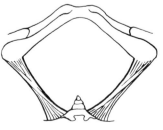

(a) Brim

(b) Lateral view

(c) Outlet

Fig. 5.26 The platypelloid pelvis

there is considerable reduction in the size of the pelvis. The android pelvis is unfavourable because of the tendency to contraction of the outlet.

ABNORMALITIES OF THE PELVIS

Abnormalities of the pelvis may be classified into three groups:

    those caused by developmental abnormalities of the pelvic bones
    those caused by disease or injury of the pelvic bones
    those caused by abnormalities of the spine, hip joints or lower limbs.

Developmental abnormalities of the pelvic bones

Developmental variations in shape have already

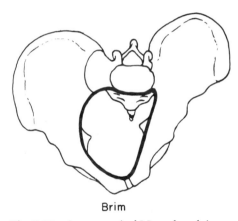

Brim

Fig. 5.27 Asymmetrical Naegele pelvis

been described and the android pelvis is the only one of these that commonly affects labour adversely. However, even a round gynaecoid pelvis may be small in size; it is then called a *generally contracted pelvis*.

The presence of a sixth segment in the sacrum, which may be found with an anthropoid pelvis, has given rise to the term *high assimilation pelvis*, but this is not of great significance.

Very rarely malformation of the pelvis may result from defective development of one side of the sacrum, which is fused with the ilium (Naegele pelvis, Fig. 5.27).

Disease or injury of the pelvic bones

The most important abnormality in this group is rickets, which causes softening of the bones in early childhood, with flattening of the pelvic brim (Fig. 5.28). Fortunately rickets is uncommon in Britain. A similar disease, osteomalacia, which may occur in adults, can cause very severe distortion of the pelvis; it is almost unknown in Britain but is still seen in Africa and Asia. In achondroplasia the pelvis is often small.

Pelvic deformity may be caused by malunited fractures, or by new growths arising from the pelvic bones.

Abnormalities of the spine and lower limbs

The shape and inclination of the pelvis may be affected by kyphosis of the spine (Fig. 5.29) or by spondylolisthesis, in which the 5th lumbar verteb-

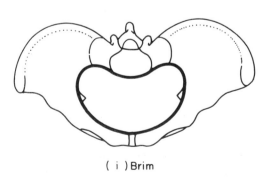

(i) Brim

Fig. 5.28 Rachitic pelvis

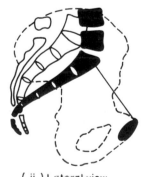

(ii) Lateral view
(Showing forward displacement
of the sacral promontory)

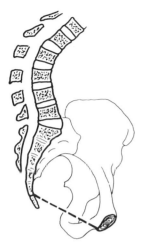

Fig. 5.29 Kyphosis with forward rotation of the lower part of the sacrum and reduction of the anteroposterior diameter of the pelvic outlet

ra slips forward on the sacrum and obstructs the pelvic inlet.

With congenital dislocation of a hip joint there may be oblique distortion of the pelvis, but this rarely causes difficulty.

LABOUR IN THE PRESENCE OF PELVIC ABNORMALITY

When the size of the fetal head exceeds the size of the pelvis even after moulding has taken place, normal vaginal delivery will clearly be impossible. If, however, there is not absolute disproportion vaginal delivery may occur if the uterine contractions are sufficiently strong to overcome the relatively increased resistance.

In practice the type of deformity is less important than the size of the pelvis relative to that of the head. The mechanism of the passage of the head through the pelvis will differ according to the shape of the pelvis, but in general there is a tendency with most pelvic abnormalities for the forepelvis to be small, thus increasing the risk of malpositions of the fetal head.

CEPHALOPELVIC DISPROPORTION

Disproportion between the size of the fetal head and that of the maternal pelvis will cause difficult labour and danger to the fetus. The size of the head at term is genetically related to the size of the maternal pelvis – small women tend to have small babies – so that in the absence of pelvic deformity the majority of labours proceed without mechanical difficulty. However, the obstetrician must always be on the lookout for possible disproportion, both in the antenatal clinic and during labour.

In cases of disproportion it is usually found that the pelvic inlet presents the chief difficulty. If the widest diameter of the head will pass through the inlet it will usually pass through the pelvic cavity and outlet. Occasionally the pelvis is to some degree funnel-shaped with a relatively narrower outlet than inlet, but even in this case the head will often pass because by the time it has reached the outlet its diameters have been reduced by moulding. In every case of disproportion the efficiency of the uterine contractions plays a major part in determining whether or not vaginal delivery will occur.

The diagnosis of disproportion

The following are the steps in the antenatal diagnosis of disproportion:

Past orthopaedic and obstetric history

A history of disease or fracture of the spine, hips or pelvis should alert the practitioner to the possibility of pelvic defomity. A distinction is made between primigravidae and multigravidae.

In a multigravidae the pelvis has been tested up to the size of the largest baby previously delivered, but in a primigravida the size of the pelvis is unknown. Disproportion in a multigravida is usually because she has a fetus larger than any she has previously borne. In dealing with a multigravida, therefore, it is important to obtain details of her previous labours, including for each the duration, the mode of delivery, the outcome and the birthweight and subsequent progress of the child.

General examination

Although it is true that small women may have small babies, it is also true that a small woman has a small pelvis, and a greater chance of disproportion. Any woman whose height is less than 150 cm or whose shoe size is below 4½ comes into this category.

Any general disease of the skeleton or disease of the lower limbs or spine should also be noted in view of any possible effect on the shape of the pelvis, which itself may have been deformed by rickets or previous fractures.

Abdominal examination

Abdominal examination in late pregnancy should indicate whether or not the widest diameter of the fetal head has passed through the pelvic inlet. In primigravidae the head normally engages between the 36th and 38th weeks. In multigravidae engagement often does not occur until labour starts.

In African women the pelvic inlet has a higher angle of inclination (*see* p. 207) than is seen in Caucasian and Asiatic women and because of this, in African women engagement of the head is uncommon before the onset of labour, even in primigravidae.

If the head is not engaged before term an attempt is made to discover if it will engage, and thus exclude inlet disproportion. This is most simply done by moderate pressure on the head in a backwards and downwards direction, or by examining the patient when she is standing.

Pelvic examination

Vaginal examination in early pregnancy is chiefly performed to assess the size of the uterus and to detect any soft tissue abnormalities. Unless the head is already deeply engaged in the pelvis examination should be repeated at the 36th week to determine the size of the pelvic cavity and outlet.

Most of the normal pelvic inlet is beyond the range of the examining fingers. The forepelvis can be reached by passing a finger behind the symphysis pubis, but the sacral promontory can only be reached in a grossly contracted pelvis. The concavity or straightness of the sacrum and the convergence or separation of the side walls of the pelvis will give some idea of the size of the pelvic cavity. The bony outlet can be readily palpated and the width of the subpubic arch and the ease with which the ischial spines can be felt should be noted. The distance between the ischial tuberosities can be measured.

The fetal head is the best pelvimeter. If it has already descended into the pelvis or can be made to do so on examination there is only the pelvic outlet left for it to pass. Pure outlet contraction is very rare, and if the biparietal diameter enters the pelvic inlet with only two fifths or less, of the head

palpable abdominally (*see* Fig. 4.19, p. 51), with the lowest point of the head at the level of the ischial spines, disproportion is extremely unlikely.

If the head will not enter the pelvis disproportion may be suspected but in many cases, with strong uterine contractions and moulding of the head, vaginal delivery will occur. Pelvic examination is of limited value in predicting the outcome as so much depends on the moulding and the efficiency of the contractions.

Diagnosis of disproportion during labour

Failure of the head to descend and of the cervix to dilate during labour may indicate unsuspected disproportion. Excessive moulding and caput formation may occur, and in some cases the caput may be felt at the level of the ischial spines even though the head has still not passed through the pelvic inlet.

In modern practice, if a partogram indicates that the cervix is not dilating normally, an oxytocin drip with good analgesia is likely to be tried, unless examination shows clear evidence of disproportion. If augmentation of the uterine action does not lead to progress in cervical dilatation a diagnosis of disproportion or some other mechanical obstruction is probable.

Radiological diagnosis of disproportion

X-rays are now used much less often to investigate suspected disproportion than they used to be. In Britain it is rare for a woman to have a pelvis which is too small to allow the passage of a normal sized fetus, provided that there are good uterine contractions. X-rays have the same inability as clinical examination to predict uterine efficiency in labour, and in addition may have undesirable effects on the maternal gonads and the fetus. Present practice is only to X-ray the pelvis when disproportion is suspected but confirmation is needed for management, and then only one lateral radiograph is taken in late pregnancy with the patient standing. This view allows measurement of the anteroposterior diameters of the pelvis but not of the transverse diameters (Fig. 5.30). The latter can be measured by taking further views of the pelvic inlet and outlet but these are not now thought to be justified in view of the limited information gained and the additional irradiation of the fetus. Apart from the anteroposterior diameters, the erect lateral radio-

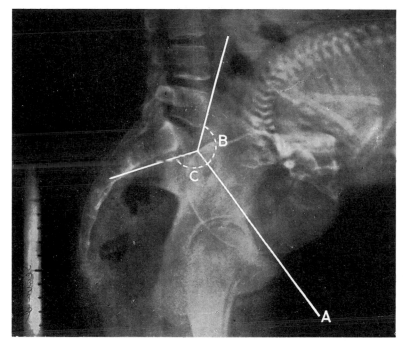

Fig. 5.30 Lateral X-ray of the pelvis, the fetus is in an occipitoposterior postion. A, plane of the inlet; B, angle between the front of the 5th lumbar vertebra and the pelvic Brim; C, angle of inclination of the sacrum

graph also shows the curve of the sacrum, the width of the sacrosciatic notches, the angle of inclination of the pelvic brim and the degree of engagement of the fetal head.

X-rays are now rarely used during labour for the diagnosis of disproportion, as they add little to the clinical assessment of progress and nothing to management.

The management of disproportion

When cephalopelvic disproportion is suspected as a result of antenatal examination a decision has to be taken whether or not to allow the patient to go into labour in the hope of vaginal delivery, or to deliver her before the onset of labour by elective caesarean section.

Indications for elective caesarean section

The indications are:

  disproportion so severe that vaginal delivery is unlikely
  lesser degrees of disproportion when there are complicating factors such as breech presenta-

tion, previous caesarean section, or a previous difficult vaginal delivery causing perinatal death or morbidity
  in older women, especially those with a long history of infertility and women with medical complications such as, for example, diabetes.

Trial of labour

Except for the cases just mentioned, patients with disproportion should be allowed a trial of labour. By this is meant that the labour is carefully watched for evidence of continuing progress as shown by dilatation of the cervix and descent of the head. The assessment of progress is made as in normal labour by repeated abdominal and vaginal examinations, and the results are recorded on a partogram.

In the majority of cases of trial of labour good uterine contractions will bring about steady progress to vaginal delivery. In multiparous patients the head may remain high until the cervix is fully dilated and then descend rapidly through the pelvis during the second stage.

Augmentation of labour in cases of suspected disproportion

Good uterine contractions are essential if mild disproportion is to be overcome. In primigravidae delay in labour caused by poor uterine action may be treated by the cautious use of an intravenous oxytocin infusion (*see* p. 177). Great care must be taken to avoid overstimulation leading to excessively strong contractions which may harm the fetus, or even rupture the uterus. Continuous monitoring of the fetal heart with a scalp electrode, as well as continuous recording of the uterine contractions by the methods described on p. 216 are essential whenever labour is being augmented, but are particularly important in cases of possible disproportion.

Deciding when a trial of labour has failed

Although no hard and fast rules can be laid down, failure to progress in a trial of labour after a period of four hours or more of good contractions suggests that the disproportion is too great to be overcome, and that caesarean section should be performed.

The trial may also have to be terminated at any time if fetal distress develops.

Uterine rupture is a rare event in primigravidae, but less rare in multigravidae. It usually only occurs after some hours of strong contractions. The development of a Bandl's ring, pain and tenderness over the lower uterine segment, or acute fetal distress are all indications that labour has been allowed to go on for too long and that rupture is impending; immediate caesarean section is required.

The management of trial of labour for suspected disproportion should be under the control of an experienced obstetrician in a fully equipped unit, as considerable skill and judgment may be needed to decide how long the labour may safely continue.

Forceps delivery and disproportion

Because pure outlet contraction is uncommon a trial of labour will usually succeed once the head has passed through the pelvic inlet and the cervix has reached full dilatation.

In women with an android pelvis disproportion is often further complicated by malposition of the head. Arrest of the head with the sagittal suture in the transverse diameter of the pelvis (deep transverse arrest) or in the occipitoposterior position may occur. In such cases forceps delivery after manual rotation, or after rotation with Kielland's forceps, requires skill and judgment on the part of the obstetrician and is best conducted in an operating theatre with everything prepared to proceed to caesarean section if difficulty arises (*trial of forceps*). The obstetrician must be careful about the force he uses to effect rotation and delivery with the forceps, as there is considerable risk of causing intracranial damage.

Most obstetricians would not use the vacuum extractor for cases of suspected disproportion, but if it is employed the same care must be exercised as with the forceps.

The risk of sepsis and anaesthetic problems occurring in caesarean section in late labour is high, but even so section is safer than difficult or prolonged forceps extraction.

Symphysiotomy

Division of the ligaments holding the pubic bones together at the symphysis through a small suprapubic incision produces an increase in the available circumference of the pelvic ring and, by widening the subpubic arch, an increase in the available anteroposterior diameter at the outlet. The operation is hardly ever performed in the UK, but has been recommended in developing countries where some women are reluctant to agree to caesarean section, and may not return to hospital for subsequent deliveries.

Craniotomy

Destructive operations on the fetal head, which were common 50 years ago, have no place in modern obstetrics except when the fetal head is hydrocephalic. In the rare event of intrapartum fetal death in the presence of disproportion caesarean section is now safer than craniotomy and extraction, procedures in which there is considerable risk of damage to maternal soft tissues (*see* p. 294).

Shoulder dystocia

Shoulder dystocia is when the shoulders remain impacted in the pelvis after delivery of the fetal head. It is a serious, but fortunately rare, complication which usually occurs with babies weighing well over 4 kg. The warning signs are unusually slow crowning of the fetal head, difficulty in delivering the baby's face by extension and slow restitution of the occiput to a lateral position. Once the condition has occurred it is important to get the patient into either the lithotomy or the left lateral position and to do an episiotomy if one has not been done already.

Examination should reveal whether or not the anterior shoulder is arrested above the pelvic brim. If it is not, it may be possible to deliver it from the pelvic cavity by a combination of suprapubic pressure and moderate lateral flexion and traction on the baby's head. If the anterior shoulder is still above the pelvic brim it will be the posterior shoulder that has descended into the sacral bay. Under these circumstances lateral flexion and traction on the baby's head will only result in tearing of the brachial plexus and an Erb's palsy, which can be a serious permanent disability for the infant. The obstetrician will therefore have to consider delivering the posterior arm and shoulder. To do

this the operator's fingers will have to be insinuated into the very restricted space available in front of the baby's chest in order to flex the posterior arm at the elbow and then bring it down. If it is possible to rotate the posterior shoulder a few degrees so that it lies in the oblique diameter of the pelvis, bringing the posterior arm down can be made a little more easy. Once the posterior arm has been brought down it will be much more straightforward to reach the anterior axilla for traction and delivery. As a last resort, and only if the manoeuvres already described have failed and the fetus has died, an experienced obstetrician would consider division of the clavicles or even symphysiotomy as a method of delivering the baby.

If a woman has had shoulder dystocia she and her attendants will be anxious to avoid this complication in future pregnancies. To this end, she should have ultrasound estimates of fetal weight at term and a caesarean section if there is evidence of a baby that is as large, or larger than the one which previously caused the problem.

OBSTRUCTED LABOUR

Labour is said to be obstructed when there is no progress in spite of strong uterine contractions. This may be shown by failure of the cervix to dilate or failure of the presenting part to descend through the birth canal. It is a most dangerous condition if it is untreated, and can be fatal to both mother and fetus.

Causes of obstructed labour

Obstructed labour may arise from maternal or fetal conditions, or both. The following list of the causes is long, but many of these operate in only a proportion of the cases in which they occur, and the causes marked with an asterisk are rare.

Maternal conditions

contraction or deformity of the bony pelvis
pelvic tumours
    uterine fibromyomata
    ovarian tumours

*tumours of rectum, bladder or pelvic bones
*pelvic kidney
abnormalities of the uterus or vagina
    *stenosis of the cervix or vagina
    *obstruction by one horn of a double uterus
    *contraction ring of uterus.

Fetal conditions

large fetus
malposition or malpresentation
    persistent occipitoposterior or transverse
        position
    *mentoposterior position
    brow presentation
    breech presentation
    *shoulder presentation (rare in Britain but
        common in countries with inadequate ante-
        natal care)
    *compound presentation
    *locked twins

congenital abnormalities of the fetus
  *hydrocephalus
  *fetal ascites or abdominal tumours
  *hydrops fetalis
  *conjoined twins.

Most of these abnormalities can and should be detected during pregnancy so that early treatment is possible, or a plan of action can be made before labour. These conditions and their management are fully described in the appropriate chapters; all that is given here is a description of the effects of obstructed labour if it is left untreated.

Symptoms and signs of obstructed labour

The importance of the early detection of possible obstruction in labour is obvious, for if labour is allowed to progress to the point of absolute obstruction the death of the fetus is almost certain and the life of the mother is endangered. In a primigravida complete obstruction leads within two or three days to a state of uterine exhaustion or secondary hypotonia; any relief which this gives to the mother and fetus is only temporary. In a multigravida obstruction becomes established much sooner and progressive thinning of the lower segment may lead to uterine rupture in a few hours.

Probably the earliest sign of impending obstruction is deterioration in the patient's general condition. She looks tired and anxious and behaves as though she is beginning to lose her ability and will to cooperate. Between the pains she seems unable to relax and her anxiety increases.

The presenting part is often above or at the level of the pelvic brim. The membranes rupture early in labour because the presenting part is badly applied to the lower segment. The liquor drains away and there is retraction of the placental site, which causes reduction in the maternal blood flow to the placenta, severe fetal distress (shown by marked slowing of the fetal heart and thick meconium in the liquor) and eventual fetal death from hypoxia.

The woman's pulse rate and temperature rise. The quantity of urine secreted diminishes and it is concentrated and deeply coloured. Ketone bodies are present in the urine and can also be smelt in the patient's breath.

The possibility of obstructed labour should be suspected when labour fails to progress. In the first stage dilatation of the cervix should be progressive,

although sometimes it is not rapid even in normal cases. A partogram will give early warning that progress has ceased. Descent of the presenting part should be continuous, especially in the second stage. Any failure in the progress of labour calls for careful abdominal and vaginal examination to exclude any possible cause of obstruction, particularly in the case of previously undiagnosed disproportion or malpresentation.

If for some reason the diagnosis of obstruction is missed for a time, the dangerous condition of over-retraction of the uterus (generalized tonic retraction) may occur. In the course of normal labour some retraction of the upper segment persists after each contraction and the upper segment becomes slightly shorter and thicker, while the lower segment becomes stretched and thinner. If the fetus is unable to descend because of obstructions the total length of the uterine cavity must remain constant, so that as uterine contractions continue progressive retraction causes abnormal stretching and thinning of the lower segment. The line of junction of the upper and lower segments becomes very evident and is known as the retraction ring of Bandl (Fig. 5.31). It can be seen or felt

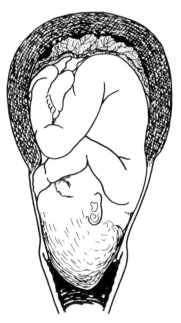

Fig. 5.31   Obstructed labour from pelvic contraction. The extreme retraction of the upper segment and the extreme stretching of the lower segment has formed a Bandl's ring. The head is greatly moulded, with a large caput succedaneum

on abdominal examination. Eventually rupture of the lower segment occurs.

In advanced obstructed labour the uterus is found, on abdominal examination, to be moulded to the shape of the fetus. It feels hard all the time and does not relax. It is tender to palpation and Bandl's ring may be evident. Fetal parts are not easily felt and the fetal heart sounds are absent. The presenting part is fixed at the level of obstruction.

On vaginal examination the vagina is found to be oedematous and feels dry. The oedematous cervix is only loosely applied to the presenting part. If the head is presenting there will be a large caput succedaneum and extreme moulding of the skull. The presenting part is tightly fixed, and even under anaesthesia it cannot be pushed upwards without the danger of uterine rupture. If there is a shoulder presentation the oedematous arm of the fetus will have prolapsed, with the hand projecting from the vulva.

Treatment

Exessive retraction of the uterus should never be allowed to develop. The cause of the obstruction should have been discovered during pregnancy or in early labour, and treatment should have been applied.

When tonic retraction is present the fetus is certainly dead and the aim of treatment is to deliver the mother immediately by the safest possible method. Intrauterine manipulations are very liable to cause rupture of the abnormally thin lower segment. Internal version is particularly dangerous. In some of the cases it is possible to deliver the fetus vaginally after a destructive operation, but (except for perforation of a hydrocephalic head) these procedures are lengthy and difficult and caesarean section is usually less hazardous. Antibiotics, blood transfusion and modern anaesthesia have combined to reduce the risks of section in these cases.

In all cases of prolonged labour, especially if operative delivery is required, there is a high risk of puerperal sepsis and appropriate antibiotics should be given.

RUPTURE OF THE UTERUS

Prolonged obstruction in a primigravida often leads to temporary cessation of uterine activity from exhaustion (secondary hypotonia), but in a multigravida it is more likely to lead to uterine rupture. In obstructed labour this usually occurs obliquely at the junction of the upper and lower segments, but occasionally the uterus splits vertically at the side near the point of entry of the uterine vessels. The peritoneum may or may not be involved. Bleeding may occur into the peritoneal cavity or may track downwards between the bladder and upper vagina. Uterine contraction may expel the fetus and placenta through the laceration into the peritoneal cavity.

The clinical picture and the treatment (which is extremely urgent) are described on page 222. If the patient survives the shock and haemorrhage there is a high risk of puerperal sepsis.

FISTULA FORMATION

In obstructed labour the fetal presenting part becomes impacted in the maternal pelvis and the result is ischaemia of the maternal soft tissues that lie between the presenting part and the walls of the maternal pelvis. If the obstruction is neglected this ischaemia can lead to tissue necrosis and the formation of vesicovaginal or rectovaginal fistulae when necrotic slough separates several days after delivery. Obstetric fistulae should not occur in countries where women have easy access to well organized hospital-based maternity services (*see* p. 227).

PRETERM LABOUR AND PREMATURE RUPTURE OF THE MEMBRANES

PRETERM LABOUR

This is arbitrarily defined as labour occurring before the 37th week of pregnancy. About 6 per cent of deliveries occur before this time.

Causes

In many cases no cause can be found.

Spontaneous premature rupture of the membranes may occur before term from a variety of causes, including incompetence of the cervix; in the majority of these cases delivery soon follows.

Preterm labour may occur in cases of multiple pregnancy, polyhydramnios and abruptio placentae. Labour usually, but not invariably, follows fetal death within three weeks.

Labour may follow direct trauma to the uterus and occasionally appears to be the result of acute emotional disturbance or severe fright. Premature labour may occur with maternal infection which causes high fever.

Artificial induction of labour before term may be necessary for a number of conditions which threaten to cause intrauterine fetal death, for example, hypertension and proteinuria, maternal diabetes, antepartum haemorrhage and haemolytic disease; it is occasionally required for maternal indications, for example rising hypertension.

Prevention

If patients with hypertension are admitted early to hospital, for rest, the need for early induction of labour may not be as great. Although it has been claimed that rest in bed will reduce the risk of preterm labour in twin pregnancies there is little statistical evidence to support this. In cases of polyhydramnios repeated paracentesis may prevent premature labour, but this measure is seldom successful.

A history of previous midtrimester abortion of a normal fetus may be an indication that the cervix is incompetent. Investigation of this possibility is more conclusive in the non-pregnant state than during pregnancy, but ultrasound examination of the internal os during pregnancy may be helpful.

In any patient with a history of repeated preterm labour or abortion the insertion of an encircling suture around the cervix during early pregnancy should be considered.

Treatment

The mother should be admitted to a hospital where there are facilities for specialized care for preterm infants. The safest method of transferring the preterm infant to the special unit is in its mother's uterus. If the mother is admitted for delivery both obstetric and paediatric facilities are immediately available. Paediatric special care units are now associated with every large obstetric unit, and the great improvement in survival of preterm infants in recent years is largely due to this.

If the mother seems to be starting labour a vaginal examination is made to determine whether liquor is escaping and whether the cervix is dilated. An external tocograph is useful for recording uterine activity.

Drugs are available which will inhibit uterine contractions. Most obstetricians would regard these as unnecessary if the pregnancy has reached the 35th week. If the membranes have ruptured there is also some risk of intrauterine fetal infection and this may sway the decision against attempting to delay delivery, unless the fetus is so small that it has a high risk of neonatal death. On the other hand, a short delay of 24 to 48 hours before delivery may permit the administration of dexamethasone to the mother with the hope of encouraging the surfactant activity of the fetal lung (p. 316).

Drugs which may be used to inhibit uterine action

Opinions differ about the effectiveness of these drugs. Some controlled trials have thrown doubt upon their value, but many clinicians believe that they are useful.

β-receptor agonists

These include salbutamol and ritodrine. Ritodrine

is added to 5 per cent glucose in water to give a solution containing 100 micrograms/ml. Intravenous infusion is started at 50 micrograms/min and increased by 50 micrograms/min every 20 min until the contractions of the uterus are inhibited or 400 micrograms/min has been reached. Infusion is continued for two hours after contractions have ceased, usually for a total of 6–12 hours. Thereafter ritodrine 15 mg 6-hourly is given by mouth for four weeks, or until the 36th week of gestation has been reached. If cardiovascular side-effects such as hypotension and tachycardia occur they may be treated with propanolol 1 mg intravenously.

Salbutamol is more potent than ritodrine. It is given intravenously at 10–45 micrograms/min until contractions cease. The subsequent dose is 4 mg by mouth every 6–8 h.

17OH-progesterones in preterm labour

Progesterone is a natural suppressor of myometrial activity, if given before labour it may postpone the start of uterine contractions. More recently, the use of β-mimetics and prostaglandin inhibitors has overtaken the use of progesterone, but in many parts of the world 17-hydroxyprogesterone hexanoate (Proluton Depot) is the drug of choice to suppress premature myometrial activity.

Management of labour

If the pregnancy has passed the 35th week, or if at an earlier stage it is evident that attempts to inhibit uterine action have failed, then prompt delivery is the aim.

During labour pain relief should be by epidural block rather than by drugs such as pethidine, which may cause respiratory depression in the newborn infant. An episiotomy is performed to minimize compression of the fetal head during delivery, and in a primigravida gentle forceps extraction with Wrigley's forceps may be advantageous. Everything must be ready for the resuscitation and care of the preterm infant.

Management of preterm labour in very small infants with cephalic or breech presentation

In very low birthweight babies the use of caesarean section has spread. Below an estimated birth weight of 1000 g, survival of fetuses with either cephalic or breech presentations is significantly

better if they are delivered by caesarean section than by vaginal delivery. From 1001–1500 g estimated birth weight, there is no added benefit from using caesarean section for those with a cephalic presentation but the survival rate is increased threefold in breeches. For infants with estimated birth weights above this level caesarean section offers a decreasing advantage, except in those presenting by the breech with proven intrauterine grown retardation (IUGR), when, at all birth weights, there is a fivefold increase in perinatal mortality for vaginal births compared with caesarean deliveries.

PREMATURE RUPTURE OF THE MEMBRANES

This refers to spontaneous rupture of the membranes before the onset of labour. Labour is likely to follow soon afterwards, and while this is of little significance if the pregnancy is near term, at an earlier stage a small fetus will be delivered, with increased perinatal mortality. If labour does not occur for some days after the membranes rupture bacteria may invade the uterine cavity and cause intrauterine infection of the fetus. There is also a risk of prolapse of the cord.

Causes

There is no evidence that the membranes are weak or abnormally developed. Sometimes there is evidence of infection of the membranes, but this may be the effect rather than the cause of early rupture.

Premature rupture of the membranes may occur in cases of multiple pregnancy and polyhydramnios. With malpresentations such as transverse lie the presenting part does not fit into the pelvic brim and premature rupture of the membranes is a theoretical possibility; in fact this seldom occurs unless labour has started.

Incompetence of the internal os of the cervix may be caused by forcible surgical dilatation of the cervix for termination of pregnancy or the treatment of dysmenorrhoea, or by obstetrical injury. The cervix dilates painlessly, the membranes bulge through it and their eventual rupture is followed by midtrimester abortion or preterm labour.

Rarely there is an intermittent escape of clear fluid in late pregnancy. In some cases this may be due to hindwater rupture, but the cause is often obscure. Exudation of fluid from the exposed but intact membranes sometimes occurs in cases of cervical incompetence. The risk of infection is not great and there is no urgency for delivery on this count.

Diagnosis

The patient notices the escape of fluid and sometimes speculum examination will show that this is coming through the cervix.

It is necessary to make sure that the escaping fluid is not urine. If it is liquor, microscopical examination may show fetal squames, lanugo hairs or vernix. If the urine is tested and contains no protein, discovery of protein in the escaping fluid suggests that it is the liquor. Liquor is alkaline, with a characteristic smell, and urine is normally acid. Cervical mucus has a different consistency.

Management

The patient is admitted to hospital. A vaginal examination is made with sterile precautions to obtain a sample of the fluid, to assess cervical dilatation, to discover the presentation and to exclude prolapse of the cord. An ultrasound scan may be required to confirm the period of gestation.

If the pregnancy has passed 32 weeks it is best to expedite labour with an intravenous oxytocin drip. Before 32 weeks it may be more prudent to delay labour until the fetus is more mature, but with good facilities for neonatal care the tendency is towards earlier delivery. The patient is kept at rest in bed and a broad-spectrum antibiotic such as ampicillin is used only if delivery is expected soon. Some liquor may be obtained by amniocentesis (rather than by testing that which is escaping) for bacteriological examination.

If there is any uterine activity this may be inhibited by giving one of the drugs mentioned above. If the fetal lung is immature the mother is given dexamethasone, 12 mg orally, then 6 mg daily in divided doses.

PRESENTATION AND PROLAPSE OF THE UMBILICAL CORD

Descent of the umbilical cord below the presenting part occurs about once in 300 births, and constitutes a grave risk to the fetus because of obstruction to the circulation in the umbilical vessels.

Two situations are described. The cord is said to be *presenting* when it lies below the presenting part in an intact bag of membranes (Fig. 5.32), and *prolapsing* when the membranes have ruptured. Sometimes the cord lies beside the head but cannot be easily felt on vaginal examination (occult prolapse). This may cause fetal distress, the cause of which is not evident at the time. Whenever unexplained fetal distress is recognized clinically or with the cardiotocograph the possibility of cord compression should be considered.

Causes

Descent of the cord is more likely to occur when the presenting part does not fit well into the lower uterine segment. In normal cases the well-flexed head engages before the onset of labour, or soon after, and tends to prevent prolapse of the cord.

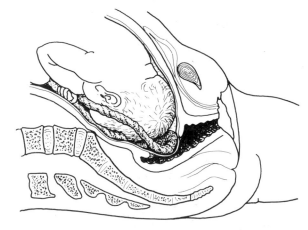

Fig. 5.32   Presentation of the umbilical cord

Prolapse is particularly likely to occur with malpresentations such as a flexed breech or a shoulder presentation, and occasionally with a brow, face or even an occipitoposterior position of the vertex. It is more likely to occur when the head is free above the pelvic brim, sometimes because of pelvic contraction. Prolapse of the cord may occur with a premature or small fetus, and in twin pregnancy.

By permitting greater mobility of the fetus an excess of liquor amnii tends to encourage malpresentation, and when the membranes rupture a sudden gush of liquor may carry a loop of cord down into the vagina. In some cases of descent the cord is unduly long, or is attached to a low-lying placenta.

Diagnosis

Presentation of the cord is seldom discovered. It is less common than prolapse of the cord and patients are not invariably examined vaginally at the onset of labour. Fetal distress does not usually occur until the membranes rupture. A presenting cord can be felt through the intact bag of membranes, and the pulsation of its vessels should be recognized. (Pulsation may also be felt in cases of vasa praevia, in which there is a velamentous insertion of the cord.) Slowing of the fetal heart may be noted when the head is pushed into the brim in cases of presentation of the cord, but slowing may also occur in cases of placenta praevia or vasa praevia, or simply as a result of compression of the head.

In prolapse of the cord the diagnosis is easy as a loop of cord is felt in the vagina, or may even present at the vulva. It should be a rule that every patient is examined vaginally as soon as possible after rupture of the membranes, whether she is having contractions or not, in order to exclude or diagnose prolapse of the cord. The loop of cord should be felt to see if pulsations are present, but even if the cord is compressed so that pulsations are absent the fetus may still be alive, and fetal heart sounds may be audible on auscultation of the abdomen.

Whenever presentation or prolapse of the cord is diagnosed, the degree of dilatation of the cervix should be noted, and the cause sought. The possibility of twins, malpresentation or contracted pelvis should be considered.

Prognosis

Presentation or prolapse of the cord does not itself increase the risk to the mother, except for any measures which have to be applied to treat the causal complications such as malpresentations or contracted pelvis. Descent of the cord often calls for speedy delivery by forceps or caesarean section, and these procedures increase the maternal risk to some extent.

The prognosis for the fetus is poor; stillbirth or neonatal death occurs in about 20 per cent of cases. It is said that the fetal prognosis is worst when the head presents, as it is more likely to compress the cord than the breech or shoulder. The outlook for the fetus has been improved by the more frequent use of caesarean section in circumstances in which the cervix is not fully dilated.

Treatment

If the fetus is alive the treatment is immediate delivery.

If the cervix is not fully dilated this will be by caesarean section. While preparations for the operation are being made immediate steps should be taken to relieve pressure on the cord. Even if pulsation cannot be felt in the cord the fetal heart may still be heard on auscultation or detected with ultrasound. Two or more fingers are inserted into the vagina and the presenting part is pushed as far out of the pelvic cavity as possible and held there. Attempts to replace the cord are usually unsuccessful and also produce spasm in the cord vessels; they should not be made.

If the cervix is fully dilated and there is a cephalic presentation with no complicating factors such as malpresentation or contracted pelvis, immediate delivery with the forceps is performed.

If there is a breech presentation the presenting part is very unlikely to be deep in the pelvis, and caesarean section may be preferable to breech extraction.

For other malpresentations which would require correction before vaginal delivery is possible, caesarean section is wisest.

If it is certain that the fetus is dead, and unless there is some other problem such as a contracted pelvis which requires treatment, labour is left to continue until eventual vaginal delivery. Analgesic drugs and epidural anaesthesia can be freely used.

FETAL DISTRESS DURING LABOUR

During each uterine contraction the maternal blood flow through the placenta is impeded; the venous outflow is obstructed before the arterial supply. The fetus is usually unaffected by this, but if uterine contractions are prolonged or if there has been previous impairment of placental function then fetal hypoxia occurs. As a result of this hypoxia the carbon dioxide concentration in the fetal blood rises and respiratory acidosis occurs, with a fall in pH. In severe hypoxia the fetal tissues meet their energy requirements by anaerobic gly-colysis, burning up glycogen but producing lactic acid in the process, and this causes further depression of the pH by metabolic acidosis. Although the fetus will withstand and recover from degrees of hypoxia and acidosis which would be fatal in an adult, if the pH falls below about 6.9 death or brain damage is almost inevitable.

The fetus also shows clinical signs of distress with the changes in hydrogen ion concentration. Distress is an ill-defined term, and may not invariably be due to hypoxia, although this is the commonest cause. The first effect of hypoxia is a rise in fetal heart rate from sympathetic action. Fetal tachycardia in cases of hypoxia is of varying degree, but a rate persisting at well above 160 beats per minute has considerable significance. Fetal tachycardia may also occur if the mother has high fever or is dehydrated, but in all other cases this sign must be regarded as evidence of fetal distress.

If the hypoxia persists and is of more severe degree the fetal heart rate will slow after each uterine contraction, and there will also be persistent bradycardia. Any case with slowing below 120 beats per minute should be carefully assessed, and urgent assessment is necessary if the rate falls below 100, or if there is cardiac irregularity.

Initial slowing of the fetal heart rate is probably a vagal effect, and vagal activity may also lead to contraction of the bowel and the passage of meconium into the liquor. However, it should be noted that premature fetuses, even if fatally hypoxic, seldom pass meconium.

Unfortunately the correlation between many of these clinical signs of fetal distress and real hypoxia is not very strong. Even the most serious combination of these signs, bradycardia with the passage of meconium, is found to be associated with a signi-ficantly hypoxic fetus in only 25 per cent of cases, so that if action were taken on these signs alone it might be unnecessary in three-quarters of the cases.

CONTINUOUS MONITORING OF THE FETAL HEART RATE

Ordinary auscultation of the fetal heart rate has several limitations. It has to be performed inter-mittently and the intervals between observations may vary. If the heart is being auscultated for 60 seconds every 15 minutes, there are 14 out of 15 minutes when changes may not be observed.

Further, the main stress that affects the fetal heart rate is a uterine contraction, yet it is at this time that many doctors and midwives fail to hear the heart. Unless auscultation takes place very soon after the contraction any change due to the stress will be missed. In consequence efforts have been made during the last 20 years to record the fetal heart rate continuously, even during contractions. This can be achieved by several methods:

Phonocardiography

In phonocardiography a carbon microphone is held on the mother's abdomen by a wide elastic belt, and picks up the fetal heart sounds. This works well enough when the patient is still, but as labour progresses and the patient moves about the microphone picks up too much background noise so that this method is now seldom used during labour.

Pulsed ultrasound

With pulsed ultrasound the fetal heart rate can be recorded using the Doppler effect when a pulse source and receiving head is placed on the mother's abdomen. An ultrasonic pulse is passed into the fetus; those waves that hit moving fluid are re-turned at a different frequency from those reflected back from static objects, and the pulsa-tions of the fetal heart can be recognized. The instrument is less affected by movements and external sounds than the phonocardiograph.

Recording electrical activity

The best method currently available is to record the electrical activity of the fetal heart. When the cervix is more than 2 cm dilated and the membranes have ruptured a scalp electrode can be fixed to the fetal scalp; this largely eliminates difficulties arising from signals from the electrical activity of the maternal heart. With a ratemeter a continuous estimate of the fetal heart rate is recorded on a trace on which the uterine contractions are also recorded with a tocometer.

A disadvantage of this method is that the electrical connection between the electrode and the recording machine restricts the mobility of the patient. This can be overcome by telemetry apparatus which transmits radio signals to the recording machine, but this is expensive and not yet widely available. The purpose of the investigation, and its possible contribution to the safety of the baby, should always be carefully explained to the mother.

Conventionally a range of 120 to 160 beats per minute is taken as the normal fetal heart rate

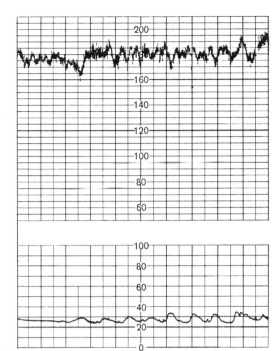

Fig. 5.34   Fetal tachycardia

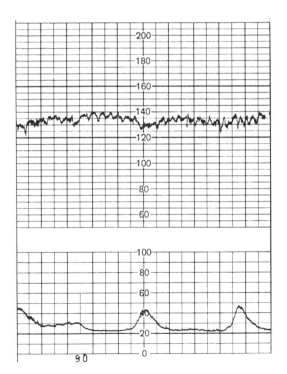

Fig. 5.33   Normal trace. The upper record is of the fetal heart rate; the lower record shows uterine activity

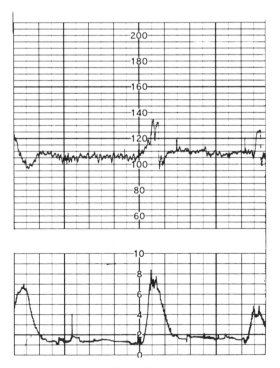

Fig. 5.35   Fetal bradycardia

during labour, but with better recording methods it is found that in most cases the rate is within a range of 130 to 150 beats per minute (Fig. 5.33). Both baseline tachycardia (Fig. 5.34) and baseline bradycardia (Fig. 5.35) have a significant association with chronic fetal hypoxia. In most instances the heart first beats faster and then slows down if the stress continues.

Continuous records of the fetal heart rate normally show continuous minor variations, with a range of about 10 beats per minute. This baseline variability is the response of the heart to a variety of factors, including vagal and sympathetic stimuli, catecholamines and oxygen tension. Loss of baseline variability (Fig. 5.36) implies that the cardiac reflexes are impaired, either from the effect of hypoxia or of drugs such as diazepam (Valium). It may be serious, but it is also a physiological phenomenon that occurs cyclically.

Stress to the fetus during labour occurs during a uterine contraction, and the response of the fetal heart rate to contractions is shown on the rate-meter trace (Fig. 5.37). With each contraction the rate often slows, but it returns to normal soon after removal of the stress. These early decelerations or

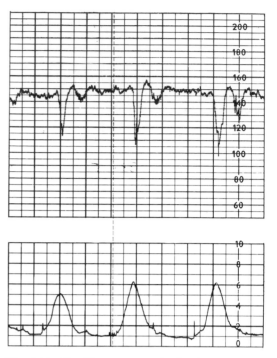

Fig. 5.37   Fetal heart rate; early decelerations

'dips' in the heart rate start within 30 seconds of the onset of the contraction and return rapidly to the baseline rate. They are due to vagal stimulation caused by head compression and are not of serious significance as a rule. They indicate that while the fetus is undergoing some stress the cardiac control mechanisms are responding normally.

Figure 5.38 illustrates a more serious condition. Here the fetal heart takes some time to respond to the stress of the uterine contraction, with the onset of late deceleration more than 30 seconds after the beginning of the uterine contraction, and a slow return to the baseline rate. Such late decelerations are commonly caused by hypoxia. They must be considered to be serious and their exact significance must be checked at once by taking a sample of fetal blood from the fetal scalp to determine its pH (*see* p. 220).

In practice variations in the fetal heart rate may be complex and difficult to interpret. Figure 5.39 shows variable decelerations with no consistent relationship to uterine contractions. These are sometimes caused by compression of the umbilical cord between the uterus and the fetal body, or because it is looped round some part of the fetus.

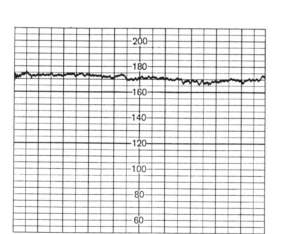

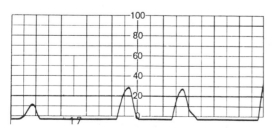

Fig. 5.36   Loss of baseline variability in fetal heart rate

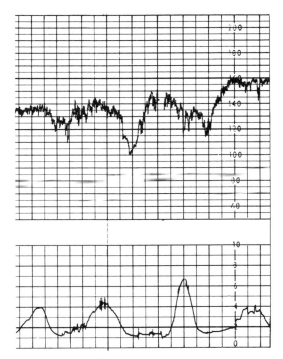

Fig. 5.38   Fetal heart rate; late decelerations

Provided that they do not persist for more than a few minutes they may have little significance, but persistence for more than 15 minutes would call for an urgent fetal scalp blood sample.

Overstimulation of the uterine muscle with oxytocin will cause prolonged uterine contractions and severe changes in the fetal heart rate (Fig. 5.40).

If the mother lies on her back compression of the inferior vena cava by the uterus may impede the venous return, depress the cardiac output and reduce placental blood flow. The effect of asking the mother to lie on her side should be observed (Fig. 5.41); if the abnormal changes in the fetal heart rate still persist myometrial overactivity may well be the cause.

A rare cause of a slow fetal heart rate is congenital heart block. It carries a bad prognosis as it may be associated with other congenital cardiac abnormalities or maternal disseminated lupus erythematosis. The condition may be recognized by noting that the rate has always been slow, even in pregnancy, and by observing that the slow rate does not vary during labour.

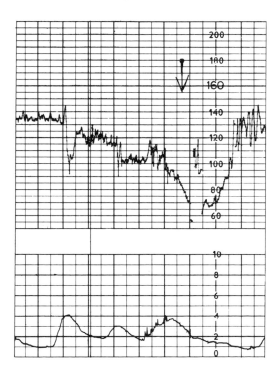

Fig. 5.40   Trace of fetal heart rate showing the effect of overstimulation of the uterus with oxytocin. The drip was turned off at the point marked with the arrow

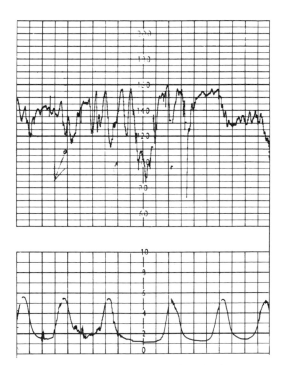

Fig. 5.39   Fetal heart rate; variable decelerations

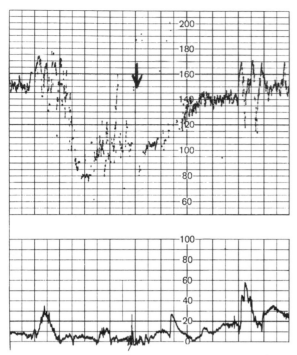

Fig. 5.41 Trace of fetal heart rate showing the effect of maternal supine hypotension. At the point marked with the arrow the mother was turned onto her side. As her blood pressure returned to normal the fetal bradycardia ceased

An increase in the fetal heart rate can occur with intrauterine infection or with maternal pyrexia from any cause.

Precise continuous recording of the fetal heart rate in relation to uterine contractions is a great advance in monitoring the fetus during labour, but it should not be assumed that such traces are absolute indications for intervention. Any suggestion that the fetus is hypoxic should be checked by determining the pH of the fetal blood before caesarean section is undertaken. The most serious pattern of heart rate changes, namely fetal bradycardia with loss of baseline variability and late decelerations, is associated with significant fetal hypoxia in about 65 per cent of cases. Even among these there will therefore be about 35 per cent of cases in which fetal blood sampling will show that immediate intervention is not necessary.

FETAL BLOOD SAMPLING

During labour, after the membranes have ruptured

spontaneously or have been ruptured artificially, a sample of fetal blood can be obtained for evaluation of its acid–base status. It is possible to measure the partial pressure of oxygen, but this fluctuates very quickly, and the pH gives a better indication of the metabolic state of the fetus. The blood is obtained by passing an endoscope through the cervix and then using a very small blade held in a suitable handle to make a small

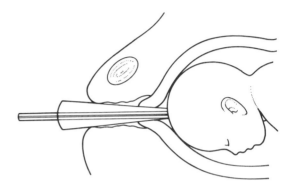

Fig. 5.42 A tapered endoscope is passed through the cervix to expose the fetal scalp. The scalp (Fig. 5.43) produces a blend of blood which is drawn off in a prelapanized tube.

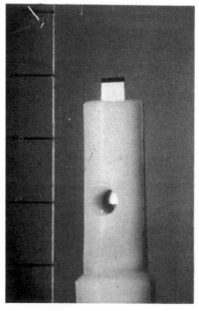

Fig. 5.43 Enlarged photograph of blade. The small rectangular blade is 2 mm long and the wide shoulder prevents deeper penetration of the scalp

incision in the fetal scalp. A drop of blood is drawn into a long fine tube. With 0.2 ml of blood the pH can be determined immediately with a micro-Astrup machine (Figs. 5.42 and 5.43).

Fetal blood sampling during labour is useful for excluding hypoxia and acidaemia in cases with clinical suspicion of fetal distress, so that unnecessary caesarean section may be avoided. If the pH is above 7.25 there is no hypoxia at the time of the observation, although the test has no predictive value. In doubtful cases a progressive fall in pH below 7.2 in successive samples during the first stage of labour is highly significant, but in the second stage a pH of 7.15 may be accepted as the lower limit of normal. Sampling is seldom performed during the second stage, because by this time it is usually simpler to deliver the fetus suspected of being hypoxic with forceps.

The state of the fetus is best monitored during labour by a combination of continuous recording of the fetal heart rate with blood sampling when necessary to confirm any suspicion of hypoxia. Obviously such monitoring is only possible in well-equipped and well-staffed units. In such units about a third of the women are usually judged to need continuous monitoring. At present continuous fetal heart rate monitoring is widely used in the UK but fetal blood sampling is less often performed. These methods do not cause an increased work load for the staff, because they may reduce the caesarean rate for unreal fetal distress. In some respects they make surveillance of the patients easier, but they must never be allowed to interfere with the close personal relationship between mothers in labour and the staff. If women who are judged to have high risk pregnancies are transferred to units with good facilities for monitoring better management of fetal hypoxia will result, with a reduction in both perinatal mortality and morbidity.

TRAUMATIC LESIONS

RUPTURE OF THE UTERUS

Rupture of the uterus is a most serious condition. It usually occurs during labour, although it can occasionally happen during the later weeks of pregnancy.

Causes

During pregnancy

During pregnancy the only common cause of rupture of the uterus is a weak scar after previous operations on the uterus. The higher the scar is placed on the uterus the greater the risk. The most dangerous scar is that of 'classical' caesarean section; this is more dangerous than a hysterotomy scar. Rupture of a lower segment caesarean scar is uncommon during pregnancy. Rupture after myomectomy, tubal reimplantation or excision of a uterine septum, or following perforation of the uterus with a curette or cannula, is rare. Rupture of the uterus during pregnancy has also followed a direct blow on the abdomen, and a perforating wound may injure the uterus.

During labour

During labour rupture may be caused by:

obstructed labour – the rupture may be spontaneous or follow manipulations carried out for the relief of the obstruction

intrauterine manipulations, such as internal version or manual removal of an adherent placenta

forcible dilatation of the cervix. Rarely, a cervical tear in a normal delivery may extend up into the body of the uterus

the injudicious use of oxytocic drugs

a weak scar in the uterus after caesarean section, or in rare instances after hysterotomy, myomectomy, tubal reimplantation or perforation of the uterus with a curette or cannula. A lower segment caesarian scar is safer than one in the upper segment

in women who have had numerous pregnancies uterine rupture occasionally occurs without any evident preceding abnormality.

Pathology

Ruptures of the uterus are divided into:

  complete or intraperitoneal
  incomplete or extraperitoneal

depending on whether the peritoneal coat is torn through or not.

Obstructed labour

In obstructed labour rupture of the uterus generally takes place in the overstretched and thinned lower segment, to which it may be limited, but sometimes it spreads upwards or downwards. The life of the mother is threatened by shock and intraperitoneal bleeding. There is also a high risk of peritonitis, especially when the accident occurs after a long labour in which repeated examinations or intrauterine manipulations have been made. In cases of obstructed labour the fetus is nearly always dead before the rupture occurs, but in any case it will perish if complete rupture occurs.

Rupture of a scar

Rupture of a scar in the uterus usually occurs during labour, but may also occur in the later weeks of pregnancy. In the UK a weak caesarean scar is now the commonest cause of rupture of the uterus. Overdistention of the uterus, by twin pregnancy for example, will increase the risk. Healing of a uterine scar may be imperfect if sepsis occurs in the puerperium, or if the edges of the incision are inaccurately sutured. If the placenta is implanted over the scar in a subsequent pregnancy the risk of rupture is increased. The scar may give way if caesarean section is repeated several times and the current operating incision is made through the scar tissue left by previous operations. A lower segment scar is unlikely to rupture during pregnancy; an upper segment (classical) scar may give way in either pregnancy or labour.

A caesarean scar in the lower segment may stretch gradually, so that the uterine wall in the region of the scar is only represented by attenuated and avascular fibrous tissue. When the weak area finally gives way during labour there is sometimes relatively little intraperitoneal bleeding. The membranes may bulge through the rent, and will eventually give way, when the fetus or placenta may pass through it.

Symptoms and signs

Rupture through a uterine scar

In cases of rupture through a uterine scar during pregnancy the history of the previous operation will be available, and the scar in the skin will be seen, although a low transverse incision may be hidden by pubic hair. The abdominal incision of a classical (upper segment) caesarean section is made one-third above and two-thirds below the umbilicus. A longitudinal incision below the umbilicus signifies a lower segment section, as does the one commonly performed across the abdomen an inch or two above the symphysis. Occasionally the attenuated scar of a classical caesarean section may be felt through a thin abdominal wall as a tender sulcus in the uterus, although nearly all caesarean sections done in the UK are lower segment. Rupture during pregnancy may be so gradual that the symptoms may be very slight at first; the description 'silent rupture' has been applied to these cases. There is abdominal pain (which may be wrongly attributed to the onset of labour) but at first there is little change in the general condition of the patient. At this stage diagnosis may be difficult and it may be necessary to observe the case for a time before a conclusion is reached. If the rupture becomes complete and part of the uterine contents are extruded into the peritoneal cavity more severe pain and shock occur.

Rupture of a scar often occurs during labour, and the scar gives way more suddenly than during pregnancy, so the symptoms are more dramatic, with severe pain, shock, fetal distress and some bleeding from the vagina. Unless the contents of the uterus pass into the peritoneal cavity uterine contractions may continue. The possibility of rupture of the scar should always be considered if a patient who has had a caesarean section suddenly complains during labour of severe pain which is not synchronous with the uterine contractions. The accident does not usually occur after a long and difficult labour, and for that reason the patient's general condition is better, and the risk of infection less, than in cases of rupture due to obstructed labour. Because pain is a good warning symptom of dehiscence of a uterine scar during labour some obstetricians hesitate to give an epidural anaesthetic to women in labour who have an increased risk of uterine rupture.

Spontaneous rupture during obstructed labour

The labour will have been prolonged, or there will have been violent uterine action almost without intermission between the pains, so that the patient may be exhausted before the rupture occurs. There may be signs of disproportion or of a malpresentation such as a transverse lie, although these signs may have been overlooked before the accident. There may be fetal distress and the fetal heart may have stopped beating. At the moment of rupture the patient cries out and complains of a sharp, tearing pain in the lower abdomen. After the rupture there is shock, with pallor, sweating and constant lower abdominal pain. The pulse becomes thready and rapid and the blood pressure falls. With an incomplete tear the signs of shock may not be so severe.

Some degree of vaginal haemorrhage is usually present. On abdominal examination there is marked tenderness over the site of the rupture. The presenting part may not be reached *pervaginam* unless it is impacted in the pelvis. If the fetus is completely extruded into the peritoneal cavity uterine contractions may cease, but in other cases they often continue. With complete extrusion the fetus may be felt in the abdominal cavity with the retracted uterus beside it.

Rupture after intrauterine manipulations

In these cases the patient is usually anaesthetized when the manipulation, such as manual removal of the placenta, is taking place, so the first evidence that anything is amiss may be a sudden deterioration in her general condition, either at the time or later when the effect of the anaesthetic wears off. In other instances the injury may be discovered while the operator's hand is still in the uterus. After any difficult manipulation the uterus should be examined carefully to exclude injury.

Extensive cervical lacerations

In some respects these injuries resemble the previous group as they are usually produced with the forceps at a difficult delivery, especially if the cervix is not completely dilated, but they seldom extend far enough to open the peritoneal cavity. Brisk external haemorrhage may occur, or a large haematoma may form in the broad ligament (*see* p. 227). Vaginal bleeding in the third stage of labour with the uterus empty and firmly retracted should always suggest the possibility of this type of injury, which can be confirmed by visual examination of the cervix. For this effective retractors and the help of an assistant will be required.

Rupture caused by oxytocic drugs

Rupture of the uterus can follow the administration of oxytocin before the delivery of the child, particularly when some obstruction prevents rapid delivery. The risk is much greater in multiparae. The danger is less if the oxytocin is given as a dilute intravenous drip and the uterine contractions are carefully observed and controlled. Several cases of rupture have followed the unmonitored use of buccal oxytocin and of prostaglandins to induce labour or a late miscarriage. In the UK the misuse of oxytocic agents is responsible for more damage to the uterus than the use of instruments or intrauterine manipulation.

Rupture caused by direct injury to the abdomen

In the rare cases of rupture from this cause severe shock and abdominal pain, together with the history of the accident, will suggest the possibility of visceral injury. Precise diagnosis may be impossible without laparotomy, and in case of doubt this would be justified.

Prognosis

Rupture of the uterus in cases of obstructed labour has a high mortality because the accident usually occurs in cases of prolonged labour with much manipulation, sometimes with inefficient obstetric aid, and often without proper aseptic precautions. The mortality after rupture of a caesarean scar is much less, as the accident does not usually follow prolonged labour, and the patient is usually confined in hospital where the rupture is more quickly detected.

In the UK the incidence of maternal death from uterine rupture has fallen from 5.7 per million maternities in 1970 to 2.1 in 1981 (four cases). Three of the four cases were traumatic ruptures associated with the administration of oxytocin in multiparous patients (in two of whom labour was being induced for intrauterine fetal death); there was no case of scar rupture.

The fetal prognosis is bad, depending on the degree of scar rupture.

Dangerous intrauterine manipulations are now rarely performed, and obstructed labour is less often seen, owing to timely caesarean section, so that the increased risk of subsequent scar rupture must be set against this.

Treatment

Prevention

Disproportion must be recognized early and labour must not be allowed to continue to the stage of obstruction. An oblique lie must be corrected early, but if the shoulder has become impacted version should not be attempted; caesarean section is the correct treatment. The cervix must not be forcibly dilated and forceps must not be applied unless it is fully dilated. Manual removal of the placenta must be carefully performed, with an external hand guarding the fundus.

A patient who has had a caesarean section, hysterotomy or any operation on the uterine wall must be delivered in a hospital where all obstetric facilities are available. However, the fact that a patient has already had one caesarean section does not mean that a subsequent pregnancy must also be treated in this way. If the first operation was not performed for disproportion but for some non-recurrent condition, such as placenta praevia, vaginal delivery should be allowed, with the proviso that if labour does not progress smoothly section will be repeated. If the patient had an upper segment operation, or if gross uterine infection occurred, elective section would be advisable, as it would be in the case of a woman who had already had two or more sections. Ultrasound scanning will show if the placenta overlies the uterine scar, when the risk of rupture is increased.

Treatment after rupture has occurred

Before operation the general condition of the patient must be improved as much as possible by giving morphine, blood transfusion and intravenous glucose solution if necessary.

Immediate laparotomy is required. In cases of scar rupture it is often possible to excise the edges of the rent and resuture the uterus. The bladder is sometimes adherent to the scar and may be torn, in which case its wall must be freed and sutured in two layers and an indwelling catheter inserted.

Many cases of uterine rupture during obstructed labour are best treated by hysterectomy, as efficient suturing of bruised and ragged tissues may be impossible. If the tear is accessible and the edges not too ragged it may be sutured, but the risk of rupture in a subsequent pregnancy is so great that it is usually wise to prevent this by ligating the fallopian tubes.

Wide-spectrum antibiotics are given and paralytic ileus is treated by giving only intravenous fluids and maintaining gastric aspiration until bowel sounds reappear.

ACUTE INVERSION OF THE UTERUS

In this condition the body of the uterus becomes, either partially or completely, turned inside out after delivery of the fetus (Fig. 5.44). It is an important but rare cause of shock in the third stage of labour and may be fatal if it is untreated. Inversion may take place before or after the delivery of the placenta. If it is complete the fundus of the uterus may be seen at the vulva.

Cause

The usual cause is mismanagement of the third stage of labour by the attendant pulling on the umbilical cord or pressing on the fundus while the uterus is not contracting and the placenta has not separated. Very rarely it occurs spontaneously.

Symptoms and signs

The chief symptoms are those of shock, with some haemorrhage, and sometimes the appearance of the uterine fundus at the vulva. As a rule shock is severe and is greater than the blood loss warrants. Pain is of variable degree. Unexplained shock during the third stage of labour should always suggest the possibility of uterine rupture or that inversion has occurred and a vaginal examination should be made. In cases of inversion the body of the uterus will not be felt in its usual position and the round mass of the uterus will be felt protruding through the cervix. Inversion has a high mortality if it is undiagnosed or left untreated.

Treatment

Shock and bleeding will continue until the uterus is

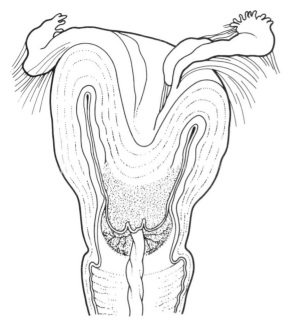

Fig. 5.44 Acute puerperal inversion of the uterus

LACERATION OF THE CERVIX

Minor lacerations of the cervix occur frequently but do not cause symptoms.

Extensive lacerations may be caused by precipitate labour, application of forceps with the cervix incompletely dilated, or rapid delivery of the head with a breech presentation. A scar in the cervix from previous injury may tear. With a deep tear there is continuing haemorrhage during or after the third stage; this goes on even when the uterus is empty and retracted. The tear must be sutured (Fig. 5.45). For this the patient is anaesthetized, a

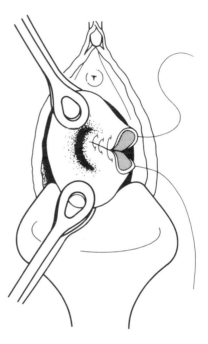

Fig. 5.45 The repair of a tear of the cervix by interrupted catgut sutures. The cervix is depicted outside the vulva for the sake of clarity

replaced, hence it is desirable that it should be replaced at once. The inverted fundus soon becomes oedematous, which makes replacement more difficult. As soon as the diagnosis is made the patient is anaesthetized and the uterus is replaced. After cleansing the vulva, vagina and inverted uterus, the placenta, if it is still attached to the uterus, is peeled off. The uterus is then squeezed in the hand and replaced, the part which became inverted last being replaced first, and the fundus last of all.

When replacement is complete further haemorrhage and recurrence of the inversion are prevented by intravenous injection of ergometrine, 500 micrograms. Treatment for shock is given concurrently.

Alternatively, replacement is possible by fluid pressure with manitol delivered through wide bore tubing from a container held at a height of about 60 cm; a surprisingly large amount of fluid is necessary.

Should inversion be discovered some days after labour reposition under anaesthesia is usually possible. Operative division of the constricting ring or vaginal hysterectomy will hardly ever be needed.

wide speculum is inserted, and the anterior and posterior lips of the cervix are held with sponge forceps and drawn well down, so that interrupted catgut or Dexon sutures can be inserted through the whole thickness of its wall. While waiting for arrangements to be made, bleeding may be temporarily controlled by applying sponge forceps to the edges of the tear.

LACERATION OF THE PERINEUM AND VAGINA

These lesions are described as being of three degrees:

the *first degree tear* involves only the skin and a minor part of the perineal body and the related posterior wall of the vagina

a *second degree tear* involves the perineal body up to (but not involving) the anal sphincter, with a corresponding tear in the vagina (Fig. 5.46)

a *third degree (complete) tear* includes the anal sphincter and usually extends for 2 cm or more up the anal canal. If a third degree tear is not repaired there will be incontinence of flatus and any loose stool.

An extensive tear of the vagina can occur without a tear in the perineum, and the vaginal walls should always be carefully inspected after delivery. Minor lacerations can also occur on the anterolateral vaginal wall.

Treatment of first and second degree tears

It is important to repair all perineal lacerations immediately, to prevent any infection of the raw surface. Deep lacerations involving the perineal

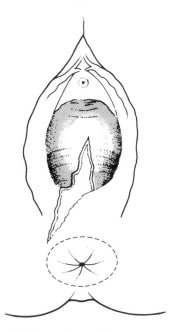

Fig. 5.46　Second degree perineal tear

body that are not sutured, or do not heal, increase the possibility of subsequent uterovaginal prolapse.

The vaginal epithelium is sutured from the apex of the tear, which must be clearly identified, down to the introitus with either a continuous suture or interrupted sutures of fine catgut or Dexon. The perineal body is repaired with stronger stitches of the same material. The skin edges are brought together without tension with fine catgut or Dexon sutures. The repair should be done carefully and accurately. Unless general anaesthesia or epidural anaesthesia is already being used local anaesthesia with 1 per cent lignocaine is employed.

Treatment of third degree (complete) tears

The operation should be done by an experienced obstetric surgeon in a properly equipped theatre with general or epidural anaesthesia. The tissues heal very well if the operation is done carefully soon after delivery, but if this is not done, or if the tissues fail to heal, the patient will have to undergo a more difficult operation later, or she will suffer from rectal incontinence.

Catgut or Dexon sutures are used throughout. The anal mucosa is first repaired with fine stitches, tying the knots inside the bowel lumen. The ends of the anal sphincter are found and carefully brought together with interrupted sutures. The other tissues are repaired as described above for second degree tears (Fig. 5.47).

After-care

Each day the perineum is washed with soap and water, and then carefully dried. Patients with extensive tears sometimes have retention of urine, for which catheterization is necessary. If the bowel has not acted by the fourth day a glycerine suppository may be used, but oral liquid paraffin should not be given.

If any perineal wound becomes infected sufficient stitches are removed to permit drainage, and antibiotics are given. Bathing, preferably in a bidet, is continued until the wound is covered with granulation tissue, when secondary suture can be performed if necessary.

FISTULAE

Fistulae may occur as a result of pressure by the

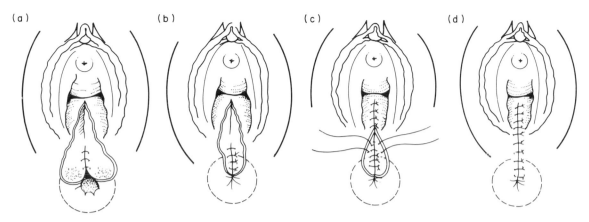

Fig. 5.47 Repair of complete perineal tear. (a) suture of the rectal mucosa; 2, suture of the ends of the anal sphincter; 3, repair of the perineal body; 4, suture of the perineal skin

presenting part in prolonged labour, or by direct injury during operative procedures such as craniotomy or caesarean section. In obstructed labour prolonged pressure between the head and the pubic bone may cause local ischaemia and the subsequent necrosis of the anterior vaginal wall and base of the bladder leads to the formation of a *vesicovaginal fistula* (*see* p. 211). With very extensive necrosis the rectum may also be involved. A much more common cause of a *rectovaginal fistula* is a complete tear of the perineum and rectovaginal septum, in which the lower part has healed but a defect remains higher up.

These varieties of fistulae are now very uncommon in the UK, but in countries with inadequate obstetric services they are still a frequent cause of distressing disability. Depending on the type of fistula the patient has urinary or faecal incontinence, and sometimes both. If the fistula is caused by operative injury the symptoms appear immediately, but if it is the result of pressure necrosis the symptoms do not appear until about the eighth day, when the sloughs separate. On examination an opening into the bladder or rectum is found.

When the wound granulates a small rectal fistula may heal, but this is unlikely with a vesicovaginal fistula. In the case of a fistula caused by direct injury immediate repair is performed, but in those caused by ischaemic necrosis repair is not attempted for two to three months, when the effects of trauma and superadded infection have subsided. Details of the surgical treatment are given in *Gynaecology by Ten Teachers*.

HAEMATOMA OF THE VULVA

This may be caused by rupture of a vulval varix, but more often it occurs after perineal repair when a vessel is not properly secured. It can occasionally occur after normal labour with an apparently intact perineum.

The haematoma appears fairly suddenly as a very tender purple swelling on one side of the vulva; it may become 10 cm or more in diameter. Sometimes the blood tracks upwards to form a swelling at the side of the vagina. The pain is severe and there is often shock. If a woman complains of severe perineal pain after delivery the perineum should always be inspected before giving her analgesics.

If the tension in the swelling is great or if the swelling is increasing in size it should be incised and the clot turned out. If the torn vessel can be found it should be ligated.

A drain is left in the cavity and a firm dressing is applied.

BROAD LIGAMENT HAEMATOMA

In this uncommon accident a deep vessel is torn and a haematoma forms above the pelvic diaphragm and spreads into the base of the broad ligament, extending between the uterus and bladder or beside the rectum. It may be caused by extraperitoneal rupture of the uterus. The bleeding most frequently occurs during or soon after labour or caesarean section and the haematoma is discovered a few hours or days later, because of pain and deterioration in the patient's general condition. The haematoma may be large enough to be palpable on abdominal examination, and it will displace the uterus upwards and to one side. The patient is often anaemic, and there may be slight fever.

A broad ligament haematoma usually undergoes gradual absorption, which will take several weeks if it is large. Infection is rare, but may occur and lead to abscess formation.

Most cases are treated conservatively. Blood transfusion may be required, and antibiotics are given. If infection occurs and an abscess forms this is opened wherever it points.

MATERNAL NERVE INJURIES DURING LABOUR

Foot-drop from paralysis of the dorsiflexor muscles of the leg may follow delivery.

In a few cases this is the result of pressure on the lateral popliteal nerve near the neck of the fibula by a leg support used to hold the patient in the lithotomy position. If the legs are placed outside the supports this cannot happen.

In the majority of cases it is a different type of injury involving the 4th and 5th lumbar nerve roots. This may be the result of sudden prolapse of an intervertebral disk, which may occur during labour, or of pressure on the lumbosacral cord by the presenting part near the brim of the pelvis. The lesion is usually unilateral, and it often follows difficult labour, especially forceps delivery. Apart from the foot-drop there is an area of sensory loss on the dorsum of the foot and lateral aspect of the ankle. The prognosis is good, although recovery may take several months. During that time a toe-spring is attached to lift the foot during walking, and regular physiotherapy is given.

Rarely, prolonged sensory loss in the leg, without foot-drop, follows epidural anaesthesia.

POSTPARTUM HAEMORRHAGE AND ABNORMALITIES OF THE THIRD STAGE

Postpartum haemorrhage (PPH) is excessive bleeding from the genital tract after the birth of the child. It is conventionally defined as a loss of more than 500 ml. The haemorrhage may be immediate (or *primary*) or if it occurs more than 24 hours after delivery it is described as *secondary*.

In England and Wales maternal deaths from PPH have been almost halved (15 to 9) from 1970 to 1981, although in the last three years of this period PPH accounted for over 60 per cent of all maternal deaths from haemorrhage. From 1970 to 1981 the number of deaths from haemorrhage (PPH, abruptio placentae and placenta praevia) fell from 11.7 to 7.3 per million maternities.

PRIMARY POSTPARTUM HAEMORRHAGE

There are two sources of primary postpartum haemorrhage, the placental site and lacerations of the genital tract. The incidence is reported to be between one and two per cent of deliveries,

although there is reason to suspect that the true rate is much higher than this.

PRIMARY HAEMORRHAGE FROM THE PLACENTAL SITE

Some blood must escape as the placenta becomes detached from its site, but usually less than 200 ml. Further loss is normally prevented by the retraction of the uterine muscle fibres which surround the vessels in the wall of the uterus and compress them until intravascular thrombosis occurs. Although a loss of more than 500 ml is arbitrarily defined as a postpartum haemorrhage, any loss which appears excessive must be treated at once. Even a small loss may be dangerous in an anaemic patient.

Causes

Ineffective uterine contraction and retraction

Weak contraction of the uterus in the third stage of

labour may fail to separate the placenta complete-ly, so that it remains in the upper segment of the uterus and prevents effective retraction of the placental site. In other cases, though the placenta has been completely separated and expelled, severe haemorrhage can occur if the uterus fails to main-tain its retraction.

If the uterus is not completely empty retraction will be ineffective. Although it is true that a very strong contraction, for example after the in-travenous injection of ergometrine, may tempor-arily control bleeding if the placenta is still in the uterus, in cases in which the contractions are less strong even a retained placental cotyledon or suc-centuriate lobe or blood clot in the uterus will interfere with retraction.

Ineffective uterine action may occur:

after a long labour caused by weak or incoordin-ate uterine action. It will also occur in cases of long labour caused by mechanical difficulty if uterine exhaustion occurs

if prolonged or deep anaesthesia has been administered

if the patient is a multipara with an atonic uterus

if the uterus has been overdistended with polyhydramnios. With twin pregnancy it is probably the increased area of the placental site rather than uterine overdistension which accounts for postpartum haemorrhage

where there has been antepartum haemorrhage. In placenta praevia the lower segment may not retract well enough to control bleeding from the placental site. In cases of abruptio placentae the damaged uterus may fail to contract (*see* also p. 76).

Mismanagement of the third stage

After a normal delivery, if ergometrine or Syntoci-non has not been injected at the end of the second stage, the uterus remains quiescent for a few minutes. The placenta is still completely attached, and no bleeding occurs. But if the uterus is man-ipulated during this interval the placenta may be partly separated, and bleeding will begin and must continue until uterine contractions complete the separation and allow proper retraction to follow. Injudicious attempts to expel the placenta before complete separation has occurred are a common cause of postpartum haemorrhage, and may even cause uterine inversion.

Abnormally adherent placenta

Sometimes part of the placenta is abnormally adherent. In rare instances most of the chorionic villi penetrate through the decidua (*placenta accre-ta*) or into the myometrium (*placenta increta*). In cases of placenta praevia the placenta may have a wider area of attachment than normal, and the lower uterine segment may fail to retract strongly enough to control bleeding effectively.

Disseminated intravascular coagulation (DIC) and other clotting disorders

These are rare causes of slow but persistent and dangerous haemorrhage. DIC is especially associ-ated with concealed abruptio placentae, but may also occur in cases of amniotic embolism and after a dead fetus has been retained in the uterus for some weeks. In cases of abruptio placentae libera-tion of thromboplastin from placental tissue into the blood stream uses up fibrinogen. In the other cases the mechanism is less certain, but there is rapid depletion of coagulation factors and platelets resulting in catastrophic bleeding (*see* p. 266).

Other rarer uterine causes

Inversion of the uterus (*see* p. 224) and hourglass constriction with placental retention may also cause PPH.

Clinical events

The escape of blood is usually obvious and the only question is whether it is coming from the placental site or from a laceration. In rare instances severe bleeding occurs into the cavity of an atonic uterus, with only some of the blood appearing externally. This should be suspected if the patient becomes shocked, the fundus of the uterus appears to be abnormally high in the abdomen and the uterus feels larger and softer than normal.

If haemorrhage continues the blood pressure falls, the pulse rate rises and in severe cases pallor and air-hunger occur.

Owing to the increase in blood volume during pregnancy, and the increase in total red cell mass, a previously healthy parturient woman stands haemorrhage comparatively well, provided that the loss is not extremely rapid. However, a patient who is already exsanguinated by an antepartum haemorrhage may die if even a relatively small amount of blood is lost after delivery, and in a similar way a comparatively insignificant secondary postpartum haemorrhage may have serious effects on a patient who has lost heavily at the time of delivery.

Postpartum necrosis of the anterior lobe of the pituitary gland is a rare sequel in cases of postpartum haemorrhage in which the blood pressure has remained at a low level for some hours (*see* p. 234).

Prevention

The prevention of postpartum haemorrhage is very important. Anaemia must be corrected during pregnancy because an anaemic patient tolerates haemorrhage badly. Any patient with a previous history of a postpartum haemorrhage, patients with twins and grand multiparae should always be admitted to hospital for delivery.

Prolonged labour which might lead to uterine exhaustion can often be prevented by the use of an intravenous infusion of Syntocinon during labour and if such an infusion is given it should not be stopped until the third stage is safely completed (*see* p. 177). The second stage of labour should be short, and if assistance with forceps is necessary general anaesthesia should be avoided whenever possible.

The correct management of the third stage of labour is the most important factor in avoiding postpartum haemorrhage. Intravenous or intramuscular Syntocinon should be given immediately after delivery of the anterior shoulder of the fetus, as described on page 171.

Treatment

Two principles govern the treatment of postpartum haemorrhage:

the bleeding must be arrested
the blood volume must be restored.

Bleeding from the placental site will stop when the uterus is empty and retracted. Treatment will differ according to whether the placenta is still in the uterus or has been delivered.

Treatment if the placenta has already been delivered

The first step is to place a hand on the abdomen, with the patient lying on her back, to ascertain whether the uterus is soft or hard. If the uterus is soft and relaxed a contraction is stimulated by rubbing the uterus gently with the abdominal hand, placing the thumb in front and the fingers behind the fundus. When the uterus contracts and bleeding is controlled any clots are expelled by fundal pressure, and an intravenous injection of ergometrine 500 micrograms is given to maintain the contraction. The placenta and membranes are examined carefully to make sure that a cotyledon or succenturiate lobe is not retained; any retained placental tissue must be removed manually under anaesthesia.

In exceptional cases the uterus is hard and firmly contracted but bleeding continues. This is likely to be from a laceration of the cervix or vagina, and management should then be as described on page 225.

Treatment if the placenta is undelivered

The first step is again to ascertain whether the uterus is soft or hard. Unless the uterus is already firm the fundus is gently rubbed as described above to stimulate a contraction. The next step is to determine whether the placenta has separated. There are two clinical possibilities:

If the placenta has separated

If the placenta has separated and then been expelled from the upper into the lower uterine segment the uterus, when it contracts, will be felt as a firm rounded mass about 10 cm in diameter, at about the level of the umbilicus. It can be moved from side to side. The umbilical cord will have lengthened as the placenta separated and the lower part of the placenta can be felt per vaginam. If these signs of separation are present the placenta is delivered by Brandt–Andrews method (p. 171). If the bleeding does not then stop an intravenous injection of ergometrine 500 micrograms is given. (Even if the patient has already received 500 micrograms of ergometrine at the time of delivery this dose can be repeated safely once.) If the uterus does not contract well in spite of the ergometrine *bimanual compression* is immediately performed. The right hand is inserted into the vagina and formed into a fist, which is placed in the anterior fornix above the cervix (Fig. 5.48). The left hand is placed on the abdomen and pressed downwards

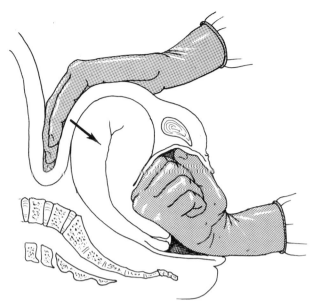

Fig. 5.48 Bimanual compression of the uterus

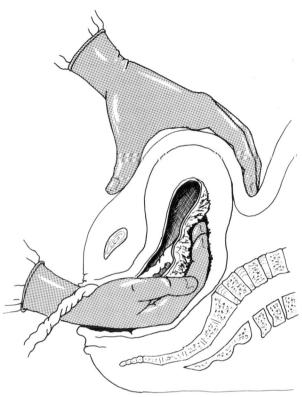

Fig. 5.49 Manual removal of the placenta

onto the posterior wall of the uterus so that it is compressed between the two hands. This is an effective but temporary method of controlling uterine bleeding, although it is uncomfortable for the patient and tiring for the obstetrician. Firm pressure must be maintained until the uterus is felt to contract.

While this is in progress the placenta should be examined by an assistant to see that it is complete. If part of it is missing that will have to be removed digitally under general anaesthesia.

If the placenta has not separated

If bleeding is taking place and clinical examination, which may include vaginal examination, indicates that the placenta has not separated and that it remains in the upper uterine segment, then *manual removal of the placenta* under general anaesthesia is performed immediately. In these cases the uterus is still enlarged and soft, well below the umbilicus and, being splinted by the pelvic brim, it is relatively immobile. On vaginal examination the cord is felt passing up into the uterus but the placenta cannot be reached. Repeated or violent attempts to express the placenta by squeezing the uterus or pressing on it are unlikely to succeed and often produce shock.

If manual removal is to be performed it is best to withhold any further injection of ergometrine until after the removal of the placenta. While the anaesthetic is being induced a catheter may be passed to empty the bladder. For manual removal the left hand is placed on the abdominal wall to locate and steady the fundus of the uterus, and then the right hand is passed into the uterus to follow the cord to the placenta. The edge of the placenta is identified, and is gradually separated from the uterine wall with the fingers, while the external hand serves as a guide and reduces the risk of tearing the uterus (Fig. 5.49). Only when the placenta is completely free should any attempt be made to remove it. The uterus is then explored carefully to ensure that no pieces of placental tissue are left behind; the beginner must realize that the site of attachment of the placenta is normally uneven and rough. The placenta is examined immediately to make sure that it is complete, which may be a difficult task as the placenta is now in pieces.

In the past manual removal of the placenta was a hazardous procedure, often performed after some delay on a shocked patient, with imperfect anaesthesia and a grave risk of infection. Today, if the operation is performed without delay, with good anaesthetic facilities, proper resuscitation, blood transfusion and antibiotic cover, the risk is slight. However, it is not an easy operation, and the beginner often diagnoses morbid adhesion of the placenta when none exists.

If bleeding still continues after removal of the placenta bimanual compression, which has already been described on page 230, may be necessary. In very exceptional cases, if bleeding continues in spite of all efforts (and is not caused by a clotting defect, *see* below) hysterectomy may be considered as a last desperate resort.

Circulatory collapse caused by haemorrhage

In all cases of postpartum haemorrhage there is the danger of circulatory collapse, and resuscitation must be started as soon as possible, preferably *before* hypotension or tachycardia appear. Immediate blood transfusion is essential to restore the blood volume, and an infusion of plasma or saline may be started while the transfusion is being arranged. In an emergency, if the patient's blood group is not known, group O rhesus-negative blood may occasionally have to be used, but in every case a direct agglutination test of the donor's corpuscles and the patient's serum is essential. Dextran may interfere with the coagulation mechanism; it should only be given after a sample of blood has been collected for cross-matching, and it should not be used if fibrinogen deficiency is suspected.

The patient is kept quiet and warm, with the foot of the bed raised. Her pulse, peripheral blood pressure and central venous pressure are monitored to assess transfusion requirements.

Problems of haemorrhage in domiciliary practice

If the patient is not delivered in a unit with full facilities for blood transfusion and emergency anaesthesia the dangers are increased, and the help of an emergency obstetric unit is essential. This 'flying squad', based on a maternity hospital, consists of an obstetrician, an anaesthetist and a midwife, and carries proper equipment for resuscitation and anaesthesia. A patient who has had a postpartum haemorrhage should not be moved until she has had a blood transfusion, the placenta

has been removed and the bleeding has been controlled. There is much higher mortality if the patient is moved to hospital with the placenta still undelivered and after inadequate transfusion.

Haemorrhage caused by clotting disorders

If bleeding persists in spite of all other treatment described, then hypofibrinogenaemia or excess fibrinolysin in the blood should be suspected. In an emergency the simple observation of failure of a sample of blood to clot in a test-tube may be sufficient to suggest the diagnosis. For discussion of investigation and treatment *see* page 262.

PRIMARY POSTPARTUM HAEMORRHAGE FROM LACERATIONS

Primary postpartum haemorrhage can occur from lacerations of any part of the birth canal during labour, the most common sites of bleeding being either the cervix or the vaginal wall. If bleeding continues after the placenta has been delivered and the uterus is firmly retracted, the vagina, cervix and lower uterine segment must be examined. This may be difficult until the patient is anaesthetized and placed in the lithotomy position. Proper retractors and instruments are needed to suture a high cervical tear. Profuse haemorrhage from a cervical tear involving a branch of the uterine artery can be temporarily controlled by clamping the highest part of the tear with sponge forceps until the patient can be taken to the operating theatre.

Bleeding from tears of the lower vagina, perineum or vulva should be controlled by pressure until the tear is sutured under local anaesthesia.

SECONDARY POSTPARTUM HAEMORRHAGE

This occurs more than 24 hours after delivery of the child, most often starting between the fifth and tenth days, although it can occur up to six weeks after delivery. It is usually caused by retention of a piece of placenta, and it is frequently complicated by intrauterine infection, with pyrexia. Ultrasound examination will show whether there is retained placental tissue. Secondary postpartum haemorrhage may also be caused by separation of an infected slough which has formed in a cervical or vaginal tear, or in a lower segment caesarean wound. A rare cause is infection and sloughing of a subendometrial fibromyoma.

Treatment

Under general anaesthesia the uterine cavity is explored with the finger or with sponge forceps to discover and remove any placental tissue; the suction curette may also be used. The cervix often remains open when there is something retained in the uterus. If there is infection a uterine swab should be taken and the appropriate antibiotic is chosen according to the result of the cultures.

DELAYED DELIVERY OF THE PLACENTA AND MEMBRANES

The normal process of separation and expulsion of the placenta has already been described (p. 156). Separation is usually complete within 10 minutes of the delivery of the baby. Retention of the placenta within the uterus for more than 30 minutes is now regarded as abnormal.

Causes

The causes of a retained placenta are:

Ineffective uterine action

If the uterine action is not sufficient to separate the placenta there will be no bleeding; the placenta is simply retained. If the placenta is partly separated and retraction is impaired there will be postpartum haemorrhage.

Contraction ring (hourglass constriction of the uterus)

In this condition a localized constriction just above the lower uterine segment prevents expulsion of the placenta; bleeding is seldom heavy. It may occur after prolonged labour with intrauterine manipulation.

Oxytocic drugs

A more generalized spasm, involving the lower as well as the upper segment may occur after administration of ergometrine, Syntometrine or Syntocinon. If one of these drugs is given in the active management of the third stage of labour, the placenta should be delivered directly it has separated to avoid any risk of its retention. The routine use of ergometrine, Syntometrine or Syntocinon in the management of the third stage of labour has reduced the incidence of postpartum haemorrhage from 7 to 0.7 per cent, but has increased the incidence of retention of the placenta from 0.4 to 5 per cent. However, no woman will die of mere placental retention, whereas a few deaths still occur from haemorrhage, and the use of these drugs is therefore fully justified.

Morbid adhesion of the placenta

The placenta normally separates in the plane of the spongy layer of the decidua. Occasionally this layer is poorly defined and the chorionic villi are adherent to the myometrium (*placenta accreta*) in part or the whole of the placental site. If the villi have penetrated even more deeply into the muscle the condition is called *placenta increta*. There is no proper line of cleavage and separation does not occur when the uterus contracts. Deficient formation of the decidua may occur over a caesarean or other scar in the uterus.

Treatment

The cause of delayed delivery of the placenta can only be ascertained by examination under anaesthesia. If the delay is accompanied by postpartum haemorrhage the treatment is urgent and is that already described above.

In the absence of bleeding intervention can be delayed for 30 minutes, but soon after that the placenta should be removed manually under general anaesthesia. If ergometrine was given at the time of delivery it is best to wait for at least this 30 minutes so that any effect of the drug will be less. Before proceeding to manual removal it is important to make sure that the bladder is empty, by catheterization if necessary, as a full bladder may cause delay in delivery of the placenta.

If a contraction ring is present this will be felt as a tight band. Inhalation of amyl nitrite (supplied in small glass capsules) or anaesthesia with fluothane or cyclopropane should relax the ring sufficiently for the placenta to be removed.

If partial placenta accreta is encountered during manual removal the placenta can usually be removed.

Placenta increta is very rare, and no plane of

cleavage will be discovered. The placenta can be left in place to separate by necrosis, but in most cases the operator will have torn the placenta and started bleeding, so that hysterectomy may be the safest course.

Antibiotics should be given and blood transfused if there is bleeding.

Retention of the membranes

Part of the membranes may be found to be missing when the placenta is examined after its delivery, but this is not a matter for concern. Even large pieces of membrane will separate and be discharged spontaneously.

SHOCK IN OBSTETRICS

Obstetric shock does not differ significantly from surgical shock. It results from the depression of many functions, in which reduction of effective circulation volume and blood pressure are of basic importance. The consequent inadequate perfusion of all the tissues leads to oxygen depletion and the accumulation of metabolites.

Most cases of shock in obstetrics are associated with severe haemorrhage, but other factors may be added; for example prolonged labour may be associated with electrolyte imbalance, general anaesthesia and trauma during operative delivery. Abruptio placentae can cause severe shock, and in the third stage of labour postpartum haemorrhage may occur. Maternal exhaustion, especially if combined with infection, will increase the effect of other factors.

Less frequent causes of shock include rupture of the uterus, acute inversion of the uterus, amniotic embolism, pulmonary embolism and adrenal haemorrhage. Bacteraemic shock is an additional form of shock.

Prolonged postpartum shock and hypotension may cause ischaemic necrosis of the anterior lobe of the pituitary gland (*see* below).

Treatment

Unless prompt resuscitation is undertaken death may occur rapidly. It is essential to restore the blood volume as quickly as possible by intravenous infusion. If blood is not immediately available transfusion with saline or reconstituted plasma should be started while it is being obtained.

Constant monitoring of the pulse rate, arterial blood pressure and central venous pressure is required to regulate the circulatory balance. Oxygen is sometimes required, and a small dose of morphine if there is severe pain. Attempts to raise the blood pressure by administration of vasoconstrictor drugs are usually ill-advised. If the limbs are pale and cold vasoconstriction is already present, and further vasoconstriction may only decrease the venous return still further. In many of these cases there is a risk of infection, and broad-spectrum antibiotics may be given intravenously.

POSTPARTUM PITUITARY NECROSIS

Severe postpartum collapse due to haemorrhage may be followed by ischaemic necrosis of the anterior lobe of the pituitary gland. Thrombosis occurs in the vessels which supply the anterior lobe, and necrosis of the whole lobe occurs, except for a thin rim of tissue which may survive at the surface of the lobe. Death may occur soon after delivery, but if the patient survives she will show the clinical picture of Simmonds' disease (sometimes also known as Sheehan's syndrome). All the endocrine functions of the anterior lobe of the pituitary gland are disturbed. There will be failure of lactation due to lack of prolactin. Because of lack of thyrotrophic hormone the patient becomes lethargic, abnormally sensitive to cold and usually gains weight. Her basal metabolic rate falls, and her glucose tolerance is increased. Because of lack of corticotrophic hormone she will also have asthenia, a low blood pressure and will respond poorly to infection. Lack of gonadotrophic hormones will lead to genital atrophy, with superinvolution of the uterus, amenorrhoea, and atrophy of the breasts.

Less severe cases may only have part of the complex clinical picture, and in very rare instances a further pregnancy has followed, with regeneration of the pituitary gland.

Prompt treatment of collapse due to postpartum haemorrhage should prevent this disastrous complication. Once the necrosis has occurred substitution therapy may maintain the patient in fair health. Thyroxine will be required for the hypothyroidism; for the failure of suprarenal function suprarenal cortical hormones are given. There is no useful purpose in giving gonadotrophic hormones, but testosterone has been found to supplement the action of cortical hormones.

6

NORMAL PUERPERIUM

THE PUERPERIUM

The puerperium is the time following labour during which the pelvic organs return to their prepregnant condition. By convention the puerperium is said to last for six weeks, although it may take much longer for some of the organs to return completely to normal.

The management of the early puerperium consists in keeping careful watch upon the physiological processes during the time, and in being prepared to intervene if they should show signs of becoming pathological. Attention is given to the general mental and physical welfare of the mother and baby. Some special points of management are set out in the following sections.

Prevention of infection

Every precaution should be taken to prevent the implantation of exogenous pathogenic organisms into the birth canal during labour and the puerperium. The vulva and perineum should be kept as clean and as dry as possible. Provided that there is no rise in temperature or pulse rate the woman may leave her bed to visit the lavatory and may have a shower or bath. There is no need to swab the vulva or to pour antiseptic solution over it during delivery or in the puerperium. The vulva is simply kept covered with a dry sterile pad; this is changed by the nurse whenever it is soaked or soiled.

Relatives, nurses, students or doctors who have septic foci due to streptococcal or staphylococcal lesions, or who may carry infection from recent contact with septic conditions must be excluded from labour and lying-in wards. Patients who develop signs indicative of sepsis must be isolated at once from the normal cases until it can be established that any infection organism is not pathogenic to others.

In order to reduce the risk of infection spreading, modern maternity units are designed with single rooms or small wards of four to six beds. Ventilation should be by a system which introduces fresh air rather than one which draws in air from other parts of the hospital. Many organisms, in particular *Staphylococcus aureus* and the haemolytic streptococcus, are found in dust and blankets in hospitals. Single rooms must be available for suspect cases. The wide range of antibiotics now available should not justify lower standards in the prevention of infection.

Time of getting up

After the physical and mental strain of pregnancy and labour a woman needs a period of rest from hard work and mental worry. The time spent in hospital varies according to the type of delivery and also the home conditions to which she will be returning. The mean stay in the UK is now five days, but providing that steps are taken for adequate supervision by a midwife and doctor there is much to be said in favour of allowing the woman to return home before this time.

If the labour has been normal and there has been no gross injury to the pelvic floor or other complications, the woman is allowed out of bed for short periods from the day after delivery, but she should limit her activities until the fifth day. This early ambulation must not be made an excuse for shortening the total time of convalescence. The period of rest will allow time for breast feeding to be comfortably established. Moderate exercise encourages recovery in the tone of the pelvic floor, the circulation is improved in the legs and the incidence of venous thrombosis is reduced.

In abnormal cases it may be necessary to keep the patient in bed for longer.

Temperature and pulse

The temperature may briefly rise to 37.9°C (100°F) in the first 24 hours, but afterwards it should fall to normal and remain so. Provided that the woman feels and looks well the temperature need only be taken morning and evening.

It is strongly emphasized that when the temperature remains raised for more than a few hours, especially if there is a corresponding rise in the pulse rate, this should be regarded as being due to infection arising in the genital tract until the contrary is proved. All cases of fever during the puerperium should be carefully investigated, as described on page 257.

For the first few hours after a normal delivery the pulse rate is likely to be raised, but it should return to normal by the second day. A rise in the pulse rate must be regarded as seriously as a rise in the temperature. It may indicate severe anaemia, venous thrombosis or infection of the birth canal, urinary tract or breast.

Onset of lactation

During pregnancy there is considerable hypertrophy of the glandular tissue of the breasts, but secretion of milk does not start until after the birth of the child. Many women who intend to breast feed put the baby to the breast within minutes of delivery. The consequent release of oxytocin may assist in keeping the uterus well contracted. With the activation of prolactin the breasts become more active, and there is increased vascularity.

Involution of the uterus

Immediately after delivery the fundus of the uterus lies about 4 cm below the umbilicus. The height of the fundus diminishes daily and it cannot normally be felt above the pubis after the 10th day. Any estimate of the height of the fundus should always be made when the bladder is empty. The uterus rapidly decreases in size for the first week, then decreases more slowly, being completely involuted in about eight weeks. At the end of labour the uterus weighs 1 kg, by the end of the first week about 0.5 kg, and by the end of the puerperium about 70 g. Involution is accomplished by autolysis of the muscle fibres, their protoplasm being broken down by enzymes, liquefied and removed in the bloodstream. The end products are excreted in the urine. Delay in involution occurs in the presence of uterine infection, retention of placental products or fibromyomata in the uterine wall, but in the absence of other signs of abnormality delay in shrinkage of the uterus is of no significance.

Retention of urine

A few women have difficulty in passing urine for the first day or two after delivery. Retention is liable to occur after a difficult labour which causes bruising or lacerations in the vulva, after epidural anaesthesia or when perineal stitches have been inserted. It is less likely with women who are ambulant.

If the bladder is atonic residual urine accumulates and may become infected. If retention occurs or residual urine in some quantity is suspected a catheter must be passed with careful aseptic precautions. Catheterization may have to be continued at regular intervals for a day or two, or a self-retaining catheter inserted.

Incontinence of urine

True incontinence, now a rare event in the UK, results from a vesicovaginal fistula, due either to a tear involving the bladder from instrumental delivery, or to pressure on the soft tissues from long labour and the formation of a slough involving the bladder. In the latter case incontinence does not appear until the slough breaks down some days after delivery.

Stress incontinence, or the leaking of urine on coughing, laughing or sneezing, is not uncommon in late pregnancy and may worsen after delivery. If it occurs soon after labour it may be only temporary, but if it persists surgical treatment is required (*see Gynaecology by Ten Teachers*). The operation is not advised until several months have elapsed because in many cases improvement occurs with the help of active pelvic floor exercises and return of tone in the pelvic floor musculature.

Cystitis and pyelonephritis

Urinary tract infection with high fever may arise in the first week of the puerperium. Symptoms such as frequency and discomfort on micturition are often absent in puerperal infections, but tenderness over the kidneys may be found, more commonly on the right than the left. The infection is usually caused by coliform organisms, and may be an exacerbation of a preceding chronic infection of the urinary tract, or it may follow catheterization. It is difficult to obtain a satisfactory midstream specimen for bacteriological examination at this time, but one may be obtained by catheter or suprapubic aspiration. Treatment is by encouraging the patient to drink adequate quantities of fluid and by giving appropriate antibiotics (e.g. ampicillin).

Constipation

This is common in the puerperium and is due to a combination of factors. The woman's food intake is interrupted, there may be dehydration during labour, the abdominal muscles are lax and perineal lacerations make defaecation painful. Constipation may be prevented by giving bran or bulk-forming drugs such as methylcellulose, ispaghula or sterculia from the first day, but if this does not act, laxatives, suppositories or an enema may be required.

The lochia

The lochial discharge comes from the placental site. For the first three or four days the lochia are red in colour. As the site begins to heal the discharge decreases in amount and its colour changes to pink and finally becomes serous. Although it is said that the lochia disappear by the 10th day the average time before they become colourless is, in fact, usually three or four weeks. Lochia which remain red and excessive in amount

indicate delayed involution, which may be associated with retention of a piece of placental tissue within the uterus, or with infection. If placental tissue is retained the uterus may be enlarged and the internal os of the cervix remains open. The retained products can be shown by ultrasound examination. Curettage is likely to be required, especially if there is an increase in red loss or the passage of clots.

Offensive lochia may indicate infection of the uterus, although the organisms may only be saprophytes. Virulent infection with haemolytic streptococci is not accompanied by an offensive smell.

Sleep and avoidance of anxiety

It is important to see that the mother not only gets a good night's rest, as free as possible from disturbance by the baby, but also that she has a rest in the afternoon. Pain from perineal stitches or engorged breasts are common causes of sleeplessness. If she is excitable and sleeping badly hypnotics such as nitrazepam (Mogadon) 5 mg should be given for the first few nights. After that sleeplessness, unless it is habitual, should arouse anxiety as it may be the first sign of the onset of puerperal psychosis.

Diet

The day after a normal delivery the woman should be given a normal diet. During lactation she will need an adequate but not excessive intake of fluid (*see p. 43*). Animal fats, fruit and vegetables will supply necessary vitamins, and protein in the diet should be increased. Milk is a very good source of nutrition and the woman should be encouraged to drink about half a litre a day.

Perineal stitches

The perineum should be washed every day with soap and water and dried. A dry sterile vulval pad is then applied, this is changed frequently. Unabsorbed stitches are removed on the fifth day.

Care of the breasts

For antenatal care *see* page 44.

During the first two or three days after delivery the breasts secrete colostrum only, but it is important that the baby is put to the breast in order to promote bonding between the mother and baby, to stimulate the secretion of milk, and to teach the baby to suck. For discussion of the details of breast feeding *see* page 248.

If the mother cannot or does not wish to breast feed, lactation is suppressed and she is helped to establish bottle feeding. Although oestrogens are effective in suppressing lactation their use has been given up because of the increased risk of thrombosis and embolism. Instead the secretion of prolactin is inhibited with bromocriptine in doses of 2.5 mg twice daily for 14 days. It has the disadvantage of being expensive. Adequate support for the breasts and the administration of analgesics for the discomfort of engorgement is often all that is required.

Postnatal exercises

In many hospitals women are given breathing exercises, exercises for the abdominal and pelvic muscles and exercises for the legs to reduce the risk of thrombosis, but for most women early ambulation has reduced the need for this. It is probably better to concentrate physiotherapy on those who have some special need for it.

Postnatal examination

This should be carried out at the end of the sixth week. Apart from discussing any problems or anxieties which the woman may present, and following up any complication of pregnancy or labour, the doctor enquires about her general health, whether the lochia have ceased, about bladder function, especially to exclude stress incontinence, and about any infant feeding problems.

The abdomen is examined and the state of the musculature noted. Pelvic examination is performed to check that any lacerations have healed normally, that there is no prolapse of the vaginal walls and that the uterus has involuted normally. The uterus is not infrequently found to be retroverted. In most cases this causes no symptoms, or the uterus is known to have been in this position before pregnancy, and no treatment is required.

A speculum is passed and if a cervical smear was not taken in the antenatal period this is done. A cervical erosion is a common finding. Many of these regress spontaneously before the 12th week and the patient should be seen again then. Only if the erosion persists and causes discharge which is sufficient to trouble the patient should it be treated (*see Gynaecology by Ten Teachers*).

Women not infrequently complain of backache at a postnatal visit. Most cases of lumbar backache are due to poor posture (persistence of the lordosis of pregnancy) or fatigue, and spontaneous recovery often occurs. Retroversion or other pelvic lesions will not cause backache at this level. Persistent backache, or any other disability discovered at the postnatal examination, may call for further investigation or treatment.

Sometimes conditions such as hypertension or urinary tract infection call for prolonged follow-up

Family planning advice

Most women are anxious to space their pregnancies if not to limit them. Practical contraceptive advice should be made easily available at the time of the postnatal visit. The choice of method lies with the patient but it is necessary to discuss with her the pros and cons of the various methods. The woman may be prepared for family planning by discussion during pregnancy, or while she is in the lying-in ward, of the methods available. If it is impossible for her to attend for advice in the postnatal period an intrauterine device may sometimes be inserted in the puerperium, or a prescription and instructions given for the use of the contraceptive pill. For a woman who has completed her family, and if she and her partner are certain that they will not change their minds later, sterilization may be performed in the early puerperium, but it is often better performed 6–12 weeks later, when the woman has had time to reflect whether or not she really wants it done, and the fallopian tubes have returned to their normal size.

Contraceptive pills containing oestrogen should not be given to women who are breast feeding because they may inhibit lactation. Progestogen-only pills do not inhibit lactation.

Details of contraceptive methods are given in *Gynaecology by Ten Teachers*.

CARE OF THE NEWBORN INFANT

At the moment of delivery the infant is launched into an independent existence and must assume the vital function of respiration, or die. The circulation has to adjust quickly to the needs of pulmonary gas exchange. The maintenance of a normal body temperature and basic metabolism must also be achieved immediately. Shortly afterwards the infant must establish an appropriate nutritional intake and digestive functions in order to maintain the new physiological equilibrium. Thus the process of birth itself is not only relatively traumatic but is a period of life in which the most profound bodily changes occur in the shortest space of time.

CHANGES IN THE RESPIRATORY SYSTEM

The fetus *in utero* demonstrates movements of breathing in a phasic manner. These movements last for varying lengths of time and are interrupted by long periods of rest. There is a net outflow of amniotic fluid from the alveolar spaces through the bronchial tree and into the upper airway. During fetal breathing this fluid is drawn in and out of the nasopharynx in volumes approximating to one tenth of that seen during the normal breathing of air after birth. These respiratory movements, although small, are an important rehearsal for what is to follow later.

During labour and immediately after birth the lungs are cleared of the fetal lung fluid. Approximately one-third is squeezed out through the mouth and nose and the remainder is absorbed directly across the alveolar walls into the pulmonary lymphatic and blood capillary systems. Meconium residues in the liquor may also be inhaled during this period and can cause inflammatory changes within the lungs.

The moderate degree of hypoxia produced in the fetus during the course of labour, with a slight fall in arterial oxygen tension and a rise in arterial carbon dioxide tension, heightens the responsiveness of the newborn infant's respiratory centres to a variety of stimuli. With increasing hypoxia these centres become depressed, leading to primary apnoea followed by release of the primitive gasping reflex as a means of initiating respiration.

The thorax is squeezed as the body passes through the birth canal, and fluid is expelled from the chest, being replaced by air during the elastic recoil after completion of delivery of the trunk. Once the baby is born the body extends from the fetal position, the spine straightens and the change in shape of the chest and descent of the diaphragm facilitate respiration.

The fall in the environmental temperature after delivery is an added stimulus to breathing, particularly if cool air impinges on the sensitive area around the mouth and nose. A combination of these factors is thought to be responsible for the establishment of full respiration. It must be remembered that any anaesthetic or sedative administered to the mother is shared by the fetus and may depress the respiratory centres.

In normal circumstances the first breath draws air into the bronchial tree, unless there is obstruction from inhaled liquor amnii or meconium. A negative intrapleural pressure is created and with successive respiratory movements the thoracic cage expands and the lung volume increases. The difference between this negative pressure and the atmospheric pressure of the air in the bronchial tree causes the fetal lungs to expand by entry of air into the alveoli. The unexpanded alveoli are filled by a thin layer of fluid and the surface tension between the walls must be overcome before full expansion can be achieved.

The maturing lung is able to produce *surfactant* from special cells (type II pneumocytes) in the alveolar wall from about 32 to 34 weeks gestation. The main constituent of surfactant is a phospholipid, lecithin, and its function is to reduce the surface tension within the alveoli and so permit easy and equal expansion throughout the lungs. If the production of surfactant is diminished by prematurity or hypoxia, or both, there is incomplete expansion of the lungs which may be the starting point of the respiratory distress syndrome (hyaline membrane disease). Normal alveolar expansion is at first rapid, but several hours elapse before complete expansion of the lungs occurs.

Although the first breath is usually taken immediately after birth, the onset of breathing is sometimes delayed. The newborn infant appears to be less susceptible to the ill effects of prolonged hypoxia than the adult, but nevertheless deep hypoxia lasting for only a few minutes can cause bradycardia with or falling blood pressure leading to impaired cerebral circulation, and can result in cerebral palsy or mental retardation.

Changes in the fetal circulation at birth

The fetal circulation has already been described on page 16. Remarkable changes occur soon after birth. The infant's first breaths expand the lungs and open up the pulmonary vascular bed. This produces a sharp fall in the pulmonary vascular resistance and a considerably increased flow of blood to the lungs, where it is oxygenated. Immediately afterwards there is contraction of the ductus arteriosus to about half its original diameter, and complete contraction of the umbilical arteries. It is thought that the ductus arteriosus and umbilical arteries have a natural tendency to contract but are prevented from doing so by prostaglandins which are circulating at high concentrations in the fetus. It is suggested that there are enzyme systems in the lungs which break down the prostaglandins once the pulmonary blood flow is established after birth. The fall in the level of circulating prostaglandins, along with the rise in the arterial oxygen saturation, allows these vessels to contract. It is possible that the use of prostaglandin inhibitors to suppress premature labour might lead to premature closure of the ductus in the fetus.

The systemic arterial pressure rises as the low resistance of the placenta is replaced by the high resistance of the peripheral circulation in the baby when the cord is clamped, and with the concomitant fall in the pulmonary artery pressure the pressure gradient across the ductus is reduced. The fall in pulmonary vascular resistance produces a fall in right sided pressures, and the increase in systemic resistance a rise in left sided pressures. These changes, together with the increased pulmonary venous return, lead to a rise in left atrial pressure over and above that in the right atrium and consequent functional closure of the foramen ovale.

Ultimately, but not for several days or weeks, the ductus becomes obliterated by endarteritis, and the final transition from fetal to adult circulation is complete. The umbilical cord dries and separates, leaving a raw area which heals by granulation and is then covered by epitheleum. The umbilical vein is now a redundant vessel and closes by aseptic thrombosis. The ductus venosus atrophies and disappears, while the umbilical vein remains as the *ligamentum teres*. The umbilical arteries show retrograde closure as far as the hypogastric arteries and persist as sclerosed remnants.

Changes in the gastrointestinal tract

Although the placenta carries out nutritional and excretory functions for the fetus, the gastrointestinal tract is active during intrauterine life. During the later months of pregnancy liquor amnii containing desquamated epithelial cells is continually being swallowed. Mucus and debrided intestinal epithelial cells are added to the gut content and, with the swallowed liquor, are digested by intestinal enzymes to form meconium, which is coloured greenish-black by bile pigments. By late pregnancy the meconium has transversed the gut as far as the rectum, and if strong intestinal contractions are stimulated by fetal distress during labour, meconium may be voided into the amniotic fluid. If premature respiration is induced by hypoxia, meconium-stained liquor may be inhaled into the bronchial tree, and this can cause respiratory difficulties after delivery.

With the first inspiration air also enters the stomach and rapidly traverses the gut, reaching the ascending colon within three hours.

Hydrochloric acid is present in the stomach in relatively high concentration on the first day of life, but in only moderate amounts during early infancy. Amylases from saliva and from the pancreas are at a low level during the early weeks of life, and this explains the difficulty in digesting certain carbohydrates which is shown by some infants. The trypsin and lipase of pancreatic secretions are present in good concentration, even during intrauterine life, and are responsible for the digestion of meconium.

The genitourinary tract

There may be delay in passing urine after birth for up to 24 hours, but this is usually not of pathological significance. Suprapubic pressure often results in the passage of urine. The first specimen may have a pinkish colour from a high concentration of urates.

Regulation of body temperature

The fetal temperature is determined by the surrounding maternal environment and the fetal heat regulating centre is relatively dormant. After birth, unless special precautions are taken, the infant's temperature falls by 1 to 3°C and external heat must be supplied. The temperature regulating centre is active immediately after birth and causes an increase in the rate of metabolism and oxygen consumption in order to maintain a constant body temperature in the face of environmental variation. Brown adipose tissue has an important role in maintenance of body temperature in the newborn, and deficiency of this tissue in preterm and small-for-dates babies contributes to their thermoregulatory difficulties.

Defences against infection

Placental transmission of maternal IgG antibodies affords the infant a non-specific, passive immunity against certain diseases. This immunity wanes after a short time, and the infant is at risk from common infections until an acquired immunity is developed. Immune protection from the mother may be specific for diseases against which she has developed an active immunity, such as diphtheria, tetanus, measles, mumps and poliomyelitis. The infant's own IgG levels are very low at birth but increase steadily during the first two to three months of life. Serum IgA levels are also low, but the infant should be receiving IgA from the mother's breast; it is in high concentration in colostrum and continues to be secreted in mature milk. This immunoglobulin plays an important part in protecting the baby against infections acquired through the alimentary tract, and possibly also against the development of hypersensitivity.

THE IMMEDIATE CARE OF THE HEALTHY INFANT

When the infant is delivered it may be limp, with only moderate muscle tone, and there is a purplish-blue cyanosis of general distribution. Liquor drains from the nose and mouth and to assist this drainage the infant should be inclined slightly head downwards. The mouth should *not* be cleaned with gauze swabs, as this will damage the delicate buccal mucosa.

The nasopharynx should be cleared of fluid with a sterile disposable mucus extractor. A mechanical sucker regulated to avoid a negative pressure of more than 30 cm of water may also be employed. Whichever method is used the procedure must be carried out with the utmost gentleness to avoid damage to the mucous membranes or the production of laryngeal spasm.

The stomach of the newborn infant, especially when delivered by caesarean section, contains large quantities of amniotic fluid which may possibly be regurgitated later and inhaled. If the infant is thought to have swallowed large amounts of blood or meconium the stomach should also be aspirated after the nasopharynx has been cleared. This can be done by passing the soft tubing of the disposable mucus extractor gently down the oesophagus into the stomach. This tubing is also sufficiently firm to permit immediate diagnosis of oesophageal atresia should this be present.

As soon as the nasopharynx has been cleared the infant will normally take a breath and give a cry and, as respiration begins, the colour of the skin rapidly changes to pink. Cyanosis of the extremities may persist for a time, but this is not usually of pathological significance.

Care of the eyes

In the past it was the practice to instil one drop of 1 per cent silver nitrate solution into each eye immediately after delivery as a prophylactic against gonococcal infection. Because there is now effective treatment, this is not advised unless there are special indications, except in countries where antenatal and postnatal supervision are lacking. Daily wiping of the eyes with cotton wool moistened with saline is a common but undesirable practice, the only result of which may be to produce pyogenic conjunctivitis.

Care of the umbilical cord

The time and method of clamping the cord is discussed on page 169. Afterwards the cord is kept dry and clean until it shrivels and comes away leaving a small area of granulation tissue, which heals over after a few days. Application of chlorhexidine or hexachlorophane powder is a good way to keep the umbilicus clean and dry.

General care of the baby

After ensuring that respiration is well established and the Apgar score (*see* p. 296) has been checked, the infant is inspected rapidly to note whether there are any obvious abnormalities before being wrapped in a warm towel and handed to the mother to be cuddled and put to the breast to suckle the colostrum.

A recent fashion is to place the naked baby on the mother's abdomen immediately after delivery so that skin to skin contact will promote emotional bonding, but there is doubt about the widsom of this. It is undesirable to place the infant above the level of the placenta before the cord is clamped (*see* p. 169), and there is some risk of heat loss. In any event the baby should be under the cover of a towel.

After this initial period of close contact, the baby is wrapped firmly in warm towels and laid prone in a cot alongside the mother with head turned to one side and facing her. Unless there is need for special care, it is important that the baby should not be removed from close proximity to the mother. Even if she falls asleep from exhaustion it is reassuring for her to find her baby beside her when she wakes.

During this initial period it is important to check the baby's axillary temperature. The rectal temperature should only be taken if the axillary temperature is low.

Details of a more complete physical examination are given below.

Identification

In institutions the infant must be identified in such a way that confusion between babies cannot arise. A plastic wrist band with the mother's name marked in indelible ink is commonly used.

The baby's bath

At birth the infant is covered with greasy vernix caseosa and blood. It is best not to bath the baby immediately but just to clean the face with sterile moistened swabs before presenting him or her to the mother. Vernix is acid and greasy and provides a natural barrier to infection, its main function is to protect the baby's skin from the effects of prolonged immersion in liquor.

Most maternity units now agree that just one bath given by the mother, under instruction, on the day before discharge is all that is required. Daily inspection of the skin, the eyes, the mouth and most particularly the umbilicus, should be carried out by experienced nursing staff. The stump of the cord desiccates and separates between the fourth and 11th days, usually by the seventh day. Until healing of the moist raw area has occurred it provides an ideal site for growth of pathogenic bacteria. Locally applied hexachlorophane powder is an effective barrier against skin sepsis, and is safe because it is not absorbed.

Examination of the newborn infant

At the earliest convenient time after the birth a systematic physical examination should be made. External examination is of great importance and attention should be paid to any minor congenital defects. Skin naevi, preauricular sinuses, branchial fistulae, supernumary digits or nipples should be noted. Defects such as cleft palate, spina bifida or club feet may escape notice if of minor degree, and especial attention should be given to possible omphalocele, penile abnormalities, cryptorchidism and imperforate anus.

The skull should be palpated and the state of the sutures noted. The circumference of the skull should be recorded. Careful examination of the skull soon after birth may yield information of which the importance is only apparent later. Widening of the sutures and an increase in the circumference of the skull may be found in cases of subdural haematoma or hydrocephalus, and an early diagnosis may only be possible because the state of the skull at birth has been recorded. Areas of softening or an encephalocele may be found.

The baby should be handled and the limbs moved to ensure that no fracture or paralysis is present. The hips should be examined for congenital dislocation (p. 313). The range of movement of the ankles must be tested to detect minor degrees of talipes.

Examination of the heart should be carried out with care, but the significance of any murmur may only become apparent after observation for several days. Palpation of the femoral pulses should always be carried out to exclude coarctation of the aorta.

The chest may show signs of incomplete expansion or the persistence of moist sounds from inhaled liquor. These conditions are discussed on page 316.

On examination of the abdomen the liver edge can usually be felt just below the costal margin, and the tip of the spleen is often palpable. In a well-relaxed abdomen the lower poles of the kidneys may be easily felt, but this is not of pathological significance.

Normal reflexes

Certain reflexes are normally only present in the newborn infant.

The Moro reflex is a startle reflex elicited by banging the table on which the infant is lying, by letting the head drop backwards by 1–2 cm or by flexing the head on the trunk. Abduction and extension of the arms is followed by adduction of the arms like an embrace, and the legs are extended. This reflex is usually symmetrical and indicates normal neuromuscular coordination. Variations from the normal response are seen when there is a nerve palsy, a fractured clavicle or long bone, or an intracranial lesion.

If the infant is touched on the area near the mouth the head will turn and the infant will try to suck the touching object. This rooting reflex is followed by the sucking reflex which seems to be designed to enable the baby to draw the nipple well back into the mouth so that the gums can gently massage the milk sinuses just below the surface of the areola and stimulate milk ejection.

A grasp reflex is seen when the palm of the hand or the sole of the foot is touched and is normal in the newborn infant. A 'walking' reflex is also usually seen in the normal infant.

Normal progress of the full term infant

During the first week of life the baby continues to adjust to the extrauterine environment.

Traumatic lesions such as a caput succedaneum, a 'chignon' after vacuum extraction, petechiae or oedema disappear rapidly. The baby begins to assume an infantile position instead of that of intrauterine folding. The feet are less dorsiflexed and the hands less firmly clenched. The chest becomes less flattened and the head is moved freely. The cry is definite and begins to assume characteristics for hunger and pain.

Weight gain

There is loss of weight for the first two or three days of up to 10 per cent of the birth weight. After feeding is established the weight increases and will usually return to birth level by the seventh to the 10th day. If this is not achieved it may indicate inadequate feeding, or some condition which is preventing normal progress, but some breast feeding mothers take longer than others to establish lactation, and their babies may take two to three weeks to regain their birth weight without any harmful effects.

Temperature

At birth the infant is thermolabile, and the temperature may fall below 36°C, but it is unwise to allow the rectal temperature to fall below this. The infant responds quickly to the application of external heat, and in a few hours temperature regulation will be stabilized in the full term infant. The temperature shows a normal daily variation from 36 to 37.2°C.

Normal stools

Meconium is normally passed within a few hours of birth, but may be delayed for 12 or even 24 hours. Although this is not necessarily pathological it demands observation, as it may indicate intestinal obstruction. The first meconium stool is often preceded by a plug of whitish mucus, a meconium plug, and if this is large the appearance of meconium can be delayed for 24 hours and the abdomen may show some distension.

In the next two or three days meconium is passed several times a day. Normal meconium is sticky, odourless and greenish-black in colour. After a few days 'changing stools' are passed. These are non-homogeneous, thin, sour, mucousy and yellowish-brown in colour. Undigested milk elements can often be seen in the stool.

Towards the end of the first week 'milk stools' are seen. The stool of the breast-fed infant is smooth, pasty, slightly sour, acid and mustard or golden-brown in colour. The motion of the artificially fed infant is paler in colour, alkaline, pasty and non-homogeneous.

The breast-fed baby may have the bowels open only once in the day, or have any number of stools, up to six or seven, in the 24 hours and yet be normal. When the stools are frequent they may be green and this should not lead to a hasty diagnosis of gastroenteritis in a baby who is otherwise well. It is usually due to a temporary excess of lactation when the milk 'comes in' and it is important to leave the baby to continue to feed normally and maintain the stimulus to lactation. Later, the maternal diet may affect the baby's bowel habit as many aperient substances are secreted in the milk.

Micturition

The baby usually passes urine shortly after delivery, but micturition may not occur until 24 hours have elapsed, especially if the infant has voided urine just before or during delivery. The bladder may then become palpable, and the genitalia must be examined to ensure that there is no evidence of congenital defect. Pressure on the abdomen will often stimulate micturition.

The urine may at first be dark in colour, but rapidly becomes colourless and of low specific gravity. During the first day or two the napkin may be stained pink from the deposit of urates.

Breast engorgement

The breasts of infants of either sex may swell and become engorged during the first week of life. Milk ('witch's milk') may be secreted and a female may bleed from the uterus. These effects are due to transfer of maternal oestrogen and require no treatment. On no account should the engorged breasts be handled or squeezed as they readily become infected to produce neonatal mastitis or breast abscess.

Skin

In Caucasian infants the colour of the skin soon changes from the ruddiness seen after birth to a paler hue. The skin may become dry and scaly as it dries out after the long intrauterine immersion. Fissures and cracks may appear in the folds of the ankles and wrists, but heal quite quickly. Milia or various non-specific rashes may be seen. It is common to observe blotchy erythematous rashes on the trunk, limbs and face. No treatment is required.

Sleep

After delivery the baby usually settles down to sleep and for the next week or so falls asleep after feeds, waking up only to protest with hunger, discomfort or thirst.

VARIATIONS FROM THE NORMAL

The variations from the normal pattern of adaptation to extrauterine life which result from birth asphyxia or congenital malformations, such as diaphragmatic hernia or major cardiac defects, are discussed in detail in Chapter 9.

INFANT FEEDING

The rate of growth during the first two years is greater than at any other stage of life after birth. The weight of a normal baby doubles in five months, trebles in 12 months and quadruples in 24 months. To achieve this the intake of food must be relatively great and of a quality that allows easy digestion. During the early months it must contain, in liquid form, a reasonably balanced mixture of protein, fat, carbohydrate, minerals and vitamins.

Discussion of infant feeding is beset with difficulties that are largely created by the use of fixed systems. No system will ever meet the needs of every infant, for each baby is an individual with its own idiosyncracies from the moment of birth; if a baby does not thrive it may be that the error lies in the system rather than the infant. However, some rules can be stated as to the quantity and quality of food needed, and these rules can do no harm so long as they are adjusted to meet the requirements of each individual.

Although the metric system is now in use in hospitals some mothers still do not understand it and some avoirdupois measurements are *given in italics*.

Daily fluid requirement

The infant needs water in relatively greater amounts than at any other period of life. The infant's kidneys are not as capable of concentrating urine as those of the adult, and to remove the waste products of metabolism the urinary output must amount to nearly half the total fluid intake. The losses of fluid from the skin, lungs and faeces are proportionately greater than in adult life. The infant needs approximately 150 ml of fluid per kg of body weight (*2½ ounces per pound*) during 24 hours. Infants below normal birth weight require even more; a baby of 2.5 kg would need 180 ml per kg (*3 ounces per pound*) in 24 hours.

Calorie requirement

The diet should provide 110 calories per kg (460 kilojoules (kJ)) in 24 hours. This calls for 70 calories (290 kJ) per 100 ml of feed (*20 calories per ounce*). Smaller infants require more calories per kg – up to 150 calories (630 kJ) per kg in 24 hours.

Protein, fat and carbohydrate

Sufficient of these are supplied in a diet of breast milk or infant milk formula.

Minerals

The only mineral which may be inadequately provided by a milk diet is iron, an element which is always jealously conserved in nature. At birth the baby has only small iron reserves. During the period of intensely rapid growth in early infancy there is a corresponding increase in the total number of red cells. The reserve stores of iron are soon exhausted in forming haemoglobin for the additional red cells, and unless adequate supplies of iron are available in the diet the infant will develop hypochromic anaemia. Breast milk supplies enough iron during the first six months, particularly as the lactoferrin content ensures rapid and complete absorption. The modern infant milk formulae contain adequate iron, but unmodified cow's milk does not, and in the premature infant it is desirable to supplement the diet with additional iron. A ferrous supplement syrup is given in doses of 2.5 to 5 ml twice daily.

Vitamins

The vitamin content of breast milk and of standard infant feeds is adequate. The optimal daily intake of vitamin C for an infant is 50 mg. The recommended intake of vitamin D to prevent rickets is 10 micrograms (400 iu) daily, and any natural source of vitamin D which yields this will also provide enough vitamin A. Milk usually contains sufficient vitamin B. Vitamin K_1 (phytomenadione) is given routinely to prevent haemorrhagic disease (*see* p. 309). Vitamin supplements should be given to preterm infants and to those who have a poor nutritional intake for any other reason, such as reduced appetite or recurrent infections. These supplements can be given as standard children's vitamin drops or any proprietary preparation which includes vitamins A, B, C and D such as Abidec. Extra vitamin C can also be given in a standard preparation of baby fruit juice.

BREAST OR BOTTLE FEEDING?

The fact that artificial feeding has become so widespread throughout the world is perhaps an indictment of the apathy of doctors, nurses and others who are in a position to give advice and education to future parents, in the face of the immense power of commerce and advertising. The trend is encouraged by the changes in society and our way of life which seem to make artificial feeding more convenient. The general public knows that when care is taken with bottle feeding the babies seem to thrive well, and the mother who is repeatedly given information on how much feed her baby should have is more content when she can see the correct quantity in the bottle.

In almost all discussions about infant feeding it is assumed that the process is solely concerned with supplying the infant with adequate nutrition, whereas anyone who has watched a successful and contented breast-feeding couple will have appreciated that it is a two-way process which was intended to provide a pleasurable experience for both parties. This 'feedback' to the mother can make the feed time something to look forward to, rather than a routine duty whose sole purpose is to make her baby grow bigger. An important part of the process is to help the mother fall in love with her baby. In this way the mother–infant attachment is made secure, so that she will not wish to be parted from her baby in the early months. Her continuous presence will give the baby security and the mother a proper understanding of its needs throughout early development. Certainly, a mother who is bottle feeding will need to work harder to establish a good relationship with her baby, especially as there is a tendency for other well-meaning helpers to interfere. Indeed, there is a curious belief, fostered by some psychiatrists, that one of the advantages of bottle feeding is that it enables the father (or other relatives) to take part in the 'mothering', thereby giving the mother more freedom and providing the baby with additional stimulation. However, experience suggests that the closest relationship is achieved by one mother receiving maximal stimulation from the baby; and the natural mother is best equipped for this purpose. Failure to recognize the importance of good mothering is undoubtedly a contributory factor in child abuse and later delinquency.

Unfortunately not all mothers enjoy breast feeding, and for some the process is painful or distasteful. For them, as well as for the small number of women who are incapable of providing adequate lactation, it is important to provide sympathy and understanding so that they are not left with feelings of guilt, but are helped to concentrate upon making a success of bottle feeding.

Modern research reveals more and more reasons why the milk from its own mother provides the baby with the best form of nutrition and the best protection against infections, especially enteric infections, and possibly against the development of hypersensitivity.

Several mechanisms are involved in protection against infections. These include maternal secretory IgA and lysozymes, which either kill organisms or prevent their adherence to the intestinal wall; lactoferrin, which ensures rapid absorption of iron so that it is not available for the essential needs of replicating organisms, and encouragement of the growth of *Lactobacillus bifidus* to the exclusion of other pathogenic organisms which flourish in the more alkaline intestinal environment provided by the ingestion of cow's milk.

While secretory IgA is thought to be an important factor against the development of hypersentivity, avoidance of the potential antigenic effect of cow's milk protein is equally important. Cow's milk antigens can also pass through into the breast milk and sensitize the baby, especially when there is a family history of atopy.

There is also cumulative evidence that the health of the breasts is best preserved when they are allowed to fulfil their physiological function. When the reasons for breast feeding are fully explained most mothers become its strong advocates. As a result of concerted efforts by many people there is at present an encouraging resurgence of enthusiasm.

ANATOMY AND PHYSIOLOGY OF THE BREAST

Anatomy and maturation

The breast is composed of about 20 segments arranged radially from the nipple, the glandular tissue being mainly peripheral. The branching duct system from each segment unites to form a single duct which opens on the nipple. Immediately before opening on the nipple each duct has a dilatation called a lactiferous sinus. This lies immediately below the areola of the nipple and is a thin-walled part of the duct which can be dilated by milk to a calibre of 0.5 to 1 cm. The ducts and alveoli of the glandular tissue are surrounded by myoepithelial contractile cells, and there are smooth muscle cells under the areola. The pectoral fascia ensheathes the whole breast and sends laminae between the lobes and alveoli. There are many fat cells and a rich supply of blood vessels.

Before puberty the nipple is flat, and the duct system is rudimentary with little glandular tissue. In the female, as puberty approaches, the nipple becomes prominent and fat is deposited. With successive menstrual cycles oestrogens cause development of the duct system, but active development of the secretory tissue does not occur until pregnancy, under the influence of oestrogens and progesterone. During pregnancy the enlargement of the breast is mainly due to hyperplasia of the glandular tissue from the 12th week onwards. From the end of the 24th week the breast is capable of secreting milk and during the last 12 weeks colostrum can be expressed from the breast, although active lactation is dormant.

Physiology of lactation

It is convenient to discuss the processes of secretion (or formation of milk) and of excretion separately.

Secretion of milk

This is the transformation of amino acids, glucose, lipids and minerals present in the blood plasma into caseinogen, lactalbumin, lactose and milk fats which are secreted into the alveoli by the activity of the alveolar epithelial cells. Only a portion of the milk yielded at a feed is preformed; the major portion is secreted during feeding.

Prolactin

Prolactin is mainly responsible for the secretion by the alveolar cells. This pituitary hormone is secreted by cells of the anterior lobe of the pituitary gland (*lactotrophs*). Oestrogens cause hyperplasia of the lactotrophs during pregnancy and prolactin levels in the blood rise. Milk secretion does not occur at this time because high levels of oestrogen also inhibit the responses of the alveolar cells to prolactin. The release of prolactin is normally held in check by a hypothalamic inhibitory factor which is probably dopamine.

After delivery the oestrogen level falls so that the alveolar cells become responsive. The basal prolactin level is lower than that of late pregnancy, but in response to stimulation of the nipple by suckling there is a surge or release of prolactin which last for about 30 minutes, presumably because discharge of prolactin inhibiting factor is inhibited. Prolactin release is also stimulated by thyroid releasing hormone, but this is not thought to be part of the normal mechanism.

After delivery colostrum is secreted for about 48 hours and then the breasts become engorged and milk is secreted.

Excretion of milk

The baby is often said to suck milk. Sucking is a relatively unimportant part of the complex process, and the word wrongly suggests that suckling is entirely dependent on an activity of the baby. When lactation is well established milk will continue to spurt or flow from the nipple if a sucking infant is removed from the breast, indicating active secretion by the breast, separate from any activity of the infant.

When the baby takes the breast the nipple is drawn into the arch of the hard palate and held there by the tongue to be exposed to suction, which clears the milk to the back of the mouth to be swallowed. The lips form a seal on the nipple and areola and the gums champ on the areola to compress the lactiferous sinuses and propel their contents into the infant's mouth.

The active secretion by the breast is due to the contractile myoepithelial network of cells which invest the alveoli and ducts. Stimulation of the nerve endings in the nipple initiates impulses which reach the posterior lobe of the pituitary gland and provoke a pulsatile release of oxytocin into the bloodstream. Release of oxytocin may begin in response to the baby crying even before stimulation of the nipple. The oxytocin causes contraction of the myoepithelial cells and propulsion of the milk along the ducts. This is called the 'let down reflex'. The reflex can be interrupted or inhibited psychologically with failure of secretion of milk. The let down reflex is known to parous women as 'the draught' and is noted as a prickly sensation in the breast after the baby has begun to feed. The practical importance of these physiological responses is considered in more detail on page 248 under frequency of feeding.

Composition of colostrum and breast milk

For the first two days colostrum is secreted and on the third and fourth days the secretion changes to normal breast milk. Colostrum is a yellow fluid containing large fat globules, the colostrum corpuscles, and it has a high mineral, moderate protein and relatively low sugar content. Colostrum has a high content of antibodies, especially secretory IgA, which play an important part in protection against infection. Colostrum may help to clear the small intestine if it becomes contaminated by infected material swallowed during the birth process. Colostrum is said to possess laxative qualities, but no laxative constituent has ever been demonstrated.

When the secretion changes from colostrum to milk its colour changes to bluish-white. With successful lactation the amount of milk increases daily, reaching about 300 ml (*10 ounces*) on the fifth day and over 480 ml (*16 ounces*) on the tenth day.

Breast milk protein contains three fractions:

caseinogen
lactalbumin
lactoglobulin.

Table 6.1   Composition of breast milk

	Protein (%)	Fat (%)	Carbohydrate (%)
Colostrum	2.25	3.15	4.00
Milk	1.25	3.50	7.25

The latter is present only in small amounts and the proportion of lactalbumin to caseinogen is 2 to 1. The calorie value of breast milk is 70 calories (290 kJ) per 100 ml (*20 calories per ounce*).

Preparation for lactation

See page 44.

MANAGEMENT OF BREAST FEEDING

The essence of the initial management of breast feeding is a gradual increase in the time at the breast and the amount which the infant is allowed to take or can obtain. The objects of this gradual approach are to stimulate lactation, to encourage the baby to suck without becoming discouraged by failure to obtain milk, and to accustom the nipples to the mild trauma of suckling. The following points should be considered:

Interval after birth when first feeding is permitted

It is to be hoped that whenever possible the mother will be encouraged to handle her baby soon after birth and that she can put the infant to the breast for a short time. This will enable the baby to obtain the valuable colostrum while starting the stimulus to lactation. After this initial contact both mother and baby rest before further feeding is attempted. Only if the infant is ill, or has suffered a difficult delivery, should it be kept from the breast for longer than 24 hours.

Frequency of feeding

In the past maternity hospitals have tended to a rather strict regimentation of baby care. Because most babies ultimately settle down to an approximate four hour interval between feeds, it has been customary to establish babies on a four-hourly regime as soon as possible. This policy was not always successful, and seldom so without recourse to a night supplement. Where there has been complete acceptance of a policy of rooming in with freedom for the mother to feed her baby on demand it has been found that there is a wide range in the frequency with which healthy babies feed during the early stages of lactation. In one investigation this varied from a minimum of six feeds per day up to a maximum of 24, with a mean of 11.

It may take two or three weeks before the baby settles down to three- to four-hourly feeds, and a further two or three weeks before the night feed is willingly foregone. The probable psychological basis for this is shown by a recent study of the frequency of spontaneous milk ejections. These were found to occur at precise and regular intervals, short at first but lengthening over the passage of days. The intervals were almost 35 minutes on day 14, 45 minutes on day 28, 90 minutes on day 56, and 120 minutes on day 112.

Animal experiments have shown that oxytocin release not only occurs in response to stimulation of the nipple during suckling, but also occurs spontaneously at precise intervals, independent of any suckling stimulus, and suckling young who are attached to the nipples are seen to suckle only after spontaneous milk ejection has occurred. The suckling reflex then stimulates further milk secretion by release of prolactin. If, as seems likely, a similar mechanism operates in women, there are sound physiological reasons for allowing the baby to be attached to the nipple frequently during the early days to take advantage of the frequent spontaneous milk ejections as a stimulus to suckling, which in turn will increase lactation by stimulating release of prolactin.

Oxytocin release occurs not only in response to stimulation of the nipple during suckling, but also to other factors such as the cry of the baby. However, it is inhibited by maternal anxiety, especially anxiety engendered by fear of being unable to feed the baby, so that encouragement and some simple explanation of these automatic responses may be helpful in some cases.

Despite fears, the completely flexible demand-feeding schedule has not been associated with an increased incidence of cracked nipples, possibly because the baby is only actively sucking when the milk is flowing freely. On the contrary, establishment of lactation is easier and engorgement of the breasts is rarely seen.

Time at the breast

Strict adherence to times is not necessary as babies tend to regulate their own time of feeding. During the first week the frequency may be increased but the time at the breast is short. Short frequent feeds of the more dilute milk which is yielded in the early part of a feed will provide the baby with a reasonable quantity of water, while the breasts are receiving the maximum stimulus to lactate. The time at each breast increases gradually as the frequency of feeds declines.

Alternation of breasts

It is customary to start feeding on the breast which was taken last at the previous feed. This is based on the idea that 'rich milk' may be left in the second breast without loss of valuable calories, since it is known that the fat content of milk increases towards the end of a feed. It was also argued that the first breast should be emptied completely to stimulate lactation. Efforts to persuade the baby to empty one breast completely are wrong, because it has been shown that the increase in fat content provides the baby with a self-regulating mechanism; if thirsty, the baby will wish to stop feeding at each breast while the milk is still dilute, perhaps after only five minutes each side, but will demand more frequent feeds.

Amount taken from each breast

As already indicated, it is best to allow the baby to regulate the supply of milk and its character according to its own needs and the mother's milk yield. The time taken for a full feed may be anything between three minutes each side to nearly 15 minutes each side.

Postition during feeding

The infant is usually nursed by the mother propped up in bed or sitting in a low armchair. The infant is held in the crook of the arm on the same side as the breast which is to be given, with the weight of the baby supported on the forearm. The head should be allowed to extend beyond the bend of the elbow as most infants feed better with the neck extended. With the baby in this position the mother should bend forward slightly and allow the nipple to fall into the baby's mouth. If the breast is large the redundant tissue can be restrained with the fingers of the other hand and the nipple allowed to protrude between the extended fingers.

Air swallowing

Most babies swallow some air with the milk. If the air remains in the stomach and the pylorus is closed the stomach becomes distended to capacity before an adequate amount of milk is taken, and the infant refuses to feed any longer. If the baby is put back into the cot the air may be expelled and carry milk with it as vomit. Although some infants do not appear to suffer discomfort from considerable gastric and intestinal distension with air, the majority are inconvenienced by it, and it is therefore desirable to bring up the wind one or more times during the feed. To do this without spilling out the milk as well calls for a certain degree of practice on the part of both the mother and the infant. The infant is sat upright to bring the air bubble to the fundus of the stomach. The mother places one hand across the upper abdomen with the baby leaning forward against this hand. With her free hand the mother rubs or pats the back of the baby; after an interval the baby will bring up wind with a loud noise. Alternatively the baby may be held face downwards against the mother's shoulder or lying across her knee. The wind should also be brought up at the end of the feed.

DIFFICULTIES IN BREAST FEEDING

Difficulties may arise from causes in the infant or in the mother.

Causes in the infant

Reluctance to feed will often indicate that the baby is ill.

A healthy baby will sometimes refuse to take one breast, but will feed if the other breast is offered first. In other cases the infant refuses to get on the breast, but may be encouraged if a few drops of milk are expressed and allowed to fall on his lips.

A baby who is suffering from an infection, cerebral trauma or a congenital heart lesion may be too weak to take the breast or may tire before a sufficient amount of milk is taken. In such cases the infant must be fed with a spoon or tube for a time.

When the baby is very small there may be disproportion between the size of the nipple and the baby's mouth, but this will be remedied as the baby grows. Cleft lip and cleft palate cause less difficulty in feeding than might be expected. Micrognathos is a much more important cause of difficulty. Difficulty will also arise if there is obstruction to nose breathing (*see* p. 260).

Causes in the mother

Anatomical

When the nipples are poorly developed or retracted the infant cannot draw them into the correct position in the mouth for satisfactory feeding. This should be detected during antenatal examination and corrected by wearing nipple shells. Sometimes the condition may improve under the stimulus of the infant's attempts to feed, or may be overcome by feeding through nipple shields, but in a number of cases inadequate development of the nipples proves to be an insuperable barrier to satisfactory feeding.

Engorgement

On the third or fourth day after delivery the breasts may become engorged and painful so that milk cannot be taken and the mother is not able to tolerate the infant at the breast. This condition can develop very rapidly, and it should be recognized before it is fully established, when it may be relieved by allowing the baby to suckle frequently. Manual expression may give relief, but often the breasts are too tender for the patient to tolerate this; some midwives become very expert at expression of the breasts by hand. The breasts may also be emptied by a breast pump. Modern electric breast pumps which provide rhythmical negative pressure in a soft rubber breast cup are most effective.

Cracked nipple

See page 260.

Acute mastitis and breast abscess

See page 260.

Deficient lactation

Adequate lactation has been defined as secretion of 300 ml (*10 ounces*) daily by the fifth day and 480 ml (*16 ounces*) by the tenth day. If these amounts are not achieved a baby of normal weight will not be adequately fed. Failure of lactation may occasionally be due to inadequate development of gland tissue, although this has nothing to do with the size of the breasts. Some women with small breasts and little breast fat produce large quantities of milk, while large fat breasts may contain little secreting tissue.

Lactation is sometimes delayed. In most instances this is due to withholding for longer than usual the natural stimulus of the baby sucking at the nipple, but there are some women in whom lactation is slow to appear. They need reassurance, and to be told that if food and fluid intake is adequate lactation will eventually be established. There is a danger that they will be wrongly advised to drink large quantities of fluid, which has been shown to *reduce* the milk yield. This may be related to inhibition of the release of antidiuretic hormone and possibly of oxytocin at the same time. Breast feeding women should drink enough to satisfy thirst and not more. The best stimulus for a mother with delayed lactation is to allow the baby to suckle more frequently.

Contraindications to breast feeding

Breast feeding may be contraindicated in HIV-positive women, in cases of severe heart or kidney disease or of open tuberculosis in the mother. The risk to the infant if the mother has active tuberculosis is of the same degree whether the mother gives feeds by bottle or at the breast. If the tuberculosis is under active treatment the baby can breast feed normally.

Secretion of drugs in breast milk

No drug should be given to a lactating mother unless there is some definite clinical indication for its use, because some of the drug, or its degradation products, is likely to be secreted in the milk. However, many drugs which are essential for the mother are only secreted in small amounts, so that breast feeding need not be discontinued except in the case of a few drugs.

Cytotoxic drugs and radioactive iodine are absolute contraindications. If a thyrotoxic mother is receiving carbimazole it is necessary to monitor the baby's thyroid function and discontinue breast feeding if it is impaired.

Warfarin, senna, phenobarbitone, phenytoin, digoxin and steroids pass into the milk in harmless amounts.

Antibiotics are excreted in extremely small amounts, but there is a theoretical possibility of sensitization of the infant.

ARTIFICIAL FEEDING

When breast milk is not available the infant is usually fed on an infant formula based on cow's milk. In rare cases of intolerance to cow's milk other milks have to be used. There are now several artificial preparations which are preferred, such as hydrolysed amino acid preparations, or vegetable milks made from soya bean. Milk allergy causes colic and frequent loose stools. Because of the risk of allergy there is an increasing tendency to use non-allergenic artificial preparations when complements or supplements to feeds have to be introduced. However, some babies have also been known to develop sensitivity to soya bean preparations.

In comparing human milk and cow's milk it has been customary to concentrate on the differences in the fat and protein content and their respective digestibility, and to suggest that all that was necessary was to modify these constituents and to add some sugar to make the cow's milk preparation a satisfactory nutritional substitute. In reality the situation is much more complex.

Table 6.2 Comparison of the composition of human and cow's milk

	Protein (%)	Proportion of caseinogen to lactalbumin	Fat (%)	Carbo-hydrate (%)
Human milk	1.25	1 to 2	3.5	7.25
Cow's milk	3.5	4 to 1	3.5	4.75

Calorific value of milk: 70 calories (290 kJ) per 100 ml (*20 calories per ounce*)

The increased risk of enteric infections in artificially fed babies has been attributed to lack of sterility in the preparation and administration of the feeds. There is much to be said for this argument, but important new discoveries about the way in which raw human milk actively maintains the stability of the small intestine, whilst cow's milk preparations have a tendency to encourage unwanted bacterial colonization, have suggested that this difference is the basic reason why cow's milk is suitable for the calf and human milk for the baby. Because the cow is a ruminant the calf requires a type of feed which encourages the formation of a rumen, which has been described as a vat full of bacterial ferments which enables the cow to subsist on a vegetable diet. Human beings are not ruminants and the fundamental difference in the character of the intestinal contents makes considerable differences to the availability of nutrients. For example, the availability of calcium depends upon the lactose content, which is high in human milk; iron is bound to lactoferrin in human milk and to transferrin in cow's milk; zinc absorption is assisted by a prostaglandin in human milk which is absent from the cow's milk. The high lactose content of human milk, by increasing the availability of calcium, makes it possible for the level of calcium and phosphate to be relatively low, thus giving human milk a lower buffering capacity so that the bactericidal action of the more acid intestinal contents is maintained. By ensuring rapid and complete absorption of iron, the lactoferrin deprives the intestinal bacteria of iron needed for their replication. Other factors which inhibit bacterial growth which are present in human milk include specific IgA, maternal lymphocytes, lysozyme and copper.

Tremendous efforts have been made to 'humanize' cow's milk and although a biochemical approximation to human milk has been obtained, the important immunological constituents are missing.

General principles of artificial feeding

Whatever the choice of feed the principles for feeding are the same. After the seventh day of life the infant takes an average of 150 ml of fluid per kg of body weight daily (*2¼ fluid ounces per pound*). Since the amount of milk provided by a lactating mother is at first quite small and gradually increases, the same principle is applied for artificial feeding. It is convenient to start with 60 ml per kg of the milk preparation on the first day, and thereafter to increase the total quantity by 30 ml per kg each day until the baby is receiving 150 ml per kg. The fully constituted artificial feed should provide 65 to 70 calories (270–290 kJ) per 100 ml (*20 calories per ounce*). If the baby seems thirsty during the early days additional water may be given, either separately or by diluting the feeds slightly. There is no need to adhere rigidly to set feed volumes in a normal healthy infant, providing the total daily intake is adequate and the weight gain is satisfactory.

Although there is no need to keep rigidly to a strict time schedule for bottle feeding, and a certain amount of flexibility is appropriate for most babies, the same frequency of feeds is not required as in the early days when lactation is being established. Babies tend to settle down to a three- or four-hourly rhythm, and some flexibility enables each infant to show its own preference. Once full feeds are established the amount offered at each feed will be 25 or 30 ml per kg of body weight, depending on whether there are five or six feeds in the 24 hours.

The cow is basically an unsuitable animal to choose for the provision of a milk substitute for the human infant, but it was originally chosen because domestic cattle had been around for centuries as milk providers in the Western world, where the habit of artificial feeding was first popularized, and so the routinely used artificial milk preparations are derived from cow's milk which is modified in one way or another. These preparations are now available in hospitals as prepacked sterilized feeds, which only require the application of a sterile teat to the bottle before being given to the baby. However, these prepacked feeds are not available for home use, where feeds are still in the form of dried milk powders or evaporated milks which need to be reconstituted by the addition of water. The dilution required for each preparation is different, and the instructions on the packet or tin must be followed carefully. Included with the powdered milk preparations are special scoops, and it is important that the powder and the water are measured accurately. The scoop should not be heaped or packed tightly as this can make up to 20 per cent difference in the composition of the feed. Some mothers find it convenient to make up all the feeds for 24 hours in a batch, and if this is done the feeds must be stored in a refrigerator. Bottles and teats are carefully washed and sterilized in dilute hypochlorite solution (Milton). In hospital bottles are usually sterilized by autoclaving.

Preparations available

The use of undiluted cow's milk (doorstep milk) is not recommended until the baby reaches the age of nine months.

Cow's milk not only contains more protein than human milk, but the protein in it is predominantly curd protein (casein), whereas breast milk protein consists of about equal parts of casein and whey protein (mainly lactalbumin). The fat content of breast milk is approximately equal to that of cow's milk, but the fat is of a different quality; it is more easily absorbed and it contains more polyunsaturated fatty acids, which are probably essential for man. All modern infant formula milk preparations are now low solute with an osmolality similar to that found in human milk.

In making a low solute preparation some manufacturers reduce the milk to a demineralized whey, containing whey protein and a low content of minerals, and then add a small amount of skim milk to provide some casein, further lactose and some minerals in their naturally occurring forms, while other minerals such as iron, copper, zinc and manganese may also be added. The fat which is added consists of a mixture of animal and vegetable fats, the composition of which approximates to that of breast milk.

Alternatively, the relative concentration of protein and minerals can be reduced by simply adding carbohydrate. This must be carefully chosen to avoid the risk of fermentation diarrhoea.

After an episode of gastroenteritis it may be found that babies on prepacked low solute feeds sometimes have a recurrence of diarrhoea, and this may be due to the presence of small amounts of lactulose in the feeds, which results from the method of manufacture. A change to one of the powdered preparations will then effectively stop the diarrhoea.

Complementary and supplementary feeds

A complementary feed is one which is given to augment a feed from the breast; a supplementary feed is one which replaces a breast feed. Complementary feeding is sometimes necessary when lactation is only slowly established. It is unnecessary before the fifth day because a thirsty baby can be given water. If the weight is still falling or is stationary, or the baby seems very hungry, test weighing may be necessary. The baby is weighed naked at the same time each day before a feed is due. This gives a good overall estimate of the trend in weight gain (or loss). Test weighing before and after each individual feed is not recommended as this has been shown to be inaccurate. If complementary feeds are given it is best to offer the infant a standard amount after each breast feed and let it take as much or as little as it wants.

7

ABNORMAL PUERPERIUM

The causes of pyrexia following delivery are:

genital tract infection
urinary tract infection
breast infection
thrombophlebitis
respiratory tract infection
other causes of pyrexia

GENITAL TRACT INFECTION (PUERPERAL SEPSIS)

Childbed fever was the scourge of the first lying-in hospitals; the mortality from it became so great that a patient was held to be fortunate if she survived her stay in hospital.

It was not realized until the middle of the nineteenth century that the cause of epidemic puerperal infection was lack of cleanliness on the part of the attendants, who carried the infection from one patient to another. It was also at this time that Semmelweis, the Austrian obstetrician working in Vienna, noticed that puerperal fever was more common among patients delivered by medical students who had attended post-mortem examinations than among cases delivered by midwives. He believed that the fever was caused by products of decomposition and showed that washing the hands in chlorinated lime water reduced the incidence of infection. Unfortunately his contemporaries did not accept his work.

Pasteur, who trained as a chemist, but whose researches in bacteriology led to inoculation against several diseases, discovered that surgical infection was caused by micro-organisms. Following this discovery antiseptics (and later asepsis) were introduced into obstetric practice and quickly diminished the risks of infection. However, infection still remained the most important cause of maternal mortality.

In 1935 the sulphonamide group of drugs was discovered and produced dramatic results in the treatment of the most lethal type of infection – infection due to the haemolytic streptococcus. Penicillin and other antibiotic drugs have further reduced the dangers of infection, and the great majority of causes occurring today are of the mild, localized type. Puerperal sepsis, once the most important cause of maternal mortality, now accounts for only 5 per cent of all direct deaths (8 per million maternities); about half of these deaths follow abortion.

Although the incidence and severity of birth canal infection has fallen dramatically in recent years there is danger in complacency. New strains of organisms, resistant to the commonly used antibiotic drugs, appear from time to time and cause outbreaks of serious infection. It is only by strict attention to asepsis and the maintenance of a high standard of obstetric practice that they can be controlled.

Aetiology

When the placenta separates from the uterine wall a raw area, which may be regarded as an extensive but superficial wound, is left on the uterine wall. Further down the birth canal other wounds may also result from delivery; thus the cervix is occasionally torn, the fourchette is commonly torn in first confinements and sometimes the perineum is also torn. These wounds may become infected, and the symptoms and physical signs resulting the infection constitute the disease *puerperal sepsis*.

Bacteriology

Organisms which may cause infection of the birth canal during labour include:

> *Endogenous*
> coliform organisms
> enterococci (*Streptococcus faecalis*)
> anaerobic streptococci
> less commonly, streptococci groups B, C, D and G
> other anaerobic bacteria (*Bacteroides* spp)
> *Clostridium perfringens.*
> *Exogenous*
> haemolytic streptococcus, group A
> *Staphylococcus aureus.*

Endogenous organisms

The endogenous organisms are present in the patient's body before the onset of labour, often in the lower intestinal tract, on the perineum and in the vagina. As many as 25 per cent of women will harbour one of these organisms in the vagina during labour, but they seldom cause more than transient and localized infection.

In exceptional cases a localized infection due to anaerobic streptococci may spread into the pelvic veins and cause lung abscesses from septic emboli, or cause thrombosis of the femoral vein.

A clostridial infection may cause collapse, jaundice and haemoglobinuria. These rare infections may be rapidly fatal. They occur when there has been much bruising and tissue damage or when there is retention of a macerated fetus.

Exogenous organisms

The exogenous organisms come from other in-fected patients or from attendants who either have an infection or are carriers of infection. The organisms may be conveyed to the birth canal of a woman in labour on the hands of birth attendants, by droplet infection or, in the case of the haemolytic streptococcus, group A, from infected dust.

Patients and attendants suffering from colds and sore throats are liable to harbour haemolytic streptococci or staphylococci in their noses and throats, and a small proportion of healthy individuals are also found to be carrying these organisms. In both types of carrier the organisms can be cultured from the hands.

β-haemolytic streptococci can be divided into several groups according to the Lancefield classification. Group A is the only group responsible for serious maternal infections; it caused severe epidemics with many fatalities in the past. Mild localized infections occur with group B organisms and uncommonly with other groups. However, some commensal organisms which cause little harm to the mother are easily transmitted to the newborn infant, in whom dangerous infection can occur. This is particularly the case with haemolytic streptococci of group B.

The virtual elimination of the haemolytic streptococcus as the cause of serious infection is the result of a probable diminution in its virulence combined with its sensitivity to penicillin. The main danger is now from *Staphylococcus aureus*, which is a penicillin-resistant strain.

After the introduction of antibiotics it was anticipated that serious infection would become a thing of the past – it would merely be necessary to administer an antibiotic to cure every type of infection. Unfortunately this has not proved to be the case. Micro-organisms have the ability to produce resistant strains, and the widespread use of antibiotics has led to the emergence of these strains.

There may be carriers of resistant strains of staphylococci among hospital staff; the organisms are harboured in dust and bedding. Staphylococci may colonize the umbilical stump of the newborn child and the organisms may be spread from this site to other infants in the nursery. Infection with penicillin-resistant strains of staphylococci is not only of importance in puerperal sepsis but also in breast infections. The organisms are also a source of danger to the newborn.

Pathology

After the organisms have entered the tissues subsequent events depend on:

the virulence of the organisms
the resistance of the patient
the amount of tissue trauma
the speed with which effective chemotherapy or antibiotic treatment is begun.

Three degrees of severity of infection may be seen:

Mild infection

In the mildest cases the infection remains localized to perineal, vaginal or cervical lacerations, to the birth canal or at the placental site.

Moderate infection

Direct spread of infection may take place from the vagina or cervix into the pelvic cellular tissue and may cause pelvic cellulitis. Infection may also spread from the uterine cavity to involve the fallopian tubes and pelvic peritoneum, giving rise to acute salpingitis and pelvic peritonitis.

Severe infection

When the organisms are particularly virulent, as in the case of the haemolytic streptococcus group A, the infection may involve the general peritoneal cavity to cause general peritonitis, or spread into the bloodstream to produce septicaemia. The pleura, pericardium or joints may also be infected. When there is an overwhelming infection of this sort the patient rapidly becomes acutely ill from the effect of toxins produced by the organisms, but the local inflammatory response at the site of entry of the organisms in the birth canal may be minimal, and a perineal laceration, for example, may look quite clean.

Symptoms and signs

The earliest and most important sign of puerperal sepsis is fever. There may be a slight and transitory rise of temperature associated with the activity of labour and also on the third postpartum day when the milk comes in causing breast engorgement. Thereafter the puerperium should be apyrexial.

The fever may appear within 24 hours of delivery, and only exceptionally does it appear later. The rise of temperature may be abrupt and is occasionally accompanied by a rigor, or it may be step-like, taking several days to reach its maximum. Coincidentally with the fever the pulse rate is raised and the patient feels hot, with headache and backache. Spread to the pelvic peritoneum is shown by lower abdominal pain and tenderness on examination of the uterus and adnexa. Pelvic cellulitis causes persistent pyrexia and a mass to one or both sides of the vagina and uterus which may take several weeks to resolve.

In cases of general peritonitis the patients are severely ill with a rapid, thready pulse; abdominal pain and distension; vomiting and diarrhoea. There is generalized abdominal tenderness and there are few, if any, bowel sounds. The fever is usually persistently high, but in the very worst cases, and terminally, it may be slight.

In septicaemia rigors are common with continuous high fever. The patients are very ill and there may be no localizing signs. A high vaginal swab and blood culture are of paramount importance in diagnosing these cases.

Diagnostic examination

Pyrexia following labour or miscarriage and persisting for more than 24 hours must always be assumed to be due to infection of the birth canal until this has been excluded by bacteriological examination. In every case a general clinical examination should be made and should include the throat, chest, breasts, abdomen, renal angles and legs. Involution of the uterus may be delayed and it is often tender on abdominal examination. The perineum should be examined to see if any lacerations or an episiotomy are infected. If infected they will not be healing normally and there will be swelling with surrounding redness and a purulent exudate. A vaginal swab should be taken and a midstream specimen of urine collected for examination and culture. In taking the vaginal swab no antiseptic cream or lotion should be applied to the vulva. Although a more accurate assessment of the bacteriology can be made from a swab taken from the cervix it may be difficult to pass a speculum to expose the cervix. Likewise, if a clean-catch specimen of urine cannot be obtained from the standard midstream sample, urine may be collected by suprapubic aspiration.

Some judgement is required in interpreting the

bacteriological findings because organisms such as coliforms and non-haemolytic streptococci are commonly found in the vagina in the absence of clinical infection, but a profuse growth of strepto-cocci must be investigated and the organisms must be typed. When coliforms and anaerobic strepto-cocci are found the lochia is often purulent and foul-smelling, but virulent haemolytic streptococ-cus group A infections may spread to the general peritoneal cavity or cause septicaemia with re-latively few local abnormal physical signs, and with lochia which is not offensive. If the severity of the illness or the type of fever leads to suspicion of septicaemia blood is taken for culture, prefer-ably when the temperature is at its highest or during a rigor. Several blood cultures are some-times needed to establish a diagnosis.

In salpingitis the fallopian tubes and ovaries are swollen and inflamed with adherent omentum and bowel, but the tenderness of these structures in the rectovaginal pouch makes them difficult to distin-guish on bimanual examination. In most cases of pelvic cellulitis a vaginal examination will show induration of the parametrium extending to the lateral pelvic side wall. If it is unilateral it may push the uterus to the other side of the pelvis. With extensive cellulitis the whole pelvis feels solid, and the induration may even be palpable in the lower abdomen.

Prevention

During labour vaginal examinations should only be made when absolutely necessary and trauma at delivery should be reduced to a minimum.

Exogenous infection

The risk of exogenous infection is diminished by the usual aseptic technique with instruments and towels, and the use of a mask, sterile gloves and gown.

Infected patients are isolated. Any member of the medical or nursing staff with any infection such as sore throat, boil or paronychia is excluded from the department. If there is more than a sporadic case of puerperal infection bacterial swabs are taken from everyone working in the unit so that the source of infection can be traced.

Endogenous infection

The prevention of endogenous infection is far more difficult. It is impossible to sterilize either the vagina or vulva completely. In normal cir-cumstances the vagina does not contain organisms of high virulence, but the vulva and perianal region are covered with intestinal organisms such as *E. coli* and *S. faecalis*. These organisms are potentially pathogenic and it is impossible to pass anything, even a sterilized instrument into the vagina with-out also conveying organisms from the introitus. To minimize this risk the vulva and perianal region are swabbed with an efficient antiseptic such as chlorhexidine before making a vaginal examina-tion. When any vaginal operation is necessary during labour the same technique should be em-ployed as in an operating theatre; after swabbing the vulva with antiseptic the surrounding skin, especially the perianal region, is covered with sterile towels.

Although the indiscriminate use of antibiotics for prophylaxis is to be condemned because it encourages the production of resistant organisms, such treatment may be considered after premature rupture of the membranes or amniotomy if labour has not started within 24 hours. Antibiotics may also be given in a case of long labour, especially if this is terminated by caesarean section. The anti-biotic chosen should be safe for mother and fetus; ampicillin, or a cephalosporin such as cephalexin, is often used.

Treatment

If the patient is not already in hospital she must be transferred there, so that all facilities for nursing, diagnosis and treatment are available. She must be made comfortable by good nursing, with analge-sics if she is in pain and sedatives to ensure rest. The fluid intake must be adequate. Haemoglobin estimations should be done every two or three days because anaemia is often associated with severe sepsis, and transfusions of fresh blood may be required. Antibiotic treatment will be chosen according to the infecting organism and its sensiti-vities. If the patient is not very ill treatment can wait for the results of the bacteriological report, but in many cases treatment is started immediately with co-trimoxazole (Septrin) or with a broad-spectrum antibiotic such as ampicillin or cephalex-in and is subsequently modified if necessary.

If there is an infected perineal wound the stitches must be removed.

Operative treatment has little place and is usually confined to exploration of the uterine cavity to remove retained pieces of placenta. It is sometimes necessary to drain a pelvic abscess by an incision in either the posterior vaginal fornix or rectum. Pelvic cellulitis may sometimes result in an abscess which points above the outer end of the inguinal ligament and needs drainage there.

URINARY TRACT INFECTION

Infection of the urinary tract is the commonest cause of puerperal pyrexia, and is generally caused by *Escherichia coli*. The infection is almost always introduced by cathetization, which is frequently necessary during labour and sometimes in the puerperium. Apart from catheterization, the bruising of the tissues during delivery may be sufficient to give rise to recurrence of a pre-existing chronic and symptomless infection.

Diagnosis

This is made by examination of a midstream specimen of urine or a specimen obtained by suprapubic bladder puncture. Part of the specimen is sent to the laboratory for bacterial culture and sensitivity tests, but immediate examination of a drop of urine under the microscope will often settle the diagnosis; a large number of pus cells in the field makes the diagnosis of a urinary infection certain. A bacterial colony count of more than 100 000 organisms/ml signifies infection. Symptoms such as dysuria and frequency are often equivocal, since they may occur after delivery when there is no infection, and may be absent in the presence of infection.

Treatment

When there is a history of recent urinary infection a prophylactic course of ampicillin or co-trimoxazole may be given during labour and the first four days of the puerperium.

In the established case the fluid intake must be at least 3 litres in the 24 hours. A full course of ampicillin or co-trimoxazole is given.

BREAST INFECTION

Acute mastitis or a breast abscess may cause puerperal pyrexia (*see* p. 260).

THROMBOPHLEBITIS

The most common time for pyrexia from this cause is from the fourth to the tenth day after delivery. The fever is slight except in cases of extensive iliofemoral thrombosis, and those cases caused by pelvic infection.

The aetiology and pathology of thrombophlebitis during pregnancy and the puerperium are described on pp. 268–270). Apart from the usual case of deep venous thrombosis, which starts in the veins of the calf and which is caused by stasis rather than bacterial infection, it is possible that in some cases of puerperal sepsis the initial thrombosis is in the deep veins of the pelvis. Anaerobic streptococci may occasionally invade pelvic veins, proliferate in blood clot, and then give rise to septic emboli which pass to the lungs or other sites with episodes of high fever.

RESPIRATORY TRACT INFECTION

When an anaesthetic has been given during labour, postanaesthetic chest complications such as basal collapse or bronchopneumonia may occur.

OTHER CAUSES OF PYREXIA

Tonsillitis, influenza, or any of the acute specific fevers may occur in the puerperium, as well as surgical conditions such as appendicitis. A general clinical examination should always be made to exclude these.

DISORDERS OF THE BREAST IN THE PUERPERIUM

ENGORGEMENT OF THE BREASTS

On the second or third day after delivery the breasts become engorged and secretion of milk begins. If the baby does not empty them sufficiently they rapidly become overdistended. The breasts are enlarged and covered with distended veins; the skin over them may be slightly congested. They are very tender and feel hard and knotty. Nodules of enlarged breast tissue may be palpable in the axilla. The pain may prevent the woman from sleeping.

Treatment

In the early stages of engorgement the baby may be able to take enough milk to relieve the congestion, but once the condition is fully established the congestion and pressure on the ducts prevent the flow of milk and the infant cannot empty the breasts. A little milk should be manually expressed before putting the baby to the breast as this will help to promote an easy flow of milk. Sometimes the mother cannot tolerate this, and an electric breast pump, which produces rhythmical negative pressure in a soft rubber breast cup, may give relief. Analgesics may be required and the breasts should be effectively supported.

CRACKED NIPPLES

The nipple may become sore and painful from two conditions. One is the loss of the epithelium covering a considerable area of the nipple, with formation of a raw area which is very tender. The other is a small deep fissure situated at either the tip or the base of the nipple, which is also very painful. The two conditions may exist simultaneously, and are referred to as cracked nipples.

After delivery a flat nipple, or one that is not kept aseptic and dry, tends to become sore. If there is not sufficient milk in the breast a hungry baby will suck too vigorously and its gums cause abrasions of the epithelium. Another cause is leaving the baby too long at the breast, but with demand feeding this does not occur so often. The nipples may also become sore if the mother does not depress the breast away from the baby's nostrils when it is suckled, because if the baby cannot breathe through its nose it has to drop the nipple repeatedly and then take it up again. Thrush (moniliasis) is another occasional cause of soreness of the nipple.

Cracked nipples cause tenderness and pain during suckling. There is also a risk of a mammary abscess forming, as the ducts are not emptied because pain and engorgement is unrelieved, and perhaps because the raw area allows access for infecting organisms.

The baby may draw blood from a fissue into its stomach with the milk. If the blood is regurgitated it may give rise to a false diagnosis of gastric haemorrhage.

Treatment

A cracked nipple will heal spontaneously if the trauma that produced it ceases. The first essential of treatment is therefore rest, and the baby must not be put to the breast on that side until the crack has healed. While the crack is healing the breast is emptied by manual expression or by an electric breast pump. When breast feeding is recommenced the baby should only be put to the breast for a few minutes at first, otherwise the nipple will crack again. If the lesion is recognized at an early stage it may heal within 48 hours, but once the crack has become extensive or indurated healing will be far more difficult, and in many cases breast feeding cannot be re-established.

Various local applications have been recommended. It is important that any such application does not stick and drag away any newly formed epithelium when it is removed, and it must not be harmful to the baby or need to be cleaned off before a feed. Flavine in liquid paraffin is a suitable and harmless antiseptic, which will not adhere.

ACUTE PUERPERAL MASTITIS

The infecting organism is almost always *Staphylococcus aureus*. All that has been said about the prevalence and problems of infection with this organism in puerperal sepsis applies equally to breast infections. In addition the baby is a frequent source of infection to its mother's breasts. It has long been known that breast infections are liable to occur in association with skin infections of the baby, and that such infections spread rapidly in a nursery unless isolation and careful aseptic techniques are practised. The umbilical cord is a common site of infection, and must be inspected daily.

Bacteriological investigations carried out in epidemics of breast infections with *S. aureus* have shown that if one baby in a nursery has the organism in its nose or mouth almost all the other babies will be similarly affected within two or three days. These infected babies, who may be thriving and not ill, are a dangerous source of infection to their mothers.

There are two main types of mastitis; *cellulitis*, when the infection enters a crack in the nipple and spreads to the interlobular connective tissue, and *adenitis*, when the infection is primarily in the lactiferous system, there being no break in the surface epithelium of the nipple. The second type is seen in epidemics and is confined to hospital practice.

Acute mastitis may arise at any time in the puerperium. The onset is rapid, with pain in the breast and fever which may rise as high as 40.5°C (105°F) within a few hours. In both types the clinical picture is the same, the infection being limited at first to one lobe. A wedge-shaped area of cutaneous hyperaemia is seen, and the affected lobe is tense and tender; there may be general malaise. Unless early treatment is successful the condition will progress to a breast abscess.

Treatment

Prophylaxis consists of scupulous attention to aseptic technique. Any mother or baby with an infection must be removed from the ward or nursery and isolated. Ideally mother and baby should always be kept together and the mother should, as far as possible, attend to her baby's needs herself, thus reducing to a minimum the risk of cross-infection from handling by other persons.

As soon as mastitis occurs breast feeding on the affected side is suspended and the breast is emptied by gentle expression or with an electric breast pump. It is firmly supported over a large pad of cotton wool. A sample of milk is sent to the laboratory for culture and sensitivity tests; it is almost always possible to grow the infecting organism from the milk. If antibiotic treatment is going to prevent an abscess forming it must be started at once. Most of the infecting organisms in hospital are likely to be penicillin-resistant, but the prevalent strain may be known so that an appropriate antibiotic can be given. If the likely strain is not known treatment with flucloxacillin (Floxapen) 250 mg orally 6-hourly may be given until laboratory reports are available.

ABSCESS OF THE BREAST

A mammary abscess follows acute mastitis. A segment of the breast becomes painful and tender, with oedema and usually redness of the overlying skin. The temperature is raised and the axillary glands become tender and enlarged. The abscess may form near the surface or in the substance of the breast. If it is neglected a deep abscess may burrow in several directions and lead to almost total disorganization of the breast.

Treatment

Breast feeding and proper treatment of the abscess are incompatible. The baby must be taken from the breast and alternative feeding must be arranged. Lactation must be suppressed with bromocriptine 2.5 mg twice daily for 14 days. As soon as an abscess forms it should be drained under general anaesthesia. It is wrong to wait for fluctuation; brawny oedema of the skin is sufficient for diagnosis.

The incision should radiate from the nipple to avoid cutting the ducts. Since these abscesses have loculi running in different directions, and not infrequently have superficial and deep portions connected by a narrow tract, the incision should be adequate and a finger inserted into the abscess to break down any septa or loculi. A drainage tube is inserted, and with large abscesses it is sometimes necessary to make a counter-incision to obtain dependent drainage. Antibiotic treatment is given.

INHIBITION OF LACTATION

Although oestrogens will inhibit lactation they are no longer used because of the risk of venous thrombosis. Bromocriptine 2.5 mg twice daily for 14 days effectively inhibits lactation, but it is expensive. In many cases all that is required is to support the breasts firmly and to await the cessation of activity. Limitation of fluid intake, but not to a degree which causes thirst, may help.

If lactation is already established weaning is achieved by omitting successive feeds, and only if there is an urgent need to suppress lactation, as in a case of breast abscess, should bromocriptine be used.

GALACTOCELE

A galactocele is a retention cyst of one of the larger mammary ducts. Its content is chiefly milk. A local fluctuating swelling is felt, and the skin over it may be reddened, but there is not severe pain and no constitutional disturbance. A galactocele that is small and deeply situated may be mistaken for a carcinoma in the breast. The cyst should be excised.

CARCINOMA OF THE LACTATING BREAST

When carcinoma occurs in the lactating breast it develops with great rapidity and spreads widely. The affected breast is larger than the other, the nipple is flattened or retracted and may be fixed, and the skin over the tumour is oedematous – the so-called *peau d'orange*. There may be redness if the growth is close to the surface.

Immediate recognition is of the utmost importance. The rapidity with which the enlargement appears and the reddening of the skin suggest mastitis, but the lack of pain and the fact that the tumour is scarcely tender to palpation should give a clue to the correct diagnosis. This must be confirmed by biopsy, and the treatment will then often be by irradiation. Results are poor.

DISORDERS OF HAEMOSTASIS IN PREGNANCY

During pregnancy there are profound physiological changes in the blood and dramatic changes in the coagulation factors and haemostatic mechanisms. These changes protect the pregnant woman from haemorrhage, particularly at delivery, and they tip the balance of haemostasis towards clotting. However, along with the beneficial effects are a number of unwanted effects; deep vein thrombosis and pulmonary embolism are found more commonly in women who are pregnant than in non-pregnant women. Haemorrhage remains a risk and, together with thromboembolic disease, deep vein thrombosis and pulmonary embolism, is a significant cause of the rare event of maternal death.

Some of the nomenclature of coagulation is confusing, especially as there are so many opposing reactions with a myriad of factors, stimulators and inhibitors. In order to understand these coagulation and related mechanisms a brief account of how haemostasis is achieved outside pregnancy is given. This will be followed by a description of the changes that occur in pregnancy and the coagulation disorders specific to pregnancy.

HAEMOSTASIS

Haemostasis is dependent on the following factors:

> the platelet–vessel wall interaction
> the coagulation system
> the natural anticoagulation system
> the fibrinolytic system.

These factors interact in a fine and balanced way. They form an intricate interlacing system that interdigitates between the coagulation, fibrinolytic, kinin and complement cascades. If the balance is upset, haemorrhage or thrombosis may result.

THE PLATELET–VESSEL WALL INTERACTION

Platelets can initiate thrombosis and can also provide a surface on which the interaction of coagulation factors may take place, by providing the necessary phospholipid.

When the vessel wall is damaged vasoconstriction occurs and any endothelial defect is bridged by the adhesion of platelets to the underlying collagen fibres. Platelets aggregate and, together with fibrin, form a haemostatic plug.

The platelets which adhere to collagen undergo a change in shape and release the contents of their dense body cytoplasmic granules. These contain adenosine diphosphate (ADP), adenosine triphosphate (ATP) and serotonin, which promote further aggregation.

Phospholipid in the platelet membrane is hydrolysed to arachidonic acid. This is converted to a labile cyclic endoperoxide called thromboxane A_2 with a half-life of only 30 seconds. It is a potent releaser of the dense granules and hence is a powerful platelet aggregator; it is also a vasocontrictor.

Phospholipid in the endothelium is also hydrolysed but a different labile endoperoxide is produced – prostacyclin. This is a powerful inhibitor of platelet adhesion and aggregation and is a vasodilator.

The balance between thromboxane and prostacyclin determines whether there is local adhesion of platelets to endothelium or not. In addition, the platelets have a negative surface charge, as does the endothelium, and the resultant electrostatic repulsion also contributes to the antithrombogenic properties of normal blood vessels.

Platelets and the coagulation cascade are interrelated. Platelet aggregation releases platelet factor 3, which in turn stimulates both the intrinsic and extrinsic coagulation pathways. Platelet factor 3 also promotes irreversible platelet aggregation and clot retraction, which reduces vessel occlusion by means of the contractile platelet protein, thrombasthenin.

MEASUREMENT OF PLATELET AND VESSEL WALL INTERACTION

Platelet function and the interaction with the vessel wall are measured by the bleeding time. There are a number of commercially available disposable devices which produce a cut in the skin of standard depth and length. Venostasis is maintained at a pressure of 40 mmHg by applying a sphygmomanometer above the elbow while cuts are made in the volar surface of the forearm. The cuts are carefully blotted with filter paper every 15 seconds and the length of time the cut bleeds is measured. This is a reflection of platelet numbers, platelet adhesion to the subendothelium and platelet

aggregation. The normal bleeding time is less than 10 minutes.

Platelet aggregation is assessed in an aggregometer. Change in the transmission of light through a suspension of platelets is measured in response to various aggregating agents such as ADP, adrenaline, ristocetin and collagen. As the platelets aggregate the light transmission increases.

Platelet turnover is usually assessed by radioisotope labelling techniques but this is not applicable in obstetric practice. An estimate of turnover can be made from platelet size; young platelets are larger. Platelet size can be measured automatically on some sophisticated cell counters but can also be assessed on a well-spread blood film. The megakaryocytes on a bone marrow aspirate may be increased if there is increased turnover.

THE COAGULATION SYSTEM

All the coagulation factors are normally present in the blood in an inert form. When there is a break in vascular integrity they are activated in the vicinity of the break. Fine control mechanisms ensure that the activation is contained within the immediate area of the wound and that the circulating blood remains fluid.

There are two pathways leading to the activation of the final common pathway. The intrinsic pathway, involving factors found in the blood and the extrinsic pathway, involving factors found in damaged tissue. They both lead to the activation of factor X. These two pathways interact with each other and to separate them is artificial but for simplicity they can be described separately (Fig. 7.1).

Intrinsic system

The intrinsic system begins with contact activation. Factor XII, prekallikrein and factor XI are activated with the participation of the cofactor, high molecular weight kininogen. It is of interest that the contact factors are also components of the fibrinolytic and kinin systems, illustrating the close interrelationships between these various physiological systems.

The activated contact factors are specific proteases and they lead to the activation of factors IX, VIII and then X. The activation of factor X probably involves the formation of a complex at the cell surface comprising activated IX, VIII, Ca^{2+} and phospholipid.

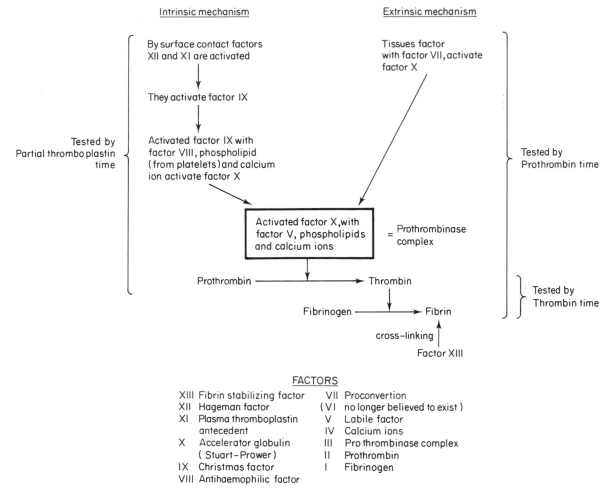

Fig. 7.1   The mechanism of clot formation

Extrinsic system

The extrinsic system bypasses the contact phase. Direct activation of factor X is achieved by a complex formed from tissue factor, phospholipid from the cell surface, Ca^{2+} and factor VII.

The activated factor X formed by either pathway then forms another complex, the so-called prothrombinase complex which consists of factor X, Ca^{2+} and factor V. This results in activation of prothrombin to thrombin, which in turn converts soluble fibrinogen to insoluble fibrin, the skeleton of a firm clot. The fibrin clot is then further strengthened by the cross-linking effect of factor XIII (Fig. 7.1).

The coagulation cascade

This is an amplifier system. The concentration of factor XII in the plasma is 20 mg/L and activation of that tiny amount of contact factor can result in the conversion of fibrinogen which has a concentration of 2 to 4 g/L.

Coagulation tests

The platelet count

This is measured electronically by modern automatic cell counters. The natural tendency of platelets to aggregate may produce falsely low counts. The interaction between the platelet and the vessel wall is best measured by the bleeding time.

The intrinsic coagulation pathway

This is measured by the activated partial thromboplastin time (APTT). Unfortunately the terminology is confusing and the test is also known as the partial thromboplastin time with kaolin (PTTK) and the kaolin cephalin clotting time (KCCT). The normal range of the APTT is 35 to 43 seconds. It is prolonged by deficiencies in factors XII, XI, X, IX, VIII, V or prothrombin and also by the presence of coagulation inhibitors such as the lupus anticoagulant. It can detect haemophilia A and B and some cases of von Willebrand's disease.

The intrinsic coagulation pathway is also affected by the presence of heparin and may be used to monitor heparin therapy. However, it may be more reliable to use the protamine sulphate neutralization test to measure therapeutic levels of heparin and the inhibition of activated factor X to measure the very small levels used in low dose heparin prophylaxis.

The extrinsic coagulation pathway

This is reflected by measurement of the prothrombin time. The title of the test is a misnomer because apart from measuring prothrombin it also measures factors V, VII and X. The normal prothrombin time is 10 to 14 seconds. The pathway may be prolonged in liver disease and by treatment with the coumarin anticoagulants such as warfarin. The results of the test are often expressed as a ratio with an international standard – the International Normalized Ratio (INR).

The thrombin time

This measures the end of the coagulation cascade with the conversion of fibrinogen to fibrin. Both the length of the test and the appearance of the clot give important information. The normal range for thrombin time is determined in each individual laboratory, but is usually about 10 seconds. Abnormalities may be due to a reduction in fibrinogen but also to the presence of interfering substances. For example the test is very sensitive to the presence of heparin and to the products of fibrin and fibrinogen degradation (FDPs). The fibrinogen level may also be measured directly.

THE NATURAL ANTICOAGULATION SYSTEM

A variety of mechanisms exist to restrict activation of the coagulation factors to the site of vessel damage and prevent their wider spread. The activation of thrombin occurs most readily where the platelet phospholipids are available, i.e. where aggregation is occurring. There are also a number of naturally occurring anticoagulants. Antithrombin III (ATIII) not only inactivates thrombin but also the activated factors IX, X, V and VIII. It is the cofactor for heparin. Protein C is another naturally occurring anticoagulant. It inactivates activated factors V and VIII and promotes fibrinolysis. Protein S is a cofactor for protein C in its effect against activated factor V.

Families with deficiencies in these factors may have a hypercoagulable state with a particular predisposition to venous thrombosis. It is interesting to note that, like factors II, VII, IX and X, proteins C and S are dependent on vitamin K for the last stage of their synthesis. They are thus similarly reduced by coumarin anticoagulant therapy and there is the possibility of increasing the hypercoagulable state in susceptible individuals in the early stages of anticoagulation. Skin necrosis has been described in protein C deficiency treated with warfarin due to the development of thromboses in the small vessels of the skin.

FIBRINOLYSIS

During fibrinolysis fibrin clots are digested, rendered soluble and vessel patency is restored. A summary of fibrinolysis is given in Fig. 7.2.

Plasmin is the effector enzyme of the fibrinolytic system but it has wide substrate specificity. There are, therefore, inhibitors to the activation of the precursor (plasminogen) and to plasmin itself, e.g. α_2-antiplasmin.

At the time of clot formation plasminogen becomes bound to fibrin where it is relatively protected from its inhibitors. Plasminogen activators diffuse from the tissues into the clot and activate plasmin, which digests fibrin to form fibrin degradation products. The uterus is particularly rich in such activators. When there is systemic overactivity of the fibrinolytic system a bleeding state may be produced. The products of fibrinolysis

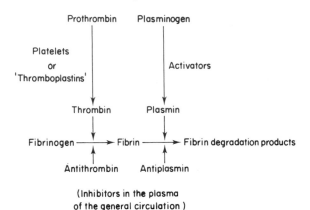

Fig. 7.2 The mechanism of fibrinolysis

may themselves act as anticoagulants, interfering with the polymerization of fibrin and prolonging the thrombin time.

Various fibrinolytic activators are used therapeutically to lyse clots. The best known are streptokinase and urokinase. However there are some newer preparations which are expensive and not fully assessed but which will probably come to have wider applications. These include single chain urokinase (SCUPA), recombinant tissue plasminogen activator (R-t-PA) and acylated plasminogen activator (APSAC).

PHYSIOLOGY OF THE COAGULATION AND FIBRINOLYTIC SYSTEM IN NORMAL PREGNANCY AND LABOUR

In pregnancy the balance of haemostasis swings towards a hypercoagulable state with increases in the coagulation factors, particularly fibrinogen, factor VIII and von Willebrand factor antigen. Allowing for the changes in plasma volume the amount of circulating fibrinogen virtually doubles by the end of pregnancy. By contrast, the fibrinolytic system is suppressed, with an increase in tissue plasminogen activator inhibitor. The source of the reduced fibrinolytic potential is thought to be the placenta because immediately after delivery of the placenta the fibrinolytic system returns to normal. The overall effect is to protect the mother from haemorrhage during labour and delivery. However, the reverse side of the coin is that there appears to be an increased susceptibility to throm-

boembolic disease and to disseminated intravascular coagulation. Apart from protein S levels, which fall in pregnancy, levels of the natural anticoagulation factors, protein C and AT III, remain approximately the same.

The number of platelets in a normal pregnancy probably does not change, although there may be a slight decrease in platelet lifespan in the last trimester. However, in pre-eclampsia there is certainly an increase in platelet turnover.

Despite the dramatic changes in the coagulation and fibrinolytic factors, probably the most important factor in preventing torrential bleeding at the time of placental separation is effective myometrial contraction. This rapidly cuts down the flow of blood to the placental site. It is facilitated by changes that occur in the structure of the spiral arteries towards the end of pregnancy. Without effective myometrial contraction all the coagulation changes that take place in pregnancy would be to no avail.

The placenta is rich in tissue factor. This activates the extrinsic coagulation cascade and results in the deposition of up to 10 per cent of the total body fibrinogen on the placental bed when the placenta has separated. At the time of delivery of the placenta the tests of coagulation and fibrinolysis show activation. Levels of fibrinogen and plasminogen fall and platelet turnover increases. After a short early puerperal increase the levels return to normal by the fourth postpartum week.

COAGULATION DISORDERS SPECIFIC TO PREGNANCY AND LABOUR

HAEMORRHAGE

Haemorrhage is an important cause of mortality in obstetric practice. The deaths directly due to haemorrhage, plus those due to ectopic pregnancy, make up 25 per cent of all direct maternal deaths.

DISSEMINATED INTRAVASCULAR COAGULATION (DIC)

The changes in the coagulation and fibrinolytic systems in pregnancy result in a tendency towards hypercoagulability but paradoxically can result in severe bleeding. Conditions associated with the systemic activation of both systems result in the deposition of multiple fibrin–platelet thrombi in the microcirculation. This results in the consumption of clotting factors and in clinical bleeding; such activation is known as disseminated intravascular coagulation (DIC).

DIC is always a secondary phenomenon, it is not a disease entity in its own right. Its treatment depends upon the alleviation of the underlying primary condition and replacement of depleted factors. Obstetric DIC is usually associated with intrauterine pathology and when the uterus is emptied the DIC fades away. It is particularly associated with abruptio placentae, retention of a dead fetus *in utero*, amniotic fluid embolism, intrauterine infection due to septic abortion, eclampsia or prolonged shock. The release of tissue thromboplastins or vascular endothelial damage by septicaemia may result in a chronic compensated DIC with an increased turnover of platelets and coagulation factors. Alternatively, there may be a rapid depletion of factors and platelets resulting in catastrophic bleeding with oozing from venepuncture sites, surgical incisions and vaginal blood loss.

In the full blown DIC syndrome the platelet and fibrinogen levels fall and all the coagulation screening tests are prolonged. The blood film shows a microangiopathic picture because red blood cells are fragmented when they are squeezed through intravascular fibrin strands. Fibrin degradation products (FDPs) are formed and these interfere with the polymerization of fibrin. The thrombin time is very sensitive to the presence of FDPs and is a quick, easy test to use in an emergency to monitor the progression of DIC. It also assays the fibrinogen level. It may be useful to monitor the platelets, although the assay of FDPs can often wait until after the cross-matching of blood and the preparation of blood products, which takes priority. The presence of FDPs cannot be taken as diagnostic of DIC because they may be raised in other circumstances such as the normal fibrinolysis of a large internal bleed.

In patients with massive bleeding, as in a failure of myometrial contraction, the coagulation factors and platelets may be depleted without there being DIC because the blood used in replacement does not contain all the coagulation factors.

Every obstetric unit should have a written code for the management of major obstetric haemorrhage. In obstetric patients with DIC the precipitant is usually easily recognized. Treatment depends on removal of the underlying cause, correction of hypovolaemia and treatment of the haemostatic disorder.

Treatment

More than one peripheral line may be required to achieve an adequate transfusion rate to maintain blood volume replacement. A central venous line can monitor replacement therapy but its insertion may need to be delayed while the coagulation defect is corrected. Transfusion of fresh frozen plasma (FFP) will alleviate hypovolaemia while blood becomes available, and will also correct coagulation deficiencies. Although FFP may be available before cross-matched blood it may take half-an-hour to thaw and it may be necessary to use albumin solution or even very large volumes of crystalloid to maintain the circulation until blood components are available. It is usual practice thereafter to replace the missing coagulation factors with a unit of FFP for every 4 to 6 units of transfused red cells. Only when hypovolaemia is corrected can delivery be expedited, although a severe coagulation defect may limit the degree of possible intervention. Oxytocics and amniotomy may be used but caesarean section may carry the risk of operative bleeding. Uncross-matched blood may be required if the loss of blood is very fast but obviously the first choice is ABO and rhesus compatible blood. Most blood issued by the transfusion service has been used in the production of blood components and is deficient in coagulation factors and platelets. FFP can be used as above to replace the depleted factors but in practice platelets are rarely necessary.

Some blood components are produced on a large scale from pooled plasma from many donors. Many of these components are heat-treated to eliminate the carriage of the human immunodeficiency virus although they can possibly still transmit certain hepatitis viruses, particularly non-A–non-B and the newly described hepatitis C. Cryoprecipitate and FFP are made from single unit donations and are not heat-treated. Both these products are good sources of fibrinogen but, not being heat-treated they carry a small risk of transmitting infection. The advantages of FFP over cryoprecipitate are that it provides a larger volume and replaces *all* the coagulation factors.

Heparin and antifibrinolytics are almost never used in the treatment of DIC. The use of heparin should not be contemplated unless the uterus is empty and the myometrium is well contracted, i.e.

only if there is an intact circulation.

Abruptio placenta

The amount of bleeding from the vagina cannot be used to predict the severity of the haemostatic defect because the bleed may be occult.

Prolonged retention of a dead fetus

If a dead fetus is retained for more than five weeks a haemostatic defect due to DIC may result. The defect should be corrected before careful induction of delivery. Although in the past this may have been an important cause of DIC, modern obstetric practice allows for the early recognition of a dead fetus and the retention of a dead fetus is now a rare cause of DIC.

Endotoxic shock

When endotoxic shock follows peripartum uterine infection the mainstay of treatment is to eliminate the cause and the underlying infection and to give supportive treatment for the coagulation defect.

Amniotic fluid embolism

This is a rare but devastating event that may occur during or just after delivery. The amniotic fluid gains access to the circulation and results in extreme shock, obstruction to pulmonary blood flow, massive depletion of coagulation factors and exsanguinating vaginal blood loss. Treatment revolves around cardiopulmonary resuscitation, supportive transfusion therapy and immediate delivery.

Pre-eclampsia

In pre-eclampsia there is an increase in platelet turnover, deposition of fibrin in the microcirculation, increased levels of FDPs and microangiopathic haemolysis. This is a chronic DIC state which increases in severity as the pre-eclampsia worsens. The differential diagnosis of the thrombocytopenia rests between autoimmune thrombocytopenia, thrombotic thrombocytopenia and DIC secondary to pre-eclampsia.

COAGULATION DISORDERS COINCIDENT WITH PREGNANCY

There are a number of bleeding diatheses which occur in women and which may complicate pregnancy. The inherited disorders of haemophilia A and B are sex-linked and female carriers may have suboptimal levels of factors VIII or IX. Von Willebrand's disease is an autosomal dominant condition which may be associated with a low factor VIII. In all these conditions it may be necessary to identify affected individuals because they may require replacement therapy or special obstetric management and also because they may need genetic counselling and antenatal diagnosis.

There are also some acquired coagulation disorders that may occur in women of childbearing age. Of these, autoimmune thrombocytopenia is the most common. It may produce a low platelet count in both the mother and the fetus, because the responsible IgG immunoglobulin can cross the placenta. Treatment strategies may include steroid and high-dose immunoglobulin therapy of the mother. Fetal blood sampling may determine whether it is safe to deliver vaginally or whether a caesarean section is indicated to protect the fetus from trauma. After delivery the infant's platelet count may continue to fall.

THROMBOEMBOLIC DISEASE IN PREGNANCY

Deep vein thrombosis (DVT) may be clinically inapparent, its first clinical sign may be an embolic complication. There must, therefore, be a high index of suspicion tempered by effective objective diagnosis because treatment carries risks for both the mother and fetus. Also, clinical diagnosis of DVT is notoriously unreliable and is wrong half the time. Recent reductions in deaths from pulmonary embolism (PE) are probably due to improved prophylaxis and the reduced use of oestrogens for suppressing lactation.

The incidence of thromboembolic disease in pregnancy lies between 0.3 and 12 per 1000 deliveries. Approximately two-thirds of cases occur postnatally. The risk of recurrence of thromboembolism in women who have had a previous episode has been estimated at 12 per cent.

While pregnancy itself is a risk factor for venous thromboembolism the risk of pulmonary embolism is increased in women of greater parity and age and in those with a previous history. The usual risk factors of obesity and any postoperative state continue to apply in pregnancy.

There is an increased risk of thromboembolism in patients with congenital deficiencies of anti-thrombin III and protein C and with some sickle-cell anaemia syndromes. The lupus anticoagulant is an acquired condition which predisposes to thrombosis. This lengthens *in vitro* tests of coagulation while causing thrombosis *in vivo*. It also causes fetal loss.

It is very important to investigate and identify thromboembolic diseases and to come to the correct diagnosis, because therapeutic and prophylactic anticoagulation in the index pregnancy and in future pregnancies carries important hazards. DVT should be confirmed by ultrasound; this can show the clot and lack of venous expansion of the affected vein during the Valsalva manoeuvre. Previously, venography was used to confirm the diagnosis with radiation limited to the midthigh and with good pelvic screening. The benefits of ultrasound over venography are that there is no exposure to radiation and it can be repeated as often as necessary to monitor progress.

In a patient who is not shocked and who has pleuritic pain but no changes on chest X-ray, the diagnosis of pulmonary embolism can be made by lung scan. Simple perfusion scans in a patient with a normal chest X-ray may show a deficit. Where there is an abnormal chest X-ray a ventilation-perfusion scan will discriminate between pneumonia which will show a matched deficit, and pulmonary embolism, where there will only be reduced perfusion. The radiation dose from such a scan is less than that given in a standard chest X-ray.

Treatment of thromboembolism

Massive pulmonary embolism may cause sudden death. If the patient survives long enough surgical embolectomy may be indicated. Fibrinolytic therapy is rarely used in pregnant patients but may be indicated in patients in the postpartum period.

Less severe cases require immediate anticoagulation with therapeutic heparin, starting with 40 000 units per day by intravenous infusion. This limits the progression of the clot and reduces mortality. Heparin does not cross the placenta. It is continued for about a week and is monitored by the APTT or the protamine sulphate test. Thereafter low-dose subcutaneous heparin is given until six weeks into the puerperium. The dose is about 10 000 units twice daily, reducing to 8000 units after delivery, and it is usually self-administered by the patient. It has no effect on the coagulation factors or on coagulation tests and it serves only to prevent the spontaneous conversion of factor X to the active form. Activation of factor X is the important link between the intrinsic and extrinsic pathways. The level of heparin achieved by this low-dose regime can only be measured by inhibition of activation of factor X.

The major short-term side-effect of therapeutic heparin is maternal bleeding. With therapeutic levels of heparin surgical delivery is contraindicated but there is no such restriction in the use of prophylactic heparin levels.

After the acute phase, the anticoagulant, warfarin, is used in some centres. It is monitored by the prothrombin time. Bleeding is the principle side-effect in the mother and this is particularly important as delivery approaches. As the effects of heparin can be reversed more quickly than those of warfarin, heparin often replaces warfarin from 36 weeks. Heparin virtually disappears from the circulation in six hours whereas it takes three days for the effects of warfarin to dissipate. However, in an emergency warfarin can be reversed with an infusion of FFP. It is not good policy to reverse the warfarin effect with vitamin K because this is said to produce a rebound effect in the mother and it may be very difficult to reinstitute warfarin therapy later. In an emergency heparin can be reversed with protamine sulphate, although in practise withholding the drug usually suffices. It must be remembered though, that protamine sulphate is an anticoagulant in its own right. Whichever drug is used it is continued until the sixth week postpartum. Women on heparin may choose to change to warfarin in the puerperium.

Warfarin carries an additional risk in pregnancy because it crosses the placenta and can cause bleeding and congenital abnormalities in the fetus in a dose-dependent fashion. It should therefore be avoided in the first trimester during the period of organogenesis. When it is used it should be well controlled and the dose should be maintained at the lower end of the therapeutic range. Its use cannot be avoided in patients with replacement heart valves because heparin cannot prevent thrombosis effectively enough in this situation.

Neither warfarin nor heparin are excreted in the breast milk and are therefore safe to use during lactation.

Prophylaxis of thromboembolism

Heparin is sometimes given to pregnant patients with a history of thromboembolism. Bone demineralization is associated with heparin treatment; the effects may be cumulative over successive pregnancies. It is likely that the risks of recurrence of thromboembolism may not be as great as was previously suspected, so that there is no need for prophylaxis in most patients with a previous solitary event. In view of the risk of bone loss, heparin may be given from delivery for six weeks in patients who have had a single episode of thrombosis. Changing to warfarin after a week further reduces the risk of bone loss.

8

OBSTETRIC PROCEDURES

CHORION VILLUS SAMPLING

Chorion villus sampling (CVS) involves taking chorionic tissue for diagnostic purposes; it may be carried out transcervically between eight and 12 weeks gestation, or transabdominally at any time from eight weeks onwards.

The main risk of the procedure is that of subsequent miscarriage, which is reckoned to be 2 per cent higher than the spontaneous miscarriage rate. For the first trimester this would mean a pregnancy loss rate following CVS of 4 per cent (2 per cent of which would be due to CVS).

Indications

Karyotyping

The most important group of mothers needing investigation are those at risk of having a fetus with Down's syndrome. This risk rises with maternal age and reaches a rate of 1 in 50 for mothers aged 40 or more, but younger mothers with a previously affected child should also be considered. Counselling usually starts with women over the age of 35 years. Alpha-fetoprotein levels in maternal serum are lower than normal in Down's syndrome pregnancies (below 0.8 times the normal median for gestational age). A low level of AFP in serum may indicate the need for CVS or amniocentesis in a younger woman.

Chorionic tissue grows rapidly. A preliminary chromosome count may therefore be obtained within 24–48 hours. If, however, a full G-banded chromosome analysis is required, the result will take two weeks.

Haemoglobinopathies

This investigation is of relevance to Negroid races (sickle-cell disease) and those of Mediterranean extract (thalassaemia). It is unusual to have a pregnant woman with the major form of either condition, but the minor forms (trait) are often encountered. If both partners are carrying the trait, the chances of any one offspring developing sickle-cell disease or thalassaemia major are 1 in 4. Such a risk is clearly an indication for CVS if the patients agree.

Biochemical abnormalities

Inborn errors of metabolism are fortunately rare, but if a family is afflicted the incidence may be as high as 1 in 4. The basic defect is an enzyme deficiency which results in an accumulation of substrate. Gaucher's disease (a disorder of glycogen storage), and Niemann–Pick disease (a disorder of lipoid metabolism), and the mucopolysaccharidoses are examples. Direct enzyme assays on the chorionic tissue will provide the diagnosis within two days.

Single gene disorders

The most common of these disorders are cystic fibrosis and Duchenne muscular dystrophy, both of which may be detected on CVS by recombinant DNA analysis. The risk for cystic fibrosis may be 1 in 4 for either sex. Duchenne muscular dystrophy, being sex-linked recessive, carries a risk of 1 in 2 for males but will not affect females. Other conditions in which the diagnosis is made by DNA analysis of chorionic villus cells include Huntington's chorea, haemophilia, myotonic dystrophy, phenylketonuria, retinitis pigmentosa and retinoblastoma.

Future considerations

New diagnostic techniques are emerging, many as a result of the recent rapid advances in DNA technology. Examples are the detection of placental (and hence fetal) infection with the rubella virus and the diagnosis of haemophilia. It is also possible to determine the rhesus status in the first trimester by direct examination of fetal red cells obtained at CVS.

Procedure

Chorion villus sampling is always carried out under ultrasound control. Sector scanners are superior to linear array for this purpose.

If the transcervical route is employed the patient is placed in the semi-lithotomy position. Following visualization of the cervix a plastic or metal catheter is introduced through the cervical canal into the chorion frondosum, and a sample of chorionic tissue is aspirated (Fig. 8.1). Sometimes biopsy forceps are used.

For the transabdominal route the patient is supine. A double needle technique is usually employed, requiring prior infiltration with local anaesthetic (Fig. 8.2).

The principle of aspirating chorionic tissue is the same. Both techniques are still being evaluated, but it would appear that the transabdominal route has the advantage of being feasible during the second and even the third trimesters. It would also seem that the pregnancy loss rate may be slightly lower with the transabdominal route, possibly due to less risk of infection. Rhesus-negative mothers should receive 250 units anti-D immunoglobulin by i.m. injection afterwards.

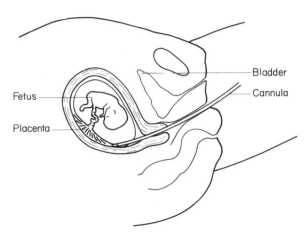

Fig. 8.1   Chorion villus sampling (Transcervical)

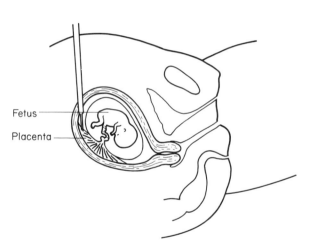

Fig. 8.2   Chorion villus sampling (Transabdominal)

CORDOCENTESIS

Cordocentesis is being more widely used now to examine constituents of the fetal blood and, in cases of fetal anaemia, for intrauterine blood transfusion. Like other invasive procedures cordocentesis is used under ultrasound guidance, using a sector scanner. The placental cord insertion is visible on ultrasound from about 15 weeks, so cordocentesis may be undertaken at any stage thereafter (*see* Procedure). The risk to the fetus appears to be 1–2 per cent.

Indications

In theory the indications for cordocentesis can be expanded to include any investigation currently undertaken on a blood sample. In practice the following are the most common indications.

Karyotyping

Fetal lymphocytes will provide a chromosome count in a few days. Such information may prove desirable if the fetus has been found to have a congenital abnormality known to be associated with Down's syndrome (e.g. exomphalos) at an ultrasound scan during the second or third trimester.

Rhesus iso-immunization

Direct assessment of fetal haemoglobin and haematocrit are better predictors of fetal outcome than liquor bilirubin, especially in the third trimester. If the haemoglobin (normally 15 g/dl) and haematocrit (normally 40–45 per cent) fall, the fetus will require transfusing with group O rhesus-negative blood via the umbilical cord.

Growth retardation

If the fetus is considered to be growth retarded, cordocentesis may be used to measure blood pH, P_{O_2}, P_{CO_2} and bicarbonate. In addition plasma levels of glucose and lactate can be estimated.

Virus infections

Rubella, cytomegalovirus and toxoplasmosis may all be detected by specific IgM radioimmunoassay of fetal blood.

Procedure

The mother is sedated and placed in the supine position, with her head slightly down. Under ultrasound control a gauge 20 needle is passed through the anterior wall of the abdomen and uterus into a cord vessel about 1 cm from its placental insertion; if the placenta is posterior the approach is transamniotic. In the event of the placenta being anterior, the approach is transplacental, but the risk to the fetus does not appear to be increased. The volume of blood withdrawn depends on the investigation required and the gestational age of the fetus. Up to 3 ml may be safely aspirated in the third trimester. Rhesus-negative mothers should receive 250–500 units of anti-D immunoglobulin by i.m. injection afterwards.

AMNIOCENTESIS

During amniocentesis a needle is inserted into the amniotic sac through the anterior abdominal wall in order to withdraw some of the amniotic fluid; it is performed after the 14th week. The risk of the procedure inducing a miscarriage in the early pregnancy is about 0.5 per cent. It has also been suggested that there is a very small risk (less than 1 per cent) of respiratory difficulties and talipes in babies following amniocentesis.

Indications

Many of the indications which prevailed a decade ago have been largely abandoned or have been superseded by chorion villus sampling or cordocentesis.

Karyotyping

This remains the main indication for amniocentesis (*see* the section on chorionic villus sampling above). Cells shed from the fetal surface and amnion may be cultured for chromosome analysis. Because the cells grow slowly it takes two to four weeks to obtain a result.

Haemolytic disease

Fetal bilirubin appears in the liquor amnii when maternal rhesus antibody (IgG) crosses the placenta and brings about haemolysis of rhesus-positive fetal red cells. By scanning the liquor with light waves at 450 mμ the concentration of bilirubin may be measured by the change in optical density and the results used as a guide to treatment.

Direct haemoglobin and haematocrit readings from fetal blood samples are now replacing this technique, see above.

Maturity of the fetal lungs

Lecithin is secreted from the fetal lungs into the

amniotic fluid during the second half of the pregnancy. Lecithin is a constituent of surfactant, which is necessary for normal lung expansion after birth, and the lecithin concentration in the liquor is an index of the maturity of the lungs. Because the total volume of the liquor varies greatly and the dilution of lecithin will therefore vary, the concentration of lecithin in the liquor is usually expressed in relation to the concentration of sphingomyelin; the ratio is fairly constant. If the lecithin-sphingomyelin ratio (L/S ratio) is greater than 2 the production of surfactant is likely to be adequate to prevent the development of respiratory distress syndrome.

Biochemical studies

Enzyme assays in fetal cells in amniotic fluid will detect inborn errors of metabolism. More often now these assays are undertaken as chorion samples obtained at CVS.

Neural tube defects

These may be suspected if the liquor level of α-fetoprotein (AFP) or acetylcholinesterase is elevated. However, the definitive diagnosis of neural tube defect is made on ultrasound scan.

Procedure

Under ultrasound guidance a spinal needle with stylet (gauge 21) is passed through the anterior abdominal wall into the uterine cavity well away from the fetus (Fig. 8.3). Local anaesthetic may be used, but for the most part it is not required. Up to 20 ml of liquor amnii may be safely withdrawn, representing 10 per cent of the liquor volume at 16 weeks gestation.

Fluid for karyotyping must be sent to the laboratory in a sterile container. If bilirubin is requested the container should be dark to protect the fluid from light. Rhesus-negative mothers should receive 250–500 units of anti-D immunoglobulin by i.m. injection afterwards.

OTHER INVASIVE PROCEDURES

These are undertaken for both diagnostic and therapeutic purposes.

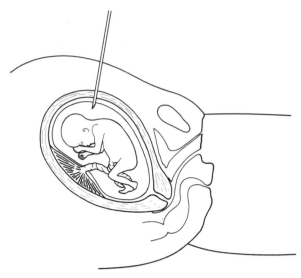

Fig. 8.3   Amniocentesis

Diagnostic

Skin biopsy

This may be performed under ultrasound control, or occasionally using the fetoscope if direct visualization of the biopsy site is required. The indications are uncommon but since many of the severe genodermatoses are fatal in infancy, the diagnosis can be important.

Liver biopsy

This may be performed under ultrasound control or fetoscopy. The indications are rare and are mainly genetic enzyme deficiencies which are detectable by other means.

Tumour biopsy

A fetal mass may very occasionally require histological diagnosis.

Therapeutic

Bladder drainage

In cases of obstructive uropathy back pressure up the ureters from chronic progressive bladder distension will lead to progressive loss of renal tissue during intrauterine life. This problem may be overcome by inserting a plastic double pig-tail catheter (shunt) through the fetal abdominal wall and into the bladder under ultrasound control. The catheter will allow urine to drain continuously into the amniotic space, restoring the liquor volume to normal and lessening the risk of the fetus developing pulmonary hypoplasia.

Aspiration of pleural or peritoneal cavities

Pleural and peritoneal effusions may be aspirated under ultrasound control. Double pig-tail catheters have been used for this purpose, especially in cases of chronic pleural effusion which, if left, leads to pulmonary hypoplasia and hydrops fetalis.

Selective fetocide

In cases of twin pregnancy when one twin is healthy but the other has a severe abnormality, air or potassium chloride may be injected under ultrasound control into the heart of the abnormal twin. This allows the development of the healthy twin to continue.

EXTERNAL VERSION

Turning the fetus by manipulation through the mother's abdominal wall is known as external version. In most cases the head is made to present (cephalic version), but occasionally, in cases of transverse lie, this is not possible and breech presentation is chosen as second best (podalic version).

Indications

External version is most commonly performed to turn a breech presentation or a transverse lie to a cephalic presentation in the antenatal clinic. It is also performed at the end of labour before the delivery of a second twin if that is found to be lying transversely before the membranes of the second sac have ruptured. The technique has already been described on page 193.

INDUCTION OF LABOUR

Indications

The indications for induction of labour include some cases of:

pregnancy-induced hypertension and other hypertensive disorders
postmaturity
intrauterine growth retardation
antepartum haemorrhage
polyhydramnios
unstable lie
diabetes mellitus
haemolytic disease
fetal abnormality
fetal death.

Details of the indications for induction in these conditions are set out in Chapters 3, 5 and 9, and yet other indications will occasionally arise. It is important that induction of labour should only be carried out for sound obstetric or medical reasons. A few patients will have exceptionally important domestic or social problems for which they request induction, and the doctor must consider such requests carefully, but in no circumstances should the operation be undertaken just for the convenience of the hospital or its staff.

Methods

Today nearly all inductions are carried out by:

administration of prostaglandins
administration of oxytocin (Syntocinon)
artificial rupture of the membranes (amniotomy).

Frequently all three methods may be combined.

Prostaglandins

In 1936 von Euler gave the name prostaglandin to a factor, found in the seminal fluid, which stimulated smooth muscle and lowered the blood pressure. It was found that this was not a single substance, but an extensive group of chemically related, long-chain hydroxy fatty acids. Prostaglandins have been found in many tissues and body fluids, and their physiological significance is still uncertain, but three (E_1, E_2 and $F_{2\alpha}$) have potent oxytocic effects on the pregnant uterus.

$PGF_{2\alpha}$ has been found in decidua and in amniotic fluid and maternal venous blood during labour. It has been suggested that it may play a physiological role during labour.

It has been shown that there is a rapid increase in plasma levels of $PGF_{2\alpha}$ after amniotomy or vaginal examination, perhaps from it's release from the adjacent decidua. Prostaglandins are also thought to play a part in the process of ovulation, in luteolysis and in the regulation of the fetal circulation by controlling the tone of the umbilical vessels and of the ductus arteriosis after birth.

Prostaglandins may be used for cervical ripening. The status of the cervix may be documented using the modified Bishop's score, as in Table 8.1. PGE_2, dinoprostone (Prostin E_2) may be used to soften and efface the unfavourable cervix (Bishop's score <4). The PGE_2 is usually administered vaginally into the posterior fornix as a sterile thixotrophic gel containing 1 mg dinoprostone, to be followed at four to six hour intervals by further doses of 1 mg, up to a maximum of four doses/24 hours.

Prostaglandins are also used in the induction of labour. PGE_2, dinoprostone (Prostin E_2) or $PGF_{2\alpha}$, dinoprost (Prostin $F_{2\alpha}$) may be used intravenously, transvaginally, extra-amniotically or by mouth. In practice the vaginal route is preferred by most obstetricians because of the troublesome diarrhoea and vomiting caused by the oral and intravenous routes. Primigravidae usually require 2 mg of PGE_2 or 5 mg of $PGF_{2\alpha}$ six-hourly until labour is established, whereas multigravidae only need half this dose.

After using prostaglandins for either cervical ripening or induction of labour the fetal heart should be monitored on a cardiotocograph to ensure that the prostaglandin-induced contractions are not distressing an already compromised fetus.

Therapeutic termination of pregnancy can be induced by prostaglandins. PGE_1, gemeprost (Cervagem) comes in a 1 mg sterile tablet and has an extremely powerful oxytocic effect on the uterus at any stage of the pregnancy. Gemeprost may therefore be used to soften the cervix prior to a suction termination during the first trimester or, with two or three doses at six hour intervals, to induce complete abortion during the second trimester. PGE_2 and $PGF_{2\alpha}$ may also be employed, either intra-amniotically or extra-amniotically through the cervix, to induce a second trimester abortion and are less painful than prostaglandin E_1.

Oxytocin

Oxytocin (Syntocinon) is best administered by intravenous infusion. Any patient receiving intravenous Syntocinon must be under continuous supervision, ideally by means of a cardiotocograph, to record simultaneously the fetal heart rate and uterine contractions. Infusion pumps regulate the flow of solution better than gravity drips. By adding 10 units of Syntocinon to 500 ml of isotonic saline, one drop of the infusion will contain approximately 1 mU of syntocinon (assuming 20 drops/ml of infusion).

The starting dose is 2 mU/min, increasing at intervals of 15 min, according to the strength and frequency of the uterine contractions, to a maximum of 32 mU/min. This may be achieved by manual control or, if an intrauterine pressure catheter has been inserted, by a monitor which has an automated feedback mechanism.

Once contractions are occurring regularly the rate of infusion can often be decreased, but it should be kept running until the third stage of labour is completed. If at any time there is evidence of fetal distress or hypertonic uterine contractions the infusion should be stopped immediately.

Table 8.1 Bishop's score for cervical ripening

Cervical state	Score			
	0	1	2	3
Dilatation (cm)	closed	1–2	3–4	5+
Length of cervix (cm)	3	2	1	0
Station of head (cm above ischial spines)	−3	−2	−1	0
Consistency of cervix	firm	medium	soft	
Position of cervix	posterior	middle	anterior	

Oxytocin has an antidiuretic effect. If a 5 per cent glucose solution is used rather than isotonic saline, water intoxication may occur if large volumes of fluid are infused.

Artificial rupture of the membranes

This is a reliable method of inducing labour even when it is used alone, but it is now common practice to combine it with the use of oxytocin or prostaglandins. Complications and failures are few if the pregnancy is near or past term, if the head is engaged in the pelvis and if the cervix is soft.

Anaesthesia is not necessary. After emptying the bladder the patient is placed in the lithotomy position and antiseptic cream is applied to the vulva. With careful antiseptic technique a finger is passed into the cervical canal and then swept round inside the uterus to separate the membranes from the lower segment as widely as possible. This in itself is an important factor in the induction, perhaps because it causes liberations of prostaglandins locally. Under the guidance of the fingers a pair of toothed forceps are passed through the cervix to seize and tear the bag of membranes. If the head is high an assistant should push it down from above; this not only makes the amniotomy easier by making the bag of membranes tense, but diminishes the risk of prolapse of the cord. Once the membranes have been ruptured the presenting part will descend as uterine contractions begin. Amniotomy is undesirable if the fetus is dead because of the possible entry of bacteria to colonize the dead tissue. Prostaglandins offer a safer method of induction.

Risks of induction

Failed induction

This term indicates that the attempt to induce labour has failed to result in full dilatation of the cervix. To all intents and purposes one sees it only in primigravidae, especially those with an unfavourable cervix (Bishop's score <4). Cervical ripening with prostaglandins has diminished the risk of failed induction.

It is important to differentiate between failed induction and failure to progress due to cephalopelvic disproportion. Should the latter be undetected there is a risk of hyperstimulation due to overdose of oxytocic drugs.

Uterine hyperstimulation

This may result from the use of prostaglandins in a multiparous patient with an already very ripe cervix (Bishop's score >8) or alternatively from the excessive use of oxytocin (Syntocinon) in a patient with cephalopelvic disproportion; either will predispose to acute fetal distress. In addition there is the risk of uterine rupture.

EPISIOTOMY

This refers to an incision in the perineum to enlarge the introitus. Although it is a minor operation it increases the safety of many obstetric procedures and can reduce the duration of the second stage of labour. There is some concern among women who have been led to believe that episiotomy is a routine practice in hospitals. It is important to explain to patients beforehand that this is not the case, but that it sometimes becomes necessary. A woman who has a perineal tear may accept the discomfort of this as a natural result of delivery, but a woman who has an episiotomy may attribute precisely the same discomfort to what she regards as an unnatural intervention unless adequate explanation is given.

Indications

The indications for episiotomy are:

When the perineum threatens to tear extensively

An uncontrolled tear may extend even to the third degree. Episiotomy is often indicated in primigravidae when the head is about to crown, and in multiparae when the perineum is scarred after suture at a previous delivery. An escape of blood from the introitus is often an indication that the vaginal wall is tearing, even if the perineal skin is still intact. Occasionally the perineum begins to split in the centre; an incision is needed even more urgently in this instance.

The perineum is more likely to tear with delivery of the head in the persistent occipitoposterior position than in the occipitoanterior position because in the former the larger occipitofrontal diameter distends the vulva (*see* Fig. 4.10, p. 161).

If there has been a previous operation for a complete perineal tear or for prolapse, episiotomy is required.

When there is delay in delivery

Episiotomy may be necessary when there is a delay in delivery with the head pressing on the perineum.

Forceps delivery

Episiotomy is commonly required for forceps delivery, but less often if the light Wrigley forceps are used. It is sometimes necessary before the introduction of the hand into the vagina to discover the cause of delay or to rotate manually a head which is in the occipitoposterior position.

Breech delivery

Episiotomy is performed when the breech is distending the perineum. The reasons are:

> to reduce the risk of intracranial haemorrhage
> to avoid the need for the breech with extended legs to undergo lateral flexion over the perineum
> to anticipate and make easier the bringing down of extended arms.

Fetal distress

Episiotomy can be life-saving for the fetus if distress occurs at the perineal stage of delivery.

Prolapse of the cord

If the cord prolapses with rupture of the membranes late in the second stage of labour, and especially if the patient is a multipara, the head may be showing when the complication is discovered. By encouraging the patient to push, and by incising the perineum, the fetus can often be delivered before forceps are available.

Premature labour

Episiotomy should be routinely performed in cases of early preterm labour to reduce the risk of intracranial injury.

Technique

The operation varies from an incision about 2 cm long to one extending the whole length of the perineum but swinging to one side to avoid the

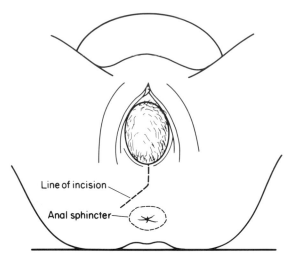

Fig. 8.4 Episiotomy. An incision is shown which starts as a median episiotomy and has then been extended laterally

anal sphincter (Fig. 8.4). The incision should be kept to the midline as far as possible because the tissues heal better there than when the incision is placed laterally, and there is also less bleeding.

The operation may be done under general anaesthesia, previously instituted epidural or pudendal block or local anaesthesia; infiltration with 10 ml of lignocaine (Xylocaine) 1 per cent is used. The incision is best made during a contraction when the presenting part is distending the perineum. Straight scissors with blunt points are used. The external sphincter ani must not be cut; if the episiotomy needs to be very extensive it should curve out laterally to avoid the sphincter.

Suturing should be done with care. The tissues are highly vascular and heal obligingly well. Every effort must be made to avoid unsutured spaces in which blood may collect and infection begin. Care must be taken to bring the upper limit of the vaginal incision into view and suture it. It is the usual practice to use fine catgut or Dexon throughout, with a continuous suture for the vagina first, then interrupted sutures for the perineal body and a subcuticular suture for the skin of the perineum. Tension stitches of nylon or thread increase discomfort, probably do not improve healing and require to be removed after five days.

Daily bathing is advised; otherwise the wound is kept as dry as possible and left alone. Sometimes local discomfort is the most irksome feature of vaginal delivery and calls for analgesics and ice-packs to the perineum.

DELIVERY WITH THE FORCEPS

The original obstetric forceps were invented by one of the two elder Chamberlen brothers, members of a Huguenot family that settled in England in about the year 1600. The invention was kept secret in the family for over 100 years and passed from the third Chamberlen brother, Peter, down to his grandson Hugh who died in 1728. For nearly another hundred years, until 1818, the original forceps lay hidden beneath the floorboards of a box-room in Woodham Mortimer Hall, Essex, which had been the family home for 80 years. Knowledge of the use of the forceps leaked out with varying degrees of completeness and accuracy during the early part of the eighteenth century.

The Chamberlen forceps consisted of two blades, curved to fit the fetal head, with short handles, the two halves being strapped together where they met because they had no lock. In 1723 Chapman improved the forceps by lengthening the shank between the blade and the handle. In 1744 William Smellie devised the double-slotted English lock which allowed easy application and gave additional strength. The pelvic curve was added by Levret of Paris in 1747.

A new type of forceps was introduced by Christian Kielland in 1915 for the purpose not only of traction, but also of rotation of the head. Lastly, light, short curved forceps were introduced by Wrigley in 1935 for the particular purpose of outlet application.

The forceps are used to apply traction to the head of the fetus in a pelvis of adequate size, never to attempt to overcome disproportion. With Kielland's forceps the head may also be rotated into a more favourable position before traction is applied. The forceps are designed to fit the head, not the breech, but forceps are usually applied to the aftercoming head in breech delivery.

The presentations suitable for the forceps operation are vertex, face with the chin anterior and the aftercoming head of the breech. The vertex may have the occiput anterior or posterior, but with the latter certain additional factors, referred to later, must be taken into account.

Indications for the use of forceps

Forceps are used in the second stage of labour for

delay
maternal distress
fetal distress
some cases of preterm delivery.
delivery of the aftercoming head of a breech presentation, even in the absence of any delay

Delay in the second stage of labour

In primigravidae the second stage of labour should not last for much over 1 hour, and in multiparae it is often much shorter, usually being less than 30 minutes. A second stage is considered to be delayed if these limits are exceeded, but this is only a general guide and if progress is not being made assistance should be given sooner.

Conditions likely to cause delay in the second stage of labour are:

inadequate uterine contractions and poor voluntary effort
resistant pelvic floor and perineum
large fetus
persistent occipitoposterior or deep transverse arrest of the head
other malpresentations such as face presentation or brow presentation
contraction of the pelvic outlet.

A common cause of delay in the second stage of labour is the resistance of the pelvic floor, but this should be treated by episiotomy rather than by the application of forceps.

Maternal distress

Maternal distress in the second stage of labour may occur because there has been a long first stage, or because there is heart disease, hypertension or pulmonary disease.

The signs of maternal distress may be broadly divided into mental and physical.

Mental distress occurs in patients who have had a long tedious first stage and are unable to cooperate in aiding expulsion during the painful second stage. This sometimes means that analgesics have been too sparingly used.

The signs of physical distress are a rising pulse rate, dehydration and a slightly raised temperature.

Fetal distress

The following conditions may cause fetal distress during the second stage of labour:

> prolapse of the cord, or a tight loop or knot in it
> placental insufficiency from hypertension, antepartum haemorrhage or postmaturity
> prolonged or difficult labour.

Prolapse or presentation of the cord is mentioned first because the threat to the fetus is serious and immediate. The subject is dealt with on page 214. If the cervix is fully dilated and the fetus is alive expeditious forceps delivery is required. Less acute cord compression may arise from tightening of a loop of cord round the neck or a knot in the cord.

Anything that interferes with fetal oxygenation will cause fetal distress. With gross placental lesions such as separation or infarction there may be severe fetal distress, but diminished uteroplacental blood flow may occur to a lesser degree in cases of postmaturity and maternal hypertension.

Each uterine contraction temporarily impedes the maternal blood flow to the placenta and in long labour, or in cases in which a great deal of retraction of the upper segment of the uterus occurs, fetal hypoxia may eventually arise.

The signs of fetal distress and the methods of monitoring the fetal heart rate are discussed in Chapter 5, page 216.

When there are signs of fetal distress in the second stage of labour delivery should be effected at once. While preparations for delivery are being made oxygen is given to the mother in the hope of improving the supply to the fetus. In forceps delivery for fetal distress episiotomy reduces the risk of adding intracranial stress to the fetal asphyxia.

Preterm delivery

When the fetus is small and the head is liable to injury during passage through the vagina a careful forceps delivery with episiotomy will reduce the risk.

Conditions necessary for the application of forceps

To apply forceps safely and successfully certain conditions must be fulfilled:

The presentation must be suitable

The forceps can only be used to extract the head of the fetus when it presents as a vertex or as a face with the chin anterior (leaving aside the use of forceps for the aftercoming head of a breech). A brow or a mentoposterior face presentation must be corrected before forceps can be used for extraction. The forceps must be applied accurately to the sides of the fetal head, otherwise dangerous compression of the head will occur causing intracranial stress and haemorrhage, and very likely the attempt to deliver will fail.

The head must be engaged

If the head is not engaged in the second stage this may be because of cephalopelvic disproportion or because the head is extended.

The pelvic outlet must be of adequate size

Even with the head engaged the pelvic outlet must be of adequate size. If the subpubic angle is narrowed there must be room in the posterior part of the pelvic cavity.

The cervix must be fully dilated

If the cervix is not fully dilated there will be difficulty in applying the forceps without including and tearing the cervix. More traction will be required to overcome the resistance of the cervix. The attempt to deliver may fail because the factor which prevented cervical dilatation may be uncorrected.

The membranes should be ruptured

If the forewaters are still present the membranes should be ruptured and only if delivery does not follow would forceps be used.

The bladder should be empty

A catheter is passed to empty the bladder before forceps delivery, not only to avoid any risk of injuring it but also to remove its inhibiting influence on retraction of the uterus after delivery, and thus to reduce the risk of postpartum haemorrhage.

The uterus should be contracting

Contractions can be stimulated with an oxytocin infusion and then delivery completed with forceps. Intravenous Syntocinon should be given as soon as the fetal shoulders are born (see p. 171).

Types of obstetric forceps

Forceps in use today are shown in Fig. 8.5:

    short curved forceps
    long curved forceps
    Kielland's forceps.

Each of these instruments consists of two halves meeting at the lock. Each half has a blade which is joined to the handle by a shank. The blades have two curves; the cephalic curve, in which the blade is curved to fit the head and a curve on the edge, the pelvic curve, to correspond with the curved axis of the pelvis. The length of the handles and shanks varies with the different forceps and the type of handle differs too. Kielland's forceps have special characteristics.

Short curved forceps

This instrument, designed by Wrigley in 1935, is for use in the low or outlet forceps operation. The shank is short (2.5 cm) and the whole instrument is light.

Long curved forceps

The total length is 35 cm, with shanks of 6.5 cm, and the instrument is relatively heavily built. It can be used for delivery of a head from the pelvic cavity.

Kielland's forceps

The advantage of this instrument is that it allows accurate cephalic application, no matter what the position or level of the head in the pelvis. If the occiput is posterior or lateral the application is made and then the head can be rotated with the forceps to bring the occiput anterior. The forceps have a lock which allows one blade to slide on the other in the long axis, and thus the blades can lie at different levels when applied to a head which is lying transversely and is tilted. The other special characteristic is the pelvic curve. This is initially in a backward direction and then it quickly begins its forward sweep, but the tips of the blades never quite reach the plane of the shanks and handles. It is this feature which makes rotation with the forceps safe without risk of injury to vagina, bladder or rectum.

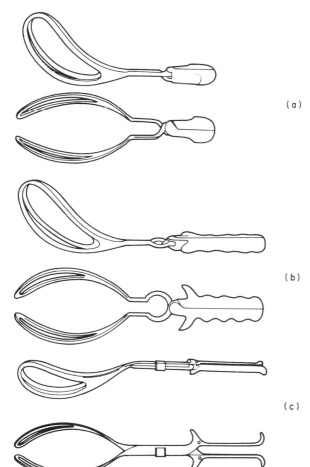

(a)

(b)

(c)

Fig. 8.5 (a) short curved (Wrigley's) Forceps; (b) long curved forceps; (c) Kielland's forceps

Preliminary steps before the application of forceps

Some form of analgesia will be required. This may take the form of pudendal block, caudal, epidural, or general anaesthesia. Pudendal or epidural block should be used whenever possible in preference to general anaesthesia. A general anaesthetic should only be given by someone experienced in dealing with the complications which may arise. Unless it is reasonably certain that the patient's stomach is empty a stomach tube must be passed before the anaesthetic is begun. It is essential that a suction apparatus is available and that the head of the obstetric bed can be lowered without delay in case of unexpected gastric regurgitation. Prolonged general anaesthesia may increase the risk of post-partum haemorrhage and depress the respiratory centre of the newborn infant.

The patient is placed in the lithotomy position with a wedge under one side of her back in order to take the pressure of the uterus off the vena cava. After swabbing the vulva and perineum with an antiseptic solution sterile towels are arranged and the bladder is emptied with a catheter.

A careful preliminary vaginal examination is made. It must first be established that the cervix is fully dilated and then the level and position of the head is determined. If the sutures and fontanelles are obscured by caput formation it may be neces-sary to insert the whole hand to feel for an ear; the pinna will be directed toward the occiput. Epi-siotomy may be needed for this. Finally the size of the pelvic outlet is assessed. This is not always easy, but the points to note are the prominence of the ischial spines, the width of the subpubic arch and the length of the sagittal diameter from the lower border of the symphysis pubis to the sacro-coccygeal joint.

If all these points are satisfactory and the occiput is near to the midline in front the forceps can be applied, but if the occiput is lying obliquely or transversely manual rotation will be needed first, unless Kielland's forceps are being used, when the head may be rotated with the forceps.

If the occiput is posterior, unless the head is so low that the perineum is already being stretched, it is almost always best to rotate the occiput to the front before the head is delivered. The disadvan-tage of not doing so is the increased risk of intracranial stress and of extensive perineal lacera-tion that goes with delivery of the head in the occipitoposterior position.

If the head has not descended to the pelvic floor then a more serious cause for delay is possible. A flattening of the sacrum might be felt, or the head may be seriously deflexed or extended. If there is doubt about the size of the pelvis with the head arrested at this level caesarean section is the safest course.

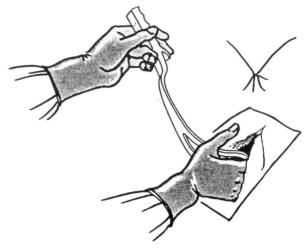

Fig. 8.6   Application of forceps; insertion of the left blade

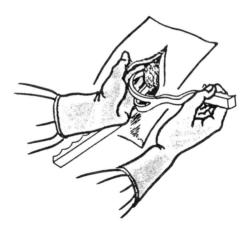

Fig. 8.7   Application of forceps; insertion of the right blade

Application of the ordinary patterns of obstetric forceps

The left blade of the forceps is applied first. The fingers of the right hand are passed into the vagina. The left blade of the forceps is held by its handle between the fingers and thumb of the left hand and is passed between the fetal head and the palmar surfaces of the fingers of the right hand (Fig. 8.6). The handle is held well over the mother's abdo-men, and inclined to the mother's right side so that it is almost parallel with her right inguinal liga-ment. As the blade passes up into the birth canal

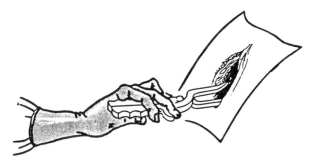

Fig. 8.8   Forceps articulated before traction

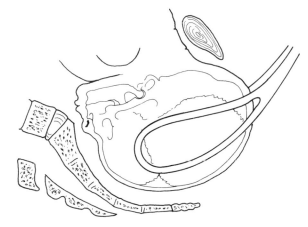

Fig. 8.9   Position of the blades of the forceps during extraction of a vertex presentation. The blades of the forceps lie in the submentovertical diameter and grasp the biparietal diameter

the handle is carried backwards and towards the midline, thus following the direction of both the pelvic and cephalic curves of the instrument. After ascertaining that the blade lies next to the head and is in the correct position the fingers of the right hand are withdrawn.

The fingers of the left hand are now introduced along the right side of the pelvis, and the right blade of the forceps is held and passed in a similar manner to the left. Its external visible portion will thus lie above and across the handle of the left blade (Fig. 8.7). The shanks are now pressed backward against the perineum and the handles should lock and come to lie in a horizontal position (Fig. 8.8).

If there is difficulty in locking the forceps it is probable that the position of the head has not been diagnosed correctly, and that the instrument has

been applied to a head in the oblique or transverse diameter of the pelvis. If the forceps will not lock, or if the handles will not close together, the blades must be removed and the position of the fetal head re-examined.

The ordinary curved forceps must always be applied correctly to the fetal head, with the parietal eminences lying within the fenestrations of the blades and the sagittal suture lying midway between the blades (Fig. 8.9). These forceps must also be correctly placed in the pelvis. It does not matter if the head is slightly oblique in the pelvis, with the occiput pointing less than 45° away from the midline. With such a slight degree of obliquity the head and forceps will turn into the midline as traction is applied (Fig. 8.10), but if the head is more oblique than this its position *must* be corrected before the ordinary type of forceps are applied to it.

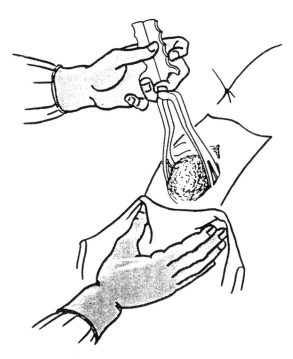

Fig. 8.10   Delivery with forceps

Application of forceps to a face presentation

If the head is delayed in the pelvic cavity and there is a mentoanterior position the forceps may be used to assist delivery (Fig. 8.11). If there is a

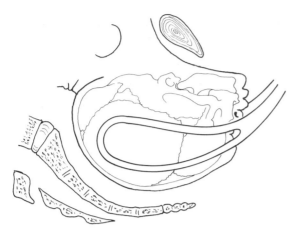

Fig. 8.11   Position of the blades of the forceps during extraction of the head in the mentoanterior position. The blades of the forceps lie in the occipitomental diameter and grasp the head in the bizygomatic diameter

mentoposterior position delivery with the forceps is only possible after the chin has been rotated forwards. This is possible manually or with Kielland's forceps, but it may be safer to treat this uncommon condition by caesarean section.

Application of forceps to the aftercoming head

The forceps are applied to the aftercoming head in breech delivery as a routine procedure.

Extraction with the forceps

The operator sits facing the perineum. Traction is applied to the handles of the forceps in a backwards and downwards direction in the axis of the birth canal. Traction is intermittent, and each pull should only last for a few seconds. As the head descends the handles are gradually raised to about 45° above the horizontal, when an episiotomy is performed through the stretched perineum (unless this has already been done). The head is then gently guided through the vulva until crowning takes place with the handles of the forceps in vertical position. The forceps blades are then removed before delivery of the face by manual extension of the head.

Excessive force should never be used. Slow intermittent traction reduces the risk of intracranial injury.

The use of Kielland's forceps (Fig. 8.12)

Kielland's forceps should only be used by those who have been trained in their use. In inexperienced hands this is a dangerous instrument, and may be the cause of severe vaginal lacerations if it is used incorrectly. The popularity of Kielland's forceps has waxed and waned; at present manual rotation of the head is often preferred to rotation with this instrument.

Before applying the forceps the exact position of the head in the pelvis must be determined. To

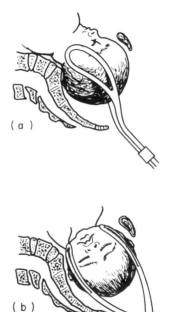

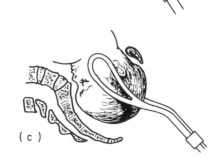

Fig. 8.12   Use of Kielland's forceps. (a) application to head in occipitoposterior position before rotation; (b) application to head in occipitolateral position before rotation; (c) position of forceps after rotation

avoid error the operator is advised to hold the articulated instrument before the vulva in the position to be taken up when it is applied to the head. The blade which is to be inserted first is selected, and the other blade is put aside. If the head lies anteroposteriorly, or only slightly obliquely, the application of the forceps is not difficult. The forceps are always applied so that, after any rotation, the pelvic curve will be positioned correctly. For example, if the occiput lies posteriorly and it is intended to rotate it with the forceps, the forceps must be applied with the pelvic curve in the reverse direction so that *after* rotation the curve will be correctly orientated to the birth canal.

Unlike ordinary forceps this instrument can be applied to a head lying transversely in the pelvis; there are special methods of application for this. In both methods the anterior blade is applied first.

Wandering method

In the wandering method the anterior blade is guided into the lateral side of the pelvis beside the head, with the cephalic surface of the blade properly facing the head. It is then slid gently round the pelvis, keeping as close as possible to the head and passing over the forehead until it comes to rest fitting the anterior parietal eminence. The posterior blade is then introduced behind the head, to fit the posterior parietal eminence.

Direct method

The direct method of application is only used when the head is low down and the fit is not too tight. The tip of the anterior blade, with the handle as far back as possible, is applied to the side of the head anteriorly and then slipped over the anterior parietal eminence behind the symphysis pubis, with the cephalic surface of the blade kept as close as possible to the head while it is in transit. The posterior blade is then inserted behind the head over the posterior parietal eminence.

Rotation of the head

Force is never used for rotation of the head, and it should be done with the fingers of one hand only. Rotation is first tried at the level of arrest, but if this is not immediately easy the head should be elevated slightly and rotation tried again. Some-times rotation will be easier after traction has brought the head down to a roomier level of the pelvis.

Traction is made in the line of the handles and is exerted with only two fingers hooked over the proximal shoulders of the handles. Rotation and traction are never done together, although spontaneous rotation sometimes occurs during traction and should not be impeded. The handles should never be compressed together, as this will have a crushing action on the head.

The dangers of forceps delivery

Some of the dangers of forceps delivery are due to the circumstances calling for the operation rather than to the operation itself. For example, delivery with forceps may be called for at the end of a long tedious first stage of labour because of maternal or fetal distress.

The risk of general anaesthesia in an unprepared patient is great if the anaesthetist is inexperienced and proper equipment is lacking.

Some of the dangers of forceps delivery may be summarized:

Mother
  dangers of general anaesthesia
  lacerations of cervix, vagina or perineum
  postpartum haemorrhage from uterine atony
    or lacerations
  puerperal genital infection.

Infant
  intracranial haemorrhage
  facial palsy
  cephalhaematoma.

Spastic diplegia in a child is sometimes attributed to instrumental delivery. It is improbable that intracranial haemorrhage will have this effect and if the haemorrhage is not fatal complete recovery is likely. On the other hand, prolonged cerebral hypoxia may well leave permanent damage; forceps may have been used in such a case but could hardly have caused the hypoxia.

Bad results from forceps delivery usually result from bad forceps delivery. The dangers will be minimal when proper regard is given to the indications for the operation; when the exact position of the head is determined by a preliminary vaginal examination and when any necessary correction of the position of the fetus is made before traction.

Failure to delivery with forceps

Fortunately failure to deliver with the forceps is now rare in Britain, for the dangers to both mother and baby are serious and are directly proportional to the lack of skill and the force employed during the unsuccessful attempts. Criticism is not so much against attempting to apply forceps or attempting traction, but against *persisting* in such endeavours in the face of obvious difficulties.

The causes of failure to deliver with the forceps are mostly commonplace; either the cervix is not fully dilated or the head is in a malposition, usually with the occiput posterior. Fortunately, attempts to apply forceps with the head not yet engaged are not often made nowadays, for the dangers are even greater. A rare cause of failure to deliver with forceps is a contracted pelvic outlet, which is often only diagnosed late in labour.

Severe laceration of the cervix may be caused by attempts to apply forceps with the cervix incompletely dilated, either because the blades are applied outside the cervix or because the head is forcibly dragged through it. Sometimes an extensive tear of the upper vagina is caused by attempts to rotate the head with the forceps. If the obstruction is at the brim the uterus itself may be perforated by a blade of the forceps. A complete tear of the perineum into the anal canal comes from a combination of roughness and misapplied force. The effect on the patient of these obstetric insults, even if she has avoided a badly given or prolonged general anaesthetic, is to cause shock from trauma or haemorrhage, or both. Sepsis is likely to follow.

The fetus may suffer intracranial haemorrhage and it may be dead before delivery is completed.

Any case of failed delivery with forceps must be carefully reassessed. Not infrequently a more experienced operator is able to effect an easy delivery with forceps after correcting a malposition. In other cases caesarean section has to be performed.

VACUUM EXTRACTOR (VENTOUSE)

The idea of extracting the fetal head by means of a vacuum cup applied to the scalp has been considered since Younge in 1706 tried a glass suction cup; an instrument was designed by Simpson in 1849, although little use was made of it. The modern vacuum extractor was introduced by Malmström in 1954. Opinions differ about the value of this method of assisting delivery. In some

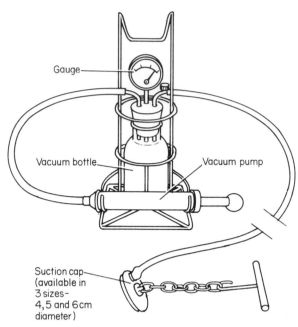

Fig. 8.13 The vacuum extractor (by courtesy of Down's Surgical PLC). The cups, which are of various sizes, are attached to a rubber tube which is connected to the reservoir, pressure gauge and hand vacuum pump. Traction is applied with chain and handle

clinics, particularly on the European continent, the vacuum extractor is preferred to the forceps, but it is chosen much less often in Britain and America.

Malmström's extractor (Fig. 8.13) consists of a metal suction cup attached by a chain to a metal handle. The cavity of the cup is connected by rubber tubing to a reservoir with a pressure gauge and a hand vacuum pump. The suction cups are made in three sizes, and the largest possible cup is used, according to the dilatation of the cervix. The modern ventouse extractor has silastic cups which not only provide better suction, but inflict less trauma to the fetal scalp.

Method of use

Local infiltration of the perineum with lignocaine 1 per cent is usually the only anaesthetic needed, and this is a great virtue to the method.

The cup is introduced sideways into the vagina by pressing it backwards against the perineum. It is then guided into place on the scalp as near as possible to the posterior fontanelle, taking care that neither the cervix nor any part of the vaginal wall comes between the cup and the scalp. While the obstetrician holds the cup in the correct position an assistant uses the pump to create a vacuum, gradually increasing the negative pressure by 0.2 kg/cm^2 at 1 minute intervals, until 0.8 kg/cm^2 is attained. Failure to maintain the vacuum indicates that either the cup is incorrectly applied or that the apparatus is faulty. The negative pressure causes an artificial caput succedaneum or 'chignon' to be formed within the cup and when the vacuum reaches 0.8 kg/cm^2 the cup is completely filled with scalp, ensuring maximum adhesion, and traction can be started.

Traction on the handle is made as nearly vertically to the cup as possible, because an oblique direction of traction will tend to pull it off. Traction is made intermittently with the uterine contractions, the direction of pull changing as the head descends through the birth canal. Unless there is obvious descent during three or four contractions the use of the ventouse should be reconsidered.

After delivery the vacuum is reduced as slowly as it was created as this tends to diminish the risk of damage to the scalp. Immediately after removal of the cup the baby has an unsightly 'chignon' where the cup was applied, but this rapidly diminishes and within a few hours only a faint ring can be seen.

Indications

These are similar to those for the use of obstetric forceps. If the occiput is not anterior the extractor may still be used. It is applied as near to the vertex as possible, and with traction forward rotation of the occiput often occurs. However, many obstetricians would prefer to use Kielland's forceps or to perform manual rotation in such a case.

Contraindication

The vacuum extractor cannot be applied to the breech or face.

The operation takes too long for urgent cases of fetal distress and forceps delivery is preferred.

There is some doubt as to its safety when used on preterm babies, when there is possibly a greater risk of intracranial haemorrhage than with forceps.

Necrosis of the scalp, cephalhaematoma, subaponeurotic haematoma and intracranial haemorrhage have all been reported after vacuum extraction, but in a number of these cases the cup had been injudiciously applied for long periods and strong traction had been applied to overcome some degree of disproportion.

INTERNAL VERSION

In internal version a hand is passed through the cervix, which must be fully dilated, or nearly so, into the uterus to turn the fetus. It is always podalic version, and one or both legs are brought down as part of the operation. The patient must be anaesthetized or have an effective epidural block. It is a difficult and hazardous procedure for both mother and child.

Before caesarean section and forceps delivery were introduced internal version was the only way out of many obstetric difficulties. Today almost the only indication is for the correction of a transverse lie of a second twin when external version has failed.

Internal version is extremely dangerous when labour has been in progress for some time and the lower segment is stretched and thin because of the risk of uterine rupture.

Figures 8.14 and 8.15 show the method of performing internal version.

CAESAREAN SECTION

Caesarean section is the operation by which a

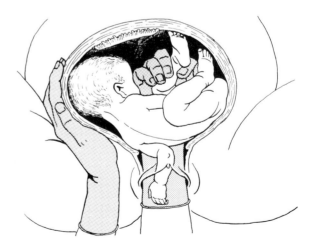

Fig. 8.14 Internal podalic version; stage 1, shoulder presentation. The operator's right hand has been introduced to grasp the leg of the fetus and bring it down. The left hand, working outside the sterile sheet, is coaxing the head out of the iliac fossa

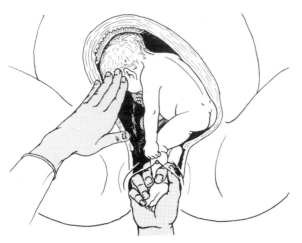

Fig. 8.15   Internal podalic version; stage 2, shoulder presentation. The leg is being brought down causing the back to rotate forwards. The head has almost reached the fundus

potentially viable fetus is delivered through an incision in the abdominal wall and the uterus. A similar procedure undertaken to terminate a pregnancy of a non-viable fetus is referred to as hysterotomy.

History

The origin of the operation is uncertain, but it is of great antiquity. There are references to it in Rabbinical writings of about 140 BC, but it is known to have been practised on the dead pregnant woman long before this. Traditional Roman history (written seven centuries later) states that the second king of Rome, Numa Pompilius (762–715 BC), forbade the burying of a woman who died during labour until the fetus had been cut out. This law later became the *Lex Caesarea*, and the term caesarean section is said to have arisen from this.

Works on caesarean section were published in the sixteenth century, but faced with the difficulties of controlling bleeding and sepsis, and in the absence of anaesthesia, the mortality remained high, and even in the beginning of the nineteenth century the Swedish obstetrician Osiander wrote: 'Of the women who undergo caesarean section more than two-thirds die. . . . Before, then, undertaking this procedure one should allow the patient to draw up her will and grant her time to prepare herself for death.'

As it was believed that sutures could not be buried in the tissues without causing sepsis, there was the problem of the open wound pouring infected lochia into the peritoneal cavity, with inevitable peritonitis. Porro, of Pavia, south of Milan, temporarily solved this problem by following section with subtotal hysterectomy and marsupializing the cervical stump in the abdominal wound. The Porro operation was abandoned when, in 1881, the German obstetrician Kehrer devised a satisfactory method of suturing the uterine wound with silk. Although the mortality fell in elective cases there was still a very high mortality after incision of the upper segment in patients who were in labour.

In 1906 Frank, of Cologne, devised an operation which not only employed transverse abdominal and lower segment incisions, but excluded the lower segment from the general peritoneal cavity by suturing the upper edge of the parietal peritoneum to the upper edge of the uterovesical peritoneum. In the next few years the lower segment operation gained popularity and it was soon found to be safe during labour, even without any attempt to close off the field from the general peritoneal cavity.

Indications

A list of indications for caesarean section can easily be devised, but in many cases there is more than one indication. As the danger of the operation has diminished there is a tendency for it to be performed more often for fetal indications such as distress during labour, placenta praevia, severe hypertension, diabetes mellitus, haemolytic disease and prolapse of the cord.

A few indications are absolute in the sense that delivery by any other method would be extremely dangerous, for example gross disproportion or placenta praevia. However, in most cases the indications are relative and caesarean section is carried out when it is thought that the balance of maternal and fetal dangers will be reduced by section rather than vaginal delivery. The indications include:

Faults in the birth canal

Cephalopelvic disproportion. Gross obstruction to delivery from pelvic contraction will obviously justify caesarean section; it is in the more common borderline cases that judgment is required.

Trial of labour is discussed on page 207. A trial often has to be terminated because of fetal distress, or because of abnormal uterine action. It is not always certain what is causing delay in labour, but when a patient has been in labour for some hours and has received cautious oxytocic augmentation of uterine action yet cervical dilatation is not progressing, but caesarean section should not be delayed.

If a trial of labour in a previous pregnancy is judged to have failed because of disproportion, delivery should be by elective section shortly before term.

In obstructed labour with a dead fetus, now fortunately very rare in Britain, caesarean section is usually safer than craniotomy.

Pelvic tumour. Impaction of an ovarian cyst or a fibromyoma in the pelvis are rare indications for section.

Cervical or vaginal stenosis are also rare indications for section.

With a *double uterus* obstruction during labour may occur because the unimpregnated horn lies below the presenting part, because the narrower part of the uterus fails to dilate or because of a vaginal septum.

Section is advised after operative repair of a fistula or successful treatment of stress incontinence, but after most repair operations vaginal delivery with episiotomy is preferable to section.

Fetal malpresentations

Caesarean section is the best treatment for a brow presentation with the head at the level of the pelvic brim.

Impacted mentoposterior face presentation is also an indication for section.

Shoulder presentation. Section is performed for a shoulder presentation if the fetus is alive in preference to internal version.

Some cases of *locked twins* are treated with caesarean section.

Section is now performed in at least 30 per cent of cases of *breech presentation*. Section would be advised if the mother is over 35 years of age, has been infertile or has an adverse obstetric history, has a small or android pelvis or

a large fetus or indeed has any additional complication. Operation would be performed during labour if the breech does not descend onto the pelvic floor after a few hours of regular contractions.

In exceedingly rare cases of *conjoined twins* section may be required.

Abnormal uterine action

In many cases of abnormal uterine action there may also be some mechanical difficulty and precise diagnosis of the cause of delay may be uncertain, but if a patient has been in labour for more than 12 hours, the membranes are ruptured and there is no progress with an oxytocic infusion, section should be considered.

A contraction ring is a very rare indication for section during the first stage of labour.

Antepartum haemorrhage

Caesarean section is the best treatment for both mother and fetus in *placenta praevia*.

Abruptio placentae. Section is seldom performed in severe cases of abruptio placentae because the fetus is usually dead. In unusual cases in which the fetus is alive but bleeding is continuing caesarean section is justified. Placental separation, even if it is slight, is a major threat to fetal survival, and during labour section may become necessary for fetal distress.

Other maternal indications

For cases of cardiac or respiratory disease, and indeed most intercurrent medical disorders, assisted vaginal delivery is preferable to caesarean section unless there is some obstetric impediment to easy delivery. Section should never be performed merely to permit sterilization; this is better done six weeks later by laparoscopy.

Fulminating pregnancy-induced hypertension. This may have to be treated by section if the chances of speedy vaginal delivery are small. The patient may not go into labour after induction, or the severity of the hypertension may demand delivery before the 34th week in a primigravida, when induction is uncertain. In other cases of hypotension or renal disease section is performed in the fetal interest, as will be mentioned in the next section.

Fetal indications

In cases of *diabetes mellitus*, when blood sugar levels have been difficult to control, complications are likely to occur. These include fetal macrosomia, polyhydramnios and pre-eclampsia. Such patients are frequently delivered before term, usually by caesarean section.

If *placental insufficiency* is suspected because of inadequate fetal growth, maternal hypertension or proteinuria, or previous fetal death, the tests described on page 130 are carried out. Many cases are treated by induction of labour before term, but if labour does not follow, if the fetus is very small, or if fetal distress occurs during the first stage of labour section is the best method of delivery.

Fetal distress may occur during labour in cases of postmaturity or hypertension, in cases of long labour or abdominal uterine action, or without explanation. Whatever the cause, if there is clinical evidence of fetal distress during the first stage of labour, confirmed by monitoring of the fetal heart rate and by scalp blood sampling, caesarean section is urgently performed.

Prolapse of the cord when the cervix is not sufficiently dilated to allow immediate vaginal delivery is treated by emergency section.

A *bad obstetric history*, when the patient has had several stillbirths or neonatal deaths, may be a sufficient indication for caesarean section. In such cases the timing of sections is very important.

Caesarean section should not be performed routinely on *older primigravidae*, but if there is an additional factor such as minor disproportion, a breech presentation, hypertension or even postmaturity, section may be indicated.

Gross prematurity is becoming a more frequent indication for caesarean section, especially in cases of breech presentation. Between weeks 26 and 32 the fetus is particularly prone to intracranial haemorrhage secondary to acute hypoxia during labour; this may be avoided by caesarean section.

Repeated caesarean section

If a patient has already had a caesarean section there is a risk of rupture of the scar in any subsequent labour. If the indication for the section persists, for example a contracted pelvis, operation should obviously be repeated. If, however, the indication was a non-recurrent one, for example placenta praevia, then the risk of a second elective operation outweighs the risk of rupture of a lower segment scar at vaginal delivery. When a patient has had more than one previous section the indication for repetition of the operation may be stronger.

The upper segment scar is less secure than the lower segment scar, and after an operation of the former type (now rarely performed) it is wise to repeat the section.

Technique of caesarean section

In the past the classical procedure was a vertical incision in the upper uterine segment. This incision was attended by free bleeding, could not be covered with a free layer of loose peritoneum and gave an insecure scar which might give way during a subsequent pregnancy or labour. It is seldom performed today.

The standard procedure is now the transperitoneal lower segment operation with a transverse incision in the uterus.

With any operation the best results are obtained when there is ample time to prepare the patient, but the need for caesarean section may only become evident during the course of labour. If section is elective it should be performed a few days before the expected date of labour, but if there is doubt about the maturity it may be wiser to wait until labour beings.

Anaesthesia for caesarean section

Caesarean section often has to be performed at inconvenient times, but the services of a skilled anaesthetist are essential. Deaths from avoidable complications of anaesthesia still make a tragic contribution to maternal mortality statistics. In emergency cases the patient may be ill-prepared for operation and it may be necessary to pass a gastric tube and empty the stomach before anaesthesia. Fifty mg of ranitidine is given intravenously together with 30 ml of a 0.3 M solution of sodium citrate minimize the risks of acid reflux.

Morphine and allied drugs which may depress the respiratory centre of the newborn infant should not be used for premedication. The patient should not be under the influence of the anaesthetic for longer than is absolutely necessary before the operation begins and all preparations for the operation must be completed before inducing anaesthesia.

The anaesthetist must be able to insert a cuffed endotracheal tube. A very common technique is to induce sleep with a small dose of intravenous thiopentone, to obtain relaxation with an injection of scoline and, after insertion of a cuffed endotracheal tube, to maintain anaesthesia with nitrous oxide and oxygen. Recently propofol (Diprivan) has tended to replace thiopentone.

An alternative method is to use a lumbar epidural block (*see* the section on relief of pain in labour, p. 173). Spinal analgesia is unsuitable because the paralysis of the vasomotor control of the lower part of the body, combined with the reduction in venous return which is a result of the pressure of the uterus on the inferior vena cava when the patient is supine, may cause dangerous hypotension.

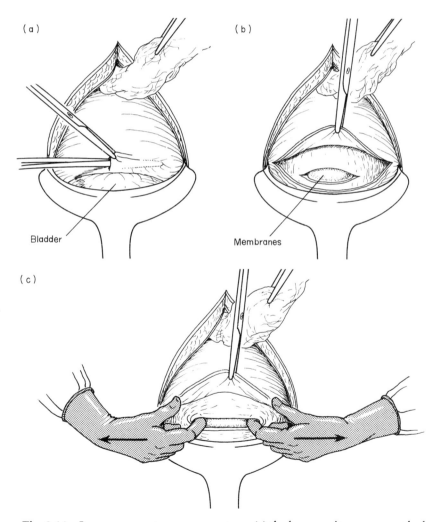

Fig. 8.16   Lower segment caesarean section. (a) the loose peritoneum over the lower uterine segment is lifted up before it is incised; (b) the lower segment is exposed and a short incision made through it down to the fetal membranes; (c) the incision in the lower segment can be enlarged by finger traction with very little bleeding

Regional infiltration of the abdominal wall and parietal peritoneum can be employed, but this method is time-consuming and is not suitable for apprehensive patients.

LOWER SEGMENT CAESAREAN SECTION

The bladder is emptied with a catheter before the operation is started. An intravenous glucose–saline drip is set up. A litre of cross-matched blood should be available (although it may not be used); in cases of placenta praevia, when blood loss may be heavy, this is essential.

The operating table is tilted laterally by 15°. This prevents the uterus from compressing the inferior vena cava and impeding the venous return.

The peritoneal cavity is opened by a low transverse or vertical subumbilical incision. A wide Doyen's retractor is inserted into the lower end of the wound. The peritoneum of the uterovesical pouch is divided transversely for about 10 cm and the bladder is pushed gently down off the lower segment. A transverse incision about 2 cm long is made in the midline of the lower segment and deepened until the membranes bulge (Fig. 8.16); the amniotic sac should be kept intact at this stage if possible. The two index fingers are slipped into the incision and by exerting finger traction the incision can be extended to about 10 cm in length.

The membranes are ruptured and the head is delivered by slipping a hand beside it and applying first one blade of Wrigley's forceps and then the other. The head is delivered gently with the forceps. As the head is delivered the anaesthetist injects 10 units of Syntocinon intravenously.

The shoulders are carefully delivered, easing them out of the wound to avoid dangerous lateral splitting of the uterine wound.

The fetus, now delivered is held head downwards at about the same level as the placenta while the mouth and pharynx are cleared of fluid with a soft catheter attached to a suction apparatus. The cord is clamped and divided and the infant is handed over to the care of an assistant.

The placenta soon separates and is delivered through the wound. The uterine incision is sutured with two layers of catgut or Dexon. It is important to secure complete haemostasis and to remove any blood, liquor and vernix from the peritoneal cavity. The abdominal wound is closed in the ordinary way.

UPPER SEGMENT CAESAREAN SECTION

Although this operation is often still described as 'classical' it has been completely replaced by the lower segment operation, except possibly for a case of transverse lie of the fetus with the arm prolapsed, or if a fibromyoma prevents access to the lower segment. A paramedian incision is made. The uterus is incised vertically in the midline of the anterior wall of the upper segment and the membranes are ruptured. The fetus is grasped by the feet and delivered in a manner similar to breech extraction. The incision in the uterus is closed with two layers of catgut, and the abdomen is closed in the ordinary way.

STERILIZATION

Sterilization may be performed at the time of caesarean section, but section should never be done just to sterilize the patient.

Sterilization is sometimes advised if a patient has had two or more sections, when the risk of further section may exceed that of normal delivery, and it may be recommended for various medical reasons.

The irreversible nature of the operation must be explained to both the patient and her partner, who should both sign consent, although the partner's consent is not necessary if there are medical reasons for the operation, but it is wise to obtain it. It is also important, because of the risk of litigation, to point out that there is a very small percentage of failures, no matter what method is used.

Because it is not possible to guarantee that any baby will survive and thrive, unless there are very strong medical reasons to advise against further pregnancy it may be wise to postpone sterilization until the baby is four to six months old and has been weaned, when sterilization can be performed by a laparoscopic method.

For sterilization at the time of caesarean section part of the tube is drawn up into a loop and a ligature is tied tightly round the base of the loop, which is then excised. Within a few days the catgut gives way and the two sealed ends of the tube separate (Pomeroy method).

CAESAREAN HYSTERECTOMY

Hysterectomy at the time of caesarean section is rarely indicated, although it carries little additional risk except on account of the condition which led to it. The technique differs little from that of an ordinary hysterectomy. The tissues are more vascular, but the tissue planes separate easily. It is occasionally indicated in cases of:

rupture of the uterus if there is gross damage to the uterine blood supply or evidence of severe infection

fibromyomata. When a patient has to be delivered by section because of multiple or large fibromyomata, hysterectomy may be considered, but it is sometimes easier to perform the hysterectomy three months later

carcinoma of the cervix. Cases that have reached late pregnancy may be treated by caesarean section followed by Wertheim's operation

abruptio placentae with concealed haemorrhage.
If persistent bleeding occurs from the uterus and from any incision or needle puncture it is likely to be caused by a bleeding diasthesis and treatment of the coagulation defect rather than hysterectomy is usually indicated.

POSTOPERATIVE CARE AFTER CAESAREAN SECTION

A patient who has had a caesarean section is looked after in the same way as any patient who has had a major abdominal operation. Possible complications will be mentioned in the next section.

DANGERS OF CAESAREAN SECTION TO THE MOTHER

It is estimated that the maternal mortality after caesarean section is four times greater than after vaginal delivery. The risk to the mother is affected by the indication for the operation, her health before and during labour, whether there have been previous attempts at delivery, the length of labour and the skill of the surgeon and anaesthetist. The risks in lower segment caesarean section performed as a planned procedure are low, but if emergency cases are considered the risk is higher.

Immediate risks

We have already emphasized the risks of anaesthesia in an unprepared patient with an inexperienced anaesthetist.

Blood transfusion must always be readily available for patients undergoing section, particularly cases of placenta praevia. When emergency section is performed anaemia and shock must first be treated by blood transfusion.

Serious infection is uncommon in planned operations, but still may occur if section is performed after labour has been in progress for some time or any other attempt at delivery has been made. Severe postoperative ileus is now rare.

Pulmonary embolism may occur after caesarean section and, together with anaesthetic complications, now accounts for most of the fatalities. It is more likely in obese and anaemic patients. Early ambulation and anticoagulant treatment will play an important part in reducing the danger.

Remote risks

Rupture of a caesarean scar is relatively rare after lower segment section, and then usually occurs during labour. An upper segment scar is much more likely to rupture, and may do so during pregnancy as well as during labour. Any patient who has had a caesarean operation should be under the care of a hospital obstetric unit for every subsequent delivery.

Intestinal obstruction from adhesions is now exceedingly rare since the upper segment operation has been largely abandoned.

DANGERS OF CAESAREAN SECTION TO THE FETUS

Caesarean section has an inherent small risk for the fetus, although the conditions for which the operation is performed may explain much of the increased perinatal mortality. Anaesthetics cross the placental barrier and may depress the respiration of the newborn; respiratory problems may also occur with premature babies or babies born to diabetic mothers.

Occasionally, when section is planned to be done near term, the duration of gestation is wrongly estimated. The routine use of ultrasound scan should eliminate this risk.

It is possible to cause intracranial damage by delivering the head without proper care when it has to be brought up from the pelvis, or even by delivering it through too small a uterine incision.

RISING INCIDENCE OF CAESAREAN SECTION

The incidence of caesarean section has been rising in the United Kingdom to around 10 per cent of deliveries partly due to the threat of litigation following the birth *per vaginam* of brain-damaged babies (see page 331) and partly due to the tendency to deliver pre-term and very small babies abdominally. It has been suggested that the increasing use of fetal monitoring in labour has been the cause of unnecessary operations which might have been avoided had the pH of fetal scalp blood been measured (see page 220).

SYMPHYSIOTOMY

See page 208.

CRANIOTOMY

Craniotomy, or perforation of the fetal head, is now hardly ever performed except for hydrocephaly (*see* p. 208).

Craniotomy used to be preferred to caesarean section in cases of obstructed labour with a dead fetus but with modern anaesthesia and the availability of antibiotics, lower segment section is now easier and safer.

9

PROBLEMS OF THE NEWBORN

ASPHYXIA AND RESUSCITATION

Pathophysiology

Before or during the process of childbirth a number of infants suffer from conditions which inhibit the onset of respiration. These babies are usually hypoxic and quickly become acidotic due to accumulation of carbon dioxide and lactic acid in the bloodstream. Unless breathing is established within the first few minutes of life there is a significant risk of cerebral damage, this risk increases as the asphyxial insult continues. A number of conditions may predispose the infant to birth asphyxia:

Maternal causes
  hypertension
  chronic cardiac or pulmonary disease
  renal failure
  diabetes
  hypotension or excessive sedation
  placental problems such as abruptio placentae,
    placenta praevia
Fetal causes
  abnormal presentation
  cephalopelvic disproportion
  multiple birth
  intrauterine growth retardation
  hydrops fetalis
  extreme immaturity
  postmaturity
  cord prolapse, fetomaternal haemorrhage and
    twin-to-twin transfusion.

preterm delivery
intrauterine fetal distress.

The typical sequence of physiological events which occurs in asphyxia is shown in Figure 9.1. Initially there is a period of gasping which is followed after 1–2 minutes by the onset of primary apnoea. At this stage the infant is blue but the blood pressure is maintained although the heart rate is falling. This is called blue asphyxia, or asphyxia livida. A further period of gasping, which lasts 8–10 minutes, occurs following which secondary or terminal apnoea ensues. The blood pressure is now extremely low and the heart rate is rapidly deteriorating. At this stage the infant is white and shocked, this is described as asphyxia pallida, or white asphyxia. Narcotic drugs such as pethidine greatly prolong the period of primary apnoea although this can be reversed by naloxone. In secondary or terminal apnoea breathing will not begin unless some form of positive pressure ventilation is provided.

ASPHYXIA NEONATORUM (FAILURE TO ESTABLISH RESPIRATION)

If the infant fails to respond to nasal or pharyngeal aspiration, and the onset of respiration is delayed, prompt action is required. In the majority of these babies the heart rate is normal, limb tone is

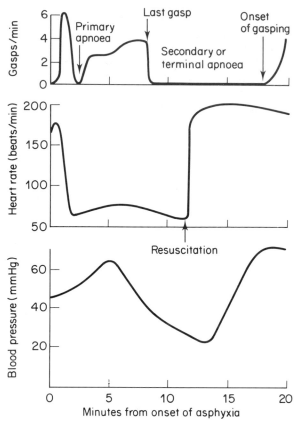

Fig. 9.1 Changes in Rhesus monkeys during asphyxia and on resuscitation by positive-pressure ventilation. Brain damage was assessed by histological examination some weeks later. (From Dawes (1968). Reproduced with permission from the author and publisher, Year Book Medical Publishers, Chicago)

present, and the failure to breathe is due to liquor or mucus blocking the respiratory tract, the respiratory centres being normally responsive. In other infants limb tone is poor or absent, the heart rate is slower or absent, and the respiratory centre

is depressed by trauma sustained during delivery or by analgesics administered to the mother.

The Apgar score is often used to evaluate the physical status of the infant at one minute after delivery and to estimate any improvement in the subsequent few minutes (Table 9.1). An Apgar score of 9 or 10 places the infant in a theoretically ideal physical state. The lower the score the worse is the condition of the baby, and the greater the urgency of resuscitation.

When the Apgar score is more than 5 (and in practice this will be a baby with a heart rate of more than 100 per minute) the infant will be in a good condition and, provided that the airways are clear, respiration is likely to begin within one minute. This is *primary apnoea*. All that is usually necessary is to stimulate the baby gently by drying with a towel and to keep a check on the heart rate. Directing a stream of oxygen towards the baby's nose and mouth can do no harm and will ensure that the first breaths take in oxygen-enriched air. Drugs have no place in treatment, with the exception of naloxone hydrochloride which is given if the mother has received morphine or pethidine within four hours of delivery. The recommended intravenous or intramuscular dose is 10 micrograms per kg, but the drug has a short half-life and may have to be repeated. It does not have any depressant effect.

If the baby remains unresponsive at the end of one minute, or if the heart rate begins to fall, the larynx must be aspirated through a catheter. This will often remove the liquor or mucus obstructing the respiratory tract and the infant will gasp, breathe and cry and rapidly become pink. Facial oxygen should be continued until regular respiration and strong crying have become established.

If the infant fails to respond to external stimulation, aspiration of the airway and facial oxygen, some form of positive pressure ventilation must be

Table 9.1 Apgar score

Sign	0	1	2
Heart rate	absent	less than 100	more than 100
Respiratory effort	absent	slow, irregular	good, crying
Muscle tone	limp	some limb flexion	active
Response to stimulus (nasal catheter)	nil	grimace	vigorous cry
Colour	blue, pale	body pink limbs blue	pink

applied. The most effective way is by intubation but a properly fitting face mask applied with an Ambu or Laerdal resuscitation bag is a satisfactory method of resuscitation for those who are not skilled in the technique of intubation. The initial puff with the bag should be held for three seconds and then 30–40 puffs per minute should be given until spontaneous breathing is satisfactorily established.

Alternatively, if aspiration is unsuccessful in initiating respiration a laryngoscope is passed and an endotracheal tube is inserted into the trachea and oxygen administered in short puffs through a T tube connected to a manometer, which ensures that the pressure is kept below 30 cm of water. This will often improve the oxygenation of the baby and start respiration after a short time. When spontaneous respiration is seen the endotracheal tube is removed and facial oxygen continued until the condition of the infant is completely satisfactory. Sometimes, especially with an initially low Apgar score, or when the infant has been narcotized, it may be necessary to continue assisted respiration through the endotracheal tube for long periods. The technique of endotracheal intubation should be learned by all doctors and senior nursing staff who are likely to attend deliveries because it is the only sure way to resuscitate the baby. Artificial respiration or mouth-to-mouth insufflation may be dangerous if performed too vigorously, and can cause a pneumothorax.

If the Apgar score is below 5 (and certainly if it is 3 or under) the baby will be pale and limp with a heart rate of less than 100 per minute. This is the condition formerly called *white asphyxia*, but which is now generally referred to as *secondary apnoea*. Such a baby is in a state of shock, with falling blood pressure, and is likely to die if nothing is done. If such babies recover they may be left with varying degrees of cerebral damage. The baby must be resuscitated with endotracheal intubation *without delay*, assisted by cardiac massage performed by gentle compression of the chest with two fingers placed in the 3rd and 4th interspaces to the left of the sternum. In these infants intermittent positive pressure ventilation at 15 to 30 puffs per minute may need to be continued for some time. Babies with severe intracranial haemorrhage may present a similar clinical picture, and the diagnosis does not become clear until resuscitation has been carried out.

The severely asphyxiated infant becomes acidotic, and when recovery is unduly delayed 10 ml of 4.2 per cent sodium bicarbonate solution may be injected slowly into the umbilical vein or into a peripheral vein. It is also suggested that 2–4 ml of 20 per cent glucose solution may be given by this route, but the injection of hyperosmolar solutions is dangerous; in particular there is a possibility of portal thrombosis if the umbilical vein is used. If the injection is made in error into the umbilical artery this may cause spasm and subsequent thrombosis of the vessel, which may spread to involve the internal or common iliac arteries with a risk of gangrene of the legs or sciatic nerve palsy by interference with the blood supply to the nerve.

The baby with secondary apnoea may have aspirated meconium into the lungs, and this should be removed by direct suction from the pharynx and the trachea via a catheter inserted down the endotracheal tube. It is important to carry out these manoeuvres before the onset of breathing, if possible, in order to prevent aspiration of meconium further down into the lungs.

After resuscitation the severely asphyxiated baby is kept in an incubator under close observation until fully recovered.

CYANOSIS

PERSISTENCE OF CYANOSIS DESPITE ESTABLISHMENT OF RESPIRATION

Generalized cyanosis, which includes cyanosis of the tongue, indicates a significantly low arterial oxygen tension. Observation of the baby during episodes of crying is helpful in differentiating the cause. Cyanosis which deepens with crying suggests intracranial damage or a congenital cardiac lesion with a right-to-left shunt. Cyanosis which is lessened by crying and which returns with shallower respiration suggests a respiratory cause such as atelectasis, or secretions remaining in the respiratory passages. A short exposure to 100 per cent oxygen through a mask applied gently to the face will provide the same information, cyanosis from cardiac and cerebral causes usually remaining unchanged.

Cardiovascular causes of cyanosis

Reference to the description of the circulatory adjustments which take place at birth (*see* p. 240) shows that the haemodynamic factors are in a delicate equilibrium which is easily disturbed if respiratory difficulties arise. For example, extensive atelectasis may result from meconium aspiration in the asphyxiated baby, and the hypoxia resulting from inadequate ventilation and from perfusion of unaerated segments of lung prevents the normal fall in pulmonary vascular resistance, so that the right atrial pressure remains elevated. The reduced pulmonary venous return diminishes the left atrial pressure and the foramen ovale is opened, permitting right-to-left shunting and a fall in arterial Po_2. The hypoxaemia leads to a fall in the systemic arterial pressure, the ductus arteriosus opens wide and right-to-left shunting through the ductus is favoured by the change in pressure gradient. If this reversion to fetal pulmonary hypertension persists, the baby will develop cyanosis, cardiac enlargement and heart failure. On auscultation there may be a systolic murmur down the left sternal border and the diagnosis of cyanotic congenital heart disease is suspected.

The advice of a paediatric cardiologist is invaluable, because it is imperative to make an accurate diagnosis of the cause of cyanotic heart disease at an early stage, so that surgical treatment can be given if necessary. Congenital heart lesions which cause cyanosis in the newborn are usually complex and severe anomalies, some of which do not produce cardiac murmurs. Expert investigation by cardiac ultrasound is likely to be required.

Other causes of cyanosis

Cyanosis may also be due to intracranial injuries, chilling, abdominal distension, and the delayed effect of anaesthetics and analgesics given to the mother.

Polycythaemia

Polycythaemia will allow the baby to become cyanosed easily since a relatively slight fall in oxygen saturation will produce the 5 g of reduced haemoglobin which is necessary to show cyanosis.

Congenital methaemoglobinaemia

Congenital methaemoglobinaemia is a rare cause of a slaty blue cyanosis in a baby with no cardiac or respiratory embarrassment; spectroscopic examination of the blood provides the diagnosis.

Acquired methaemoglobinaemia

Acquired methaemoglobinaemia can occur if artificial feeds happen to be made up with water containing an excess of nitrites.

THE VERY SMALL INFANT

Infants who are born early (preterm), who are very small, have a low birth weight or who are light-for-dates have a number of potential problems which usually necessitate their transfer to a transitional, special or neonatal intensive care unit. The definition of these terms is important and is as follows:

> preterm babies; born at less than 37 completed weeks of gestation from the first day of the last menstrual period
> low birthweight babies; those whose birthweight is 2500 g or less
> light-for-dates or small-for-dates babies; those whose birthweight is below the 10th centile for gestation.

Two other terms are in common use. Babies weighing less than 1500 g at birth are called very low birthweight babies and those weighing less than 1000 g at birth are described as extremely low birthweight babies.

In clinical practice it is usually babies under 35 weeks gestation and those weighing less than 1700 g at birth who develop significant problems. Those who are more mature, or heavier, can usually be nursed by their mother on a specially designated postnatal ward which serves as a transitional nursery. This has the advantage of allowing close supervision but does not separate mother and baby in the immediate postnatal period.

About 30 per cent of babies who are born early are also small for gestational age. There is often uncertainty about gestational age. Methods of attempting to assess fetal maturity are discussed on pages 57, 61 and 131.

After the baby is born gestational age may be assessed by using tables which include such factors as body proportions, presence or absence of lanugo hair, genital development, auricular cartilage formation and neonatal reflexes; these are claimed to be accurate to within two weeks. A rapid and almost equally accurate assessment can be made from the time at which the neonatal reflexes appeared.

When intrauterine malnutrition starts early in pregnancy the head circumference and weight are in their normal proportions, but when the onset is late in pregnancy the head is disproportionately large because of relatively normal growth of the brain at the expense of the rest of the body. It is particularly important to recognize the latter type of case in which there is depletion of glycogen stores in the liver and heart, and depletion of fat stores, because these depletions make such babies more susceptible to intranatal hypoxia, hypothermia and hypoglycaemia.

In general, if the birth weight of the baby falls below the 10th centile of the expected weight for the gestational age the baby is assumed to be small-for-gestational age, but the appearance is often characteristic, with dry folds of lax skin.

The aetiology of intrauterine malnutrition is not well understood, and may be multifactorial. Placental insufficiency, including cases of maternal hypertension and proteinuria, is generally accepted as the most important single factor, although infections, endocrine and chromosomal aberrations have been incriminated, especially when growth is affected throughout pregnancy. Excessive smoking is an important cause of growth failure. Excessive consumption of alcohol and drug addition affect the growth and development of the fetus and produce recognizable neonatal syndromes.

PRINCIPLES OF SPECIAL CARE

The purpose of special care is to control the environment according to the special needs of the baby, to monitor all the important bodily functions in order to detect any signs of illness immediately and to treat them without delay, and to use special feeding techniques if necessary. It is important to remember that preterm infants have contributed significantly to the number of babies

suffering non-accidental injury so that it is essential to involve the mother in the care of her baby, including handling under supervision, as much as possible. Prematurity is rarely a bar to breast feeding. In several maternity units it has been shown that with encouragement breast feeding can be established with most low birth weight babies, and this is the best way of keeping the mother closely integrated with her child.

Temperature

Small infants become hypothermic very quickly. They have a large surface area relative to their weight which permits rapid heat loss, and there is deficiency of subcutaneous fat for insulation. There is also a deficiency of brown adipose tissue which is present in significant amounts in term infants, and which can metabolize rapidly to produce heat. It is therefore necessary to provide a high and constant environmental temperature. If it is decided to nurse the baby naked in an incubator to improve observation, excessive heat loss by radiation can be reduced by placing a Perspex heat shield (with one end closed to prevent a cooling through draught) over the baby. However, there is no reason why the infant should not be clothed. The covering provided by a thin cotton gown and a stockinette hat incorporating a layer of gamgee is sufficient to maintain the body temperature. Heat loss is also minimized by maintaining a high environmental temperature. With the room temperature at 27°C the infant's core temperature should remain at about 37°C if the incubator temperature is as show in Table 9.2.

The temperature of the incubator is reduced by 1°C weekly. The larger babies stabilize their temperature quite quickly and can soon be transferred to a cot and then to a cooler room (24°C). For infants weighing less than 1 kg it may be necessary to make special adjustments to the incubator to raise the temperature further. The regular use of humidifiers in incubators is no longer

Table 9.2 Incubator temperature (at room temperature 27°C) required to keep rectal temperature at 37°C

Weight of infant	Temperature of incubator
1 kg	35°C
2 kg	34°C
3 kg	33°C

recommended because of the increased risk of infection. Very low birthweight babies (<1000 g at birth) do, however, require special insulation and high humidity to prevent excessive heat loss.

It must be remembered that infants can lose heat during resuscitative procedures so that these are best carried out under a heat shield or canopy. When transferring a baby to hospital it should be well wrapped in gamgee, or preferably transferred in a special ready-warmed portable incubator. Swaddlers made of aluminium foil are effective in retaining the baby's own heat, but can prevent heat reaching a baby who is cold.

Infection

Low birthweight babies are particularly susceptible to infection, which can be carried from one baby to another on the hands of an attendant or doctor. The most scrupulous care must be taken with hand washing, using special washing solutions containing a suitable antiseptic such as chlorhexidine. It is not necessary to wear masks, but any member of the staff with a respiratory infection should be excluded from the unit. Infection is considered in detail later in the chapter (*see* p. 322).

Feeding

Preterm infants have poor swallowing and coughing reflexes and methods of feeding must prevent aspiration into the lungs. At first it will be necessary to give tube feeds. Small frequent feeds will not lead to over distension of the stomach, and therefore there will be less risk of aspiration and of apnoea due to embarrassment of respiration. The present consensus opinion is that an attempt should be made to keep up with the rapid rate of weight gain which normally occurs *in utero*. With milk feeds this entails giving quite large volumes throughout the 24 hours. If the infant is unable to tolerate bolus feeds this can be achieved by continuous infusion through a nasogastric tube. The method is safe and trouble-free, provided that certain basic rules are followed.

The infant is nursed prone on a firm mattress. This position reduces regurgitation and makes sure that no milk is aspirated. A moderately fine PVC tube is passed through the nose into the stomach. The correct distance is gauged by measuring the distance from the tip of the nose to the lower end

of the sternum – usually about 20 cm. The part of the tube adjacent to the nose is then marked with strapping. Fluid is withdrawn with a syringe, and if it is colourless and acid to litmus the tube is in the correct position and is then taped firmly to the cheek. If green fluid is obtained the tube is withdrawn 2 cm and aspiration is repeated. Once the infusion has been started the position of the tube is checked by aspiration at least three times in each 24 hours, and the tube is changed every third day. The milk is given through a constant infusion pump, especially when very small volumes are being used. In the infusion pump the syringe is tipped up at an angle. This ensures that the fat, which floats on the top, is always delivered first and not allowed to remain in the syringe, with the loss of valuable calories. Breast milk is best given this way.

One hour after birth, feeding is started with milk. If expressed breast milk is not available a special low birthweight formula is used. The initial volume of feed is 60 ml/kg per 24 hours, which is increased by 30 ml/kg per 24 hours up to a maximum of 180 ml/kg per 24 hours, provided that it is well tolerated. A careful watch is kept on the baby's abdomen and if this is unduly distended the infusion is discontinued to allow the distension to subside, and the daily rate is put back to that of the previous 24 hours. By using the technique described these large volumes of feed have not been associated with aspiration pneumonia or an increased tendency to necrotizing enterocolitis.

Continuous infusion is usually maintained until the infant develops a sucking reflex. If the mother intends to breast feed the baby can be put to the breast for short periods while the infusion is temporarily stopped, thereby providing a stimulus to lactation. When intermittent feeding is started the feeds are given frequently at first and then gradually the intervals are increased to a three-hourly regime.

Intravenous feeding with glucose, amino acids and lipid has a place in the management of infants with necrotizing enterocolitis or after intestinal resection, but there is no convincing evidence that it improves the prognosis for other infants of very low birth weight.

Early and adequate feeding prevents hypoglycaemia and reduces the maximum serum bilirubin level. Vitamin K_1 (phytomenadione) is given routinely to prevent haemorrhagic disease.

From the second week vitamin supplements are

added, such as Abidec 0.6 ml daily, which would provide vitamin A 4000 units, vitamin D 400 units and vitamin C 50 mg, with small amounts of vitamin B complex. In addition iron is given as ferrous fumarate or ferrous sulphate in a dose to provide approximately 10 mg of elemental iron daily. Preterm babies are also given regular folic acid supplements.

Other hazards

Respiratory distress syndrome, hyperbilirubinaemia, hypoglycaemia and hypocalcaemia are special hazards in low birth weight babies that are discussed on pages 316, 310, 308.

Prognosis

The prognosis for the very small infant has improved dramatically in recent years. The number of infants surviving has steadily increased. The major outstanding question is whether the rate of handicap has decreased. Although it has undoubtedly decreased among those of birth weight 1000–1500 g the total numbers may not have done so, since there are now more survivors in the extremely low birth weight group (<1000 g). As these infants have the greatest number of problems in the neonatal period the potential for handicap is considerable. A number of long-term follow-up studies are in progress to answer this important question.

Overall, survival rates for infants 1000–1500 g at birth are of the order of 70–80 per cent, although the best units can achieve survival rates of greater than 90 per cent. The survival of infants <1000 g at birth is 35–45 per cent overall, with the best units achieving up to 50 per cent. The handicap rate is determined not only by birth weight, being greater in the smallest infants, but also by the number of neonatal complications which occurred, especially if these involved hypoxic–ischaemic insult from birth asphyxia, respiratory distress syndrome or intracerebral haemorrhage.

The type of handicap can be broadly divided into four categories:

intellectual impairment
visual deficit
hearing deficit
cerebral palsy.

Cerebral palsy is the most common deficit after intracerebral haemorrhage but those who have suffered from hypoxic–ischaemic insult are more likely to have intellectual and sensory impairment in addition to cerebral palsy. Overall handicap rates for those babies weighing between 1000 g and 1500 g at birth are of the order of 10–15 per cent, this figure includes major and minor degrees of deficit. Infants under 1000 g at birth have an overall handicap rate of 15–20 per cent. Despite these problems an increasing number of very low and extremely low birthweight infants are surviving with an excellent quality of life and a good prognosis for the future.

DISEASES OF THE NEWBORN

BIRTH TRAUMA

Birth injuries vary from minor skin abrasions to severe internal haemorrhage. Their prevention depends on the art of obstetrics, and a balance must be struck between the safety of the mother and that of the child in a difficult labour. It is a reflection of the improvement in antenatal and perinatal care in recent years that serious birth trauma is now uncommon.

BIRTH INJURIES TO THE SCALP AND SKULL

Caput succedaneum

This is caused by oedema of the subcutaneous layers of the scalp (Fig. 9.2). It lies over whatever part of the head presents through the cervical opening. The swelling is maximal at birth and resolves within a few days. A localized caput,

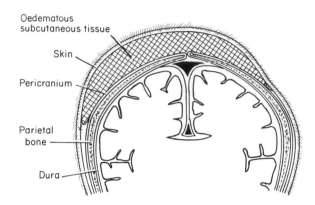

Fig. 9.2 Caput succedaneum. The swelling is formed by oedema of the structures lying superficial to the pericranium. Note that it is not limited to one bone

referred to as the 'chignon', is produced by the vacuum extractor.

Cephalhaematoma

This is a subperitoneal haematoma which most commonly lies over one of the parietal bones (Fig. 9.3). It never extends beyond the limits of a single bone, and it is fluctuant but incompressible. It never varies in tension with crying, thus differing from the less common encephalocele. Spontaneous absorption occurs, but this may take several weeks. Ossification may take place round the periphery and create a raised rim which can be mistaken for a depressed fracture. The edge of the lesion gives a cracked eggshell sensation on palpation.

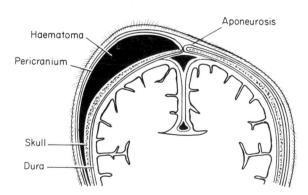

Fig. 9.3 Cephalhaematoma. The swelling consists of blood lying between the pericranium and the skull and is limited to the area of bone on which it started because the pericranium is attached to sutures around the bone

No treatment is necessary; aspiration invites infection. There may be asymmetry of the skull which persists for many months, but ultimately this resolves completely.

Subaponeurotic haematoma

After vacuum extraction a few cases of sub-aponeurotic haematoma have occurred. The blood lies in the loose areolar layer between the aponeurosis and the periosteum. The haematoma is not limited to a single bone, and a large collection of blood may even extend as far as the cervical region. Slow absorption takes place.

Sometimes an extremely large cephalhaematoma or subaponeurotic haematoma may cause anaemia or moderately severe jaundice.

Skull fractures

These are now rarely seen. They may be depressed, linear or stellate. They usually occur over a parietal or frontal bone as a result of difficult forceps delivery. Often there are no symptoms and even depressed fractures may resolve spontaneously. If there are signs suspicious of underlying haemorrhage or pressure on the brain a neurosurgical opinion should be obtained, in case elevation of a depressed fracture is required.

Craniotabes

Although it is not caused by injury this condition is mentioned here for convenience. The skull may show areas of softening near the suture lines, especially in the parietal region, and the bone in these areas can be indented like a table tennis ball. Craniotabes is of no significance, and the bones develop and thicken normally as the infant grows.

INTRACRANIAL INJURIES

Intracranial haemorrhage, especially when it is combined with hypoxia, causes a number of stillbirths and neonatal deaths. Such haemorrhage may occur in any difficult, instrumental or breech delivery, and especially with preterm birth. It may even occur occasionally during normal delivery or caesarean section.

The cerebrospinal fluid acts as a cushion to the brain and permits some mobility of the intracranial contents, but injury occurs when excessive moulding or sudden changes in pressure occur during delivery. The site of the haemorrhage may be extradural, subdural, subarachnoid, intraventricular or intracerebral.

Extradural haemorrhage

Caused by rupture of the middle meningeal artery or the veins near the sigmoid sinus, extradural haemorrhage is rare in the newborn infant. It may occur with a fracture through the middle temporal fossa or from forcible separation of cranial sutures. In cases of tearing of the tentorium cerebelli or falx cerebri there may be extradural bleeding, but the blood also escapes into the subarachnoid space, and the symptoms produced are chiefly caused by this.

Subdural haemorrhage

This takes the form of slow bleeding into the space between the dura and pia-arachnoid, and is due to rupture of small veins crossing this space. A haematoma usually forms slowly over a period of some days, but may develop more quickly. *See* page 304.

Subarachnoid haemorrhage

This is most commonly seen in association with prolonged or traumatic delivery, but hypoxia plays a part in causing it. It can arise from a tear of the tentorium or falx, with rupture of small vessels or of a dural sinus. With gross tentorial tearing there may be fatal rupture of the great cerebral vein of Galen.

Intraventricular haemorrhage (IVH)

This occurs most frequently in preterm babies and is the result of hypoxia. The bleeding follows rupture of poorly-supported blood vessels in the highly vascular germinal layers of the brain close to the ventricles. The blood then breaks through into the ventricle. Significant haemorrhage may also arise from the choroid plexus. The largest degrees of IVH are associated with dilatation of the ventricles and with intracerebral haemorrhage. Many of these infants do not survive the neonatal period and the majority of those who do are left with permanent brain damage, usually resulting in cerebral palsy. Hydrocephalus is another common complication of this condition. Ultrasound scanning has shown that many infants, especially preterm ones, have much lesser degrees of IVH which is usually associated with complete recovery. This complication is seen during the first week of life in approximately 40 per cent of babies who weigh less than 1500 g at birth.

Intracerebral haemorrhage

This is often only petechial but it is distributed throughout the substance of the brain. Such haemorrhage is usually the result of severe asphyxial episodes. Although the haemorrhage may be small and not fatal it may be associated with cerebral palsy, mental retardation and a high incidence of morbidity.

Clinical signs

Minor intracranial haemorrhages must often escape recognition, but massive haemorrhages cause stillbirth or almost immediate death. Lesions of intermediate severity create intricate diagnostic problems, in which physical signs are often misleading or difficult.

General signs and symptoms may occur, including convulsions, asphyxia pallida, depression of respiration and heart rate, which are associated with alterations in muscular tone. Cyanosis or unusual pallor, fever, a shrill cry, excessive restlessness or somnolence may all occur. An anxious facial expression, adder-like movements of the tongue and unusual yawning may suggest the diagnosis. With an extensive haemorrhage the fontanelle may become tense or even bulge.

The clinical picture may be differentiated according to the site of the bleeding.

Supratentorial bleeding

This usually affects the surface of the hemisphere and the basal ganglia. The picture is one of irritation, with fullness of the fontanelle, convulsions which may be unilateral, and excessive response to stimuli of sound, light and touch. The eyes may roll upwards and the face twitch during the clonic contractions, and adductor spasm may be demonstrated. The vital centres are involved in the terminal stages.

Infratentorial bleeding

This is often associated with early neck rigidity, opisthotonus and alteration in the rate and depth of respiration. Cyanosis is common. The baby tends to be limp and toneless; the vital centres are affected early.

Treatment

The infant must be kept quiet, warm and sheltered from any noise or disturbance which might induce further restlessness or convulsions. Unnecessary handling should be avoided. Respiration and oxygenation must be maintained. These conditions are achieved by nursing the baby in an incubator in which optimal conditions of warmth, humidity and oxygen concentration can be provided. The incubator should be kept in a quiet, darkened area of the nursery where the baby receives minimal disturbance until recovery has occurred. The infant can be fed in the incubator and need not be removed for any nursing services. If the baby sucks badly or refuses to feed, tube feeding is given at intervals of up to four hours.

Phytomenadione (vitamin K_1) 1 mg should be given by intramuscular injection to prevent the risk of any further bleeding from haemorrhagic disease (*see* p. 309).

An infant who has convulsions should be given sedatives until the convulsions are controlled, as they may provoke further bleeding. An intravenous loading dose of Phenobarbitone 12–20 mg/kg is given initially followed by a maintenance dose of 5 mg/kg per 24 hours, which is usually effective.

Lumbar puncture will prove the diagnosis by demonstrating blood in the cerebrospinal fluid, and it will also exclude a diagnosis of meningitis.

The prognosis in cases of cerebral haemorrhage is always in doubt and is often poor. The infant may survive to show cerebral palsy, convulsions or mental retardation; but complete recovery may follow a subarachnoid haemorrhage.

Subdural haematoma

These cases may be described separately as the clinical signs often develop more slowly. There is slow bleeding into the space between the dura and the pia-arachnoid. The haematoma increases in size because of further small haemorrhages or because of lysis of the clot and accumulation of serum.

Symptoms may occur soon after birth or may be delayed for 24 hours or more. Early symptoms are those of the supratentorial irritation (*see* above, p. 303) but more delayed symptoms are failure to gain weight, irregular fever, vomiting and irritability. Coma or convulsions may occur at this stage, but it is more common to find fits with enlargement of the skull simulating hydrocephalus during the first few months of life. The diagnosis is made by ultrasound or CT scan. Treatment is by needling the subdural space through the lateral angles of the fontanelle, when blood-stained or xanthochromic fluid may be found. Repeated aspiration is performed until the cavity is emptied. Surgery is rarely indicated, and has not been found to reduce the occurrence of sequelae due to cortical atrophy, namely convulsions, spasticity and mental retardation.

Real-time ultrasound scanning and CT scanning are proving increasingly helpful in the early diagnosis and response to treatment of intracranial conditions in the newborn.

FRACTURES OF THE LONG BONES

These are now uncommon. They were more often seen when breech extraction was practised more frequently.

Clavicle

This is the bone which is most frequently broken during delivery. The injury is usually detected when the infant fails to raise his arm above his head, or there is an absent Moro reflex in one arm, or callus formation is noticed. X-ray shows an oblique fracture. Healing occurs without treatment.

Humerus

Epiphyseal detachment or fracture of the shaft may occur. The injury is often difficult to detect clinically. The usual symptom is failure to move the arm. Splinting the arm and bandaging it to the trunk gives sufficient fixation for healing.

Femur

Fractures have occurred in breech extraction.

Orthopaedic advice should be sought for proper splinting and support to ensure satisfactory healing. In nearly all fractures of the long bones healing is rapid, and subsequent growth of the bone corrects any angulation and deformity.

VISCERAL INJURIES

Rupture of the liver, spleen or kidney may occur in difficult deliveries, especially breech extraction. There will be signs of shock, and enlargement of the viscus may be observed. The diagnosis is difficult, but ultrasound or CT scanning makes it easier. If the diagnosis is confirmed the infant is given a blood transfusion, if necessary, and laprotomy is performed to repair the injury. The mortality is high.

Haemorrhage may rarely occur into the adrenal glands.

PERIPHERAL NERVE INJURIES

Facial nerve

The nerve may be damaged by pressure of a blade of the forceps, but palsy has also occurred after normal delivery.

On the affected side the eye does not shut, the corner of the mouth drops and the nasolabial fold is less marked than on the other side. When the child cries the mouth is drawn to the normal side. In the vast majority of cases recovery occurs spontaneously within a few days.

Brachial palsy

This may occur from overstretching or tearing of the nerves by lateral traction on the neck, usually during a difficult extraction of the shoulders. The clinical picture depends on the nerve roots involved. If the roots of C5 and C6 are damaged (Erb's palsy) the arm lies at the side of the trunk with internal rotation at the shoulder, inability to bend the elbow, and clenched fingers. If the roots C7, C8 and D1 are involved there is paralysis of the muscles of the forearm with wrist drop (Klumpke's palsy). In fact Klumpke's palsy is very rare and most cases of wrist drop are caused by compression of the radial nerve against the humerus during labour. In such cases the discovery of a nodule of fat necrosis at the site of compression is diagnostic.

If the nerves have merely been compressed or stretched recovery occurs, but in the rare case of rupture of a nerve spontaneous recovery is much less likely.

DIGESTIVE DISTURBANCES DURING THE NEONATAL PERIOD

VOMITING

Vomiting is a relatively frequent symptom during the neonatal period. While most cases are not serious, this symptom sometimes has grave significance and it must never be treated lightly.

Vomiting of mucus

Many infants vomit mucus, which may be blood-stained, during the first few hours after delivery. This may persist after feeding has started, and the probable explanation is that the gastric mucosa has been irritated by material swallowed during delivery with the production of gastritis. If the vomiting is severe or persistent a lavage with normal saline is performed.

Overfeeding

Vomiting is sometimes due to the taking of more food than can be retained in the stomach, and the excess is regurgitated. Failure to help the baby bring up wind after feed often causes vomiting as the milk is brought up with the swallowed air after the baby is laid in the cot.

Obstructive vomiting

Vomiting which begins shortly after birth and is persistent raises the possibility of an obstructive lesion of the gastrointestinal tract. The vomiting is frequent, non-projectile, copious and usually bile-stained, unless the obstruction is above the level of the ampulla of Vater. Bile-stained vomit always demands consideration as a symptom of an obstructive lesion. Abdominal distention, visible peristalsis and failure to pass meconium are usually present, and are associated with a progressive loss of weight and deterioration in the general condition. These symptoms demand immediate radiological investigation and surgical consultation. A plain erect radiograph of the abdomen should be taken. If the infant is unwell, a lateral film taken with the infant lying supine in the incubator will usually give all the information required, and it has the advantage of showing whether there is gas in the rectum. The films will show dilatation of the gut, with characteristic fluid levels if there is obstruction. It is not usually necessary to use contrast media as these may complicate surgical treatment. Possible causes of obstruction include oesophageal atresia with or without tracheal fistula, duodenal stenosis or atresia, jejunal or ileal atresia, meconium ileus and Hirschprung's disease. These surgical conditions are discussed in detail on pages 327–328.

Other causes of vomiting

Vomiting may be a symptom of increased intracranial pressure or cerebral irritation. It may be the initial and sometimes the only sign of an infection in any system during the neonatal period, and is then often accompanied by diarrhoea. It cannot be too strongly emphasized that vomiting and reluctance to feed may be the earliest signs of infection such as pyelonephritis, meningitis, septicaemia or other severe illness, and such symptoms must never be lightly disregarded.

DIARRHOEA

Diarrhoea is sometimes diagnosed without justification because of ignorance of the normal variation in bowel habit of healthy infants. Frequency of stool is not necessarily pathological.

The passage of frequent loose and watery stools, usually containing curds of undigested milk and often green in colour with unchanged bile, is evidence of hurry through the gut. The presence of mucus suggests irritation of the intestinal mucosa, and blood in the stool is suggestive of infection. Colic and screaming often accompany the diarrhoea, and signs of dehydration such as loss of skin turgor, loss of weight and sunken fontanelle occur early.

The most common cause of diarrhoea are:

errors in feeding, either in the quality of the food or in the amount
lactose intolerance
infection of the gastrointestinal tract by bacteria or viruses
necrotizing enterocolitis.

Feeding irregularities

In breast fed babies there may be some intestinal hurry at the time when lactation is becoming established between the third and fifth days. The stools are frequent and greenish in colour and may contain a moderate amount of mucus. No ill effects result, and after a few more days the stools become less frequent, are pasty in consistency and yellow in colour. Sometimes in artifically fed babies there may be a similar hurried transit of gut contents if the amount of the feeds is increased too rapidly in the first few days. It is then advisable to reduce the quantity of milk until the frequency of the stools diminishes, but it may be necessary to maintain the fluid intake by adding more water to the feeds for a day or two.

Infection of the gastrointestinal tract

Diarrhoea caused by the dysentery group of organisms is uncommon in the neonatal period. Occasionally infections with pathogenic coliforms and other organisms of relatively low pathogenicity may occur. Contamination of feeds with staphylococci is possible, and if fresh milk is not sterilized infection with a great variety of bacteria may occur. In nurseries epidemics of diarrhoea among newborn infants may be caused by virus infection (*see* p. 307).

Bacterial infection

This is usually accompanied by vomiting, diarrhoea and failure to feed. The infant is usually, but not always, febrile; a few babies may be prostrated with subnormal temperatures. The stools are watery, loose and undigested. They may contain mucus, pus and red cells. The infant will either fail to gain or will lose weight. In severe cases dehydration occurs rapidly and the condition of the infant is poor. Metabolic acidosis occurs.

Infants with these symptoms must be isolated from all other babies immediately, and in institutions they must be nursed with full barrier precautions. Milk feeding is stopped until the diarrhoea improves. Sodium chloride solution 0.18 per cent, with glucose 4 per cent, and with potassium chloride 2 g per litre, is given frequently in small amounts at intervals of two or three hours. The total daily intake should be approximately 175 ml per kg of body weight, the excess being necessary to make good the additional fluid loss caused by the diarrhoea. Should vomiting persist, or the baby become further dehydrated despite this treatment, it will be necessary to give fluid by intravenous infusion, the type of fluid being dictated by electrolyte estimations.

Stool cultures are taken at the onset to determine the infecting organism and its sensitivities to antibiotics. Antibiotic therapy will not usually influence the symptoms. The prognosis must always be guarded until the response to treatment is seen.

Epidemic diarrhoea of the newborn

In other cases a baby with symptoms of gastrointestinal infection may fail to show pathogenic bacteria on stool culture, and a virus infection must be suspected, this will commonly be a rotavirus and its presence can be confirmed by electron microscopy. The symptoms may not be severe, but the loose stools and low grade fever with failure to gain weight may persist for more than a week. The stools are voided in explosive fashion and tend to be watery, yellow and acid, but seldom contain mucus, pus or blood. The condition of the infant may deteriorate rapidly, and the need for rehydration may become urgent. The condition may improve only to relapse during treatment, and the infant may develop intercurrent infections of the lungs, ears or septicaemia. The infectivity is high, and the disease may spread in nurseries in epidemic form.

Isolation and full barrier nursing is essential as soon as the diagnosis is suspected. The treatment consists of the cessation of milk feeding and oral or intravenous administration of electrolyte-containing fluids to combat dehydration and acidosis.

Necrotizing enterocolitis

Necrotizing enterocolitis (NEC) is a severe illness usually seen in preterm infants. The exact cause is not known but it is probably due to a combination of factors including gut ischaemia, infection and the effects of hypoxia from birth asphyxia or secondary to respiratory distress syndrome. Sporadic cases are not infrequent in neonatal intensive care units especially in very small preterm infants and from time to time epidemic outbreaks also appear. NEC is occasionally seen even in healthy infants.

The baby presents with shock, lethargy, poor feeding, abdominal distension and the passage of blood-stained stools. Abdominal radiograph usually shows distended oedematous loops of bowel and in severe cases intramural gas bubbles in the bowel wall (pneumatosis intestinalis).

Treatment is to stop oral feeds and commence nasogastric suction. The baby will need intravenous fluids and parenteral nutrition. Antibiotics including penicillin, gentamicin and metronidazole are given. Shock and acidosis should be treated with blood, plasma and sodium bicarbonate. Surgery is required for those who deteriorate further or who develop perforation of the gut. This is a high risk procedure, especially in very preterm infants. NEC has a significant mortality and morbidity at all gestations and some infants who survive the intial illness go on to have malabsorption syndromes or develop late strictures of the gut.

COLIC

Colic is manifest by screaming, flushing of the face, clenching of the fists, flexing of the arms and legs and tenseness of the abdominal wall. The common causes are distension of the gut with wind or spasmodic contractions of the gut due to some irritative stimulus. Swallowing of air and failure to help the baby bring it up is the most common cause, but improper feeding techniques may be responsible. When it is obvious that the colic is severe, or the baby has screaming attacks, the possibility of some mechanical obstruction such as volvulus or intussusception must be considered.

Elimination of the cause, whether it is aerophagy or improper feeding will relieve most cases.

CONSTIPATION

True constipation in the newborn infant is comparatively uncommon. Cases of obstruction such as gut atresia have already been mentioned. Hirschprung's disease does not usually give rise to marked symptoms in the neonatal period, although delay in the passage of the first meconium may be the earliest sign of this condition. Constipation in young infants is usually a variation in normal bowel habit, and the passage of hard motions at irregular intervals is most commonly the result of insufficient intake of food or fluid, or the use of artificial feeds which are too rich in protein or too low in sugar content. Treatment consists in correction of the dietary error and giving extra water.

Once lactation is fully established in breast fed babies stools may be passed infrequently. It is not unusual for two or three days to elapse without a stool being passed, but when it appears it is yellow and pasty. Obviously no treatment is required.

METABOLIC DISTURBANCES

Hypoglycaemia

Hypoglycaemia in the newborn is present when the true plasma glucose concentration is below 1.1 mmol/L (20 mg/100 ml). It is particularly likely to occur in the first 72 hours of life in babies who are small-for-gestational-age, but it may develop in any baby under stress, for example in the respiratory distress syndrome, in congestive cardiac failure or following exchange transfusion. It may be found in infants of diabetic mothers and in other infants who are large-for-gestational-age. The diagnosis should be considered in any baby who exhibits a sudden fall in temperature, twitching, convulsions, eye-rolling, apathy, refusal to feed, apnoeic spells or, in extreme cases, coma. Consideration of the likely causes is important in management.

In the light-for-dates baby, or the baby who has suffered from placental insufficiency, there has been depletion of the glycogen stores and the aim must be to replenish them. In these babies, although they have no symptoms, three-hourly Dextrostix tests on blood from a heel stab may reveal low levels of glucose. Such asymptomatic hypoglycaemia has an excellent prognosis and symptoms can be prevented by early and frequent feeding. If symptoms have already occurred nasogastric feeding is started at once without waiting for laboratory confirmation of the plasma glucose level and the Dextrostix is rechecked. If there have been convulsions intravenous glucose solution, 5 ml per kg of 20 per cent solution, is given *immediately*. Thereafter Dextrostix tests are carried out to confirm that the hypoglycaemia has been relieved. Only in a resistant case is it necessary to administer 10 per cent glucose solution intravenously. The advantage of intragastric infusion is the ease of administration, and the avoidance of the risk of reactive hypoglycaemia if the intravenous infusion stops for one reason or another.

The baby is also receiving valuable nutrients.

The problem in the large-for-dates babies or the babies of diabetic mothers is different. In these infants the liver is likely to be full of glycogen, but hyperplasia of the islet cells in the pancreas results in high blood insulin levels, particularly in response to glucose administration. The widespread practice of giving intermittent glucose drinks to these babies can sometimes provoke hypoglycaemia. In practice early milk feeding has proved most successful. Glucose can be released from glycogen stores by administering glucagon, but it is more practical to give small doses of hydrocortisone (5 mg six-hourly) if hypoglycaemia proves to be persistent in these babies.

Hypocalcaemia

Some preterm or small-for-dates babies develop tetany or other symptoms from hypocalcaemia after birth. These infants show twitching and neuromuscular irritability, increased muscular tone, and are often vomiting. If the plasma calcium level is lower than 1.8 mmol/L (7 mg/100 ml) treatment will depend on whether convulsions are continuing. If they have ceased it is sufficient to add 3 ml of 10 per cent calcium gluconate solution to each feed. The total daily dose of calcium gluconate solution should not exceed 20 ml, otherwise diarrhoea may occur. If convulsions are continuing the calcium gluconate solution is diluted to 2.5 per cent concentration with 5 per cent glucose solution and injected *slowly*, intravenously, until the convulsions cease. Not more than 4 ml/kg body weight of this solution should be given at one time. The heart rate is monitored during the injection, which is stopped if bradycardia occurs. Thereafter calcium gluconate is added to the feeds until the plasma calcium concentration rises to normal. In infants with hypocalcaemia it is always important to check the magnesium as well as the calcium levels. Hypocalcaemia is difficult to correct unless the magnesium levels are normal.

Inborn errors of metabolism

Many of these are not detected until after the neonatal period. Phenylketonuria and galactosaemia deserve mention as their early detection will lead to dietary measures which will reduce their ill effects.

Phenylketonuria

Phenylketonuria is inherited as a recessive condition. There is inability to convert phenylalanine to tyrosine. Phenylalanine accumulates in the body fluids, and when the blood level rises to a dangerous point alternative metabolic pathways convert it to phenylpyruvic acid and other substances which are excreted in the urine.

The infant appears normal, and is often strikingly blond with blue eyes. Deterioration occurs as the child grows, with progressive neurological disease and mental retardation. Phenylalanine is not excreted in the urine until the blood level reaches 1.8 mmol/L (30 mg per 100 ml) which is a toxic level, but the renal threshold for phenyl ketones is about half this. However, testing for phenylpyruvic acid in the urine with ferric chloride has not proved to be a satisfactory screening test in newborn infants, and the Guthrie microbiological test for the blood level of phenylalanine must be performed. For the test one drop of blood is taken on the seventh day (i.e. after at least six days of milk feeds). The test gives early warning of the disease, and if treatment with a diet low in phenylalanine is started in early infancy mental retardation can be prevented.

Galactosaemia

Galactosaemia is inherited as a recessive trait. There is a defect in the metabolism of galactose, which is derived from the lactose in milk. Enzyme lack prevents the conversion of galactose to glucose-1-phosphate, which is necessary if galactose is to be utilized by the tissues. Galactose accumulates in the body and appears in the urine. The infant appears normal at birth, but listlessness, vomiting, anorexia and weight loss soon appear, with jaundice and hepatomegaly. Cataracts, mental retardation and cirrhosis of the liver develop in untreated cases.

Galactose in the urine is detected by Clinitest strips, but not by Clinistix. Routine testing of the urine of babies with jaundice, especially those with hepatomegaly, will detect the condition. The diagnosis is confirmed by urine chromatography and deficiency of the enzyme (galactose-1-phosphate uridyl transferase) can be confirmed by testing the infant's red blood corpuscles. Treatment consists of withdrawing all dietary lactose and feeding synthetic galactose-free milk.

Neonatal cold injury

Babies are sometimes admitted after cold injury. They are cold to touch, apathetic and immobile. They may refuse to feed. The colour may be pink, but there is oedema of the hands and feet, and a firm texture to the subcutaneous fat. The rectal temperature may be 27–32°C and the respiration and pulse rate are slow. They must be warmed very gradually to a normal temperature while glucose solution is given intravenously.

HAEMORRHAGIC STATES IN THE NEWBORN

Haemorrhagic disease

In this condition there is a tendency to spontaneous and prolonged bleeding in the first week of life, usually from the second to the fifth day. The common site of bleeding is the gut, causing vomiting of blood or melaena, but the lungs, skin, brain or mucous membranes may be affected. The bleeding coincides with the period of low prothrombin level which occurs in the newborn infant from the second to the seventh day, when the level of prothrombin may fall to 20 per cent of normal, but some other factors may also be involved. Bleeding and clotting times and the platelet count may be abnormal. The prothrombin level may be raised to normal by administration of vitamin K_1, but not every case responds to this treatment. In such unresponsive cases infusion of fresh-frozen plasma arrests the haemorrhage. An intramuscular injection of 0.5–1 mg of phytomenadione (vitamin K_1) is usually sufficient. Normal infants are given oral vitamin K at birth as routine prophylaxis.

Disseminated intravascular coagulation

A more serious disorder may occur, especially in sick babies of low birth weight, as a complication of septicaemia. Disseminated intravascular coagulation (DIC) is due to widespread intravascular coagulation and consumption of available clotting factors. Severe bleeding may occur from almost any site, and there is widespread purpura because of the low platelet count. There is an increase in fibrin degradation products and blood films show numerous fragmented red cells. The only effective treatment is replacement of red blood cells and clotting factors with appropriate blood products; fresh platelets may also be required. The condition will resolve only if the underlying infection is controlled. Exchange transfusion is sometimes life-saving. Heparin is of little value because the coagulation has already occurred.

Umbilical bleeding

This may occur from a slipped ligature in the first 24 hours, or from infection of the stump after the cord has separated. The baby may be shocked as 30 ml of blood lost is equivalent to about 10 per cent of the baby's total blood volume. A fresh ligature must be applied, or if the cord has separated the bleeding point must be controlled by pressure from a mattress suture or application of artery forceps. Blood transfusion may be required urgently.

Thrombocytopenic purpura

Congenital thrombocytopenia may cause a petechial rash, ecchymoses and bleeding from various sites. It is to be distinguished from simple traumatic purpura of the head and neck caused by pressure; in the latter the platelet count is not reduced. The infant is frequently affected if the mother has had thrombocytopenic purpura during pregnancy. Most cases resolve quickly, but it may be necessary to treat the infant with platelets or steroids if there is severe thrombocytopenia.

Anaemia

The most common cause of anaemia at birth is haemolytic disease; otherwise it is usually the result of haemorrhage. Haemorrhage may occur from tearing of the cord during delivery, incision of the placenta during caesarean section, or from bleeding from the fetal side of the placenta during delivery. The infant may be pale at birth with a low haemoglobin level. Immediate transfusion may be required.

Bleeding from the fetal into the maternal circulation may occur and can be proved by the demonstration of fetal cells in the mother's blood (*see* p. 319) but is hardly ever of such an amount as to cause fatal anaemia. Occasionally in twin pregnancies with a shared placenta one twin may lose blood into the circulation of the other. At birth one twin may be pale and anaemic, while the other is polycythaemic. Death *in utero* of one or both twins may occur.

Vaginal bleeding

Slight bleeding from the endometrium occasionally occurs as a result of withdrawal of maternal oestrogens.

JAUNDICE IN THE NEWBORN INFANT

Jaundice (icterus) in the neonatal period may be due to a variety of causes. Breakdown of red blood cells results in the production of indirect, non-conjugated bilirubin, which is insoluble in water and is carried in the serum bound to albumin. Normally this type of bilirubin is conjugated in the liver to form water-soluble bilirubin glucuronide which is excreted in the bile. Conjugation is effected by the glucuronyl transferase system of enzymes. In the newborn infant this enzyme system is at first inadequate, and the concentration of unconjugated bilirubin may rise in the serum for a few days and cause physiological jaundice. In cases of haemolytic disease and in some premature infants excess bilirubin may cross the blood–brain barrier and damage the basal ganglia. This is called kernicterus (*see* page 320).

Physiological jaundice

This does not begin before the second day; it may last for only a few days or until the 10th day. The skin is lemon yellow in colour, so are the conjunctivae. The liver and spleen are not increased in size and the stools remain normal in colour. There is no fever or constitutional upset, although the infant may be sleepy and less eager for food. No special treatment is required and the prognosis is entirely favourable, except in premature infants in whom kernicterus can occur if the bilirubin level is high. The exact level at which this occurs varies with the baby's gestation and general condition. In the term infant levels in excess of 360 μmol/L for prolonged periods are dangerous. In the preterm infant much lower levels are potentially toxic to the brain and can cause hearing impairment, even in the absence of kernicterus itself. Treatment is with phototherapy using special light units. In severe cases exchange transfusion may be needed.

Jaundice in the neonatal period may have many pathological causes:

Haemolytic disease

See page 319.

Congenital spherocytosis (acholuric jaundice)

This is a rare cause of familial haemolytic anaemia and jaundice.

Congenital atresia of the bile ducts

This rare anomaly may be partial or complete. Jaundice appears at the end of the first week of life or later. The liver enlarges progressively and becomes firm, the stools become white and the urine contains bile. Special investigations including ultrasound and radioisotope liver scan are required. Fifteen per cent of the infants have extrahepatic atresia which can be treated surgically. A few cases of successful liver transplant have also been reported.

Sepsis

Sepsis, especially when accompanied by septicaemia, may cause anaemia and jaundice after the first few days of life. A urinary tract infection may be associated with jaundice of hepatic origin.

Syphilis

Congenital infection may cause skin rashes, nasal obstruction and hepatosplenomegaly.

Toxoplasmosis

Mothers who have suffered an occult infection with the protozoon *Toxoplasma gondii* may give birth to infants affected by the disease. Internal hydrocephalus, choroidoretinitis, fits and mental retardation may result. If infection occurs shortly before birth the infant may have hepatosplenomegaly and jaundice. Diagnosis is made by complement fixation tests and tests for dye-modifying antibodies. Treatment is available but is not always effective.

Viral infections

Intrauterine infection with rubella or cytomegalovirus may cause neonatal jaundice associated with thrombocytopenic purpura and hepatosplenomegaly. In both cases estimation of the titre of antibodies, especially specific IgM, will assist in the diagnosis. It is important to remember that affected infants excrete live virus.

Infection with herpes virus is another cause of neonatal hepatitis with jaundice. The infection is usually acquired from the mother during delivery. In severe cases signs of general infection appear during the latter part of the first week or during the second week. The disease is often fatal. Treatment with acyclovir may modify the infection.

Neonatal infection caused by the hepatitis viruses may also occur, with hepatic enlargement, jaundice, and often splenomegaly. The jaundice may be prolonged, with obstructive features clinically indistinguishable from those of congenital atresia of the bile ducts. Infants at risk should be given hepatitis vaccine.

Coxsackie B group virus may rarely cause generalized infection of the newborn, with myocarditis, encephalitis and hepatitis. There is a high mortality.

Glucose-6-phosphate dehydrogenase deficiency (G-6-PD)

The genetically determined deficiency of this enzyme, which is essential for the survival of erythrocytes, is not uncommon in Asiatic and Mediterranean races, and a less severe form occurs in Africa. Spontaneous destruction of red cells in the neonatal period may cause haemolytic jaundice, and later this may be precipitated by various drugs.

Galactosaemia

This inherited metabolic disorder usually presents with persistent jaundice and hepatomegaly (*see* p. 309).

Congenital hypothyroidism

Prolonged neonatal jaundice without any obvious cause, especially in an apathetic anorexic infant, should raise the suspicion of hypothyroidism.

All neonates are screened for this during the first

week of life by the measurement of TSH on the dried blood spot (Guthrie) card which is also used to screen for phenylketonuria.

Management of neonatal jaundice

The most important question to ask is when the jaundice appeared. Jaundice appearing within the first 24 hours of life is almost certainly pathological and due to rhesus or ABO incompatibility. A Coombs' test, ABO and rhesus grouping of the infant, and examination of a blood film for spherocytes are obligatory.

Jaundice appearing from the second to the fifth days of life is often physiological, whereas jaundice appearing for the first time after this is usually pathological. Significant jaundice at any age requires a careful search for infection, exclusion of haemolytic disorders and measurements of enzymes such as G-6-PD in susceptible infants.

In cases of early jaundice caused by haemolysis the bilirubin can be reduced by phototherapy with a specially constructed light unit that avoids overheating. The baby's eyes must be covered to avoid conjunctival reaction. Blue light converts bilirubin in the skin to other compounds which are not harmful to the brain. Those with rapidly rising bilirubin levels will need exchange transfusion.

CONGENITAL MALFORMATIONS

The cause of many congenital malformations is unknown. Some are genetically determined; others have been attributed to pressure effects related to the intrauterine posture of the fetus, to the adverse effects of drugs, radiation, fetal infections or metabolic disturbances. The fetal tissues which are most actively growing at the time when the adverse factor operates are most likely to show the defect.

The malformations which may occur are numerous and varied. Some are incompatible with life and no treatment is possible. The lesions which are especially important to recognize in the neonatal period are those which endanger life but which, with prompt intervention, can be treated. Other lesions can be treated later in infancy. An increasing number are now recognized prenatally by ultrasound.

Rubella syndrome

See page 113.

Congenital heart disease

Precise diagnosis is difficult at this age but the presence of cardiac disease should be recognized in most cases by careful examination. During the routine examination the apex beat and femoral pulses should be palpated. Since it is not always easy to feel the apex beat in the newborn it is useful to place a finger just below the xiphisternum to assess the strength of epigastric pulsation; this will be increased if there is cardiac enlargement.

Absent or weak femoral pulses will suggest the diagnosis of coarctation of the aorta. The blood pressure in all four limbs can be measured by the 'flush' method. A cuff is inflated after the limb is squeezed until it is blanched. As the pressure is slowly released the limb will suddenly flush. The pressure reading at that moment gives the mean systolic pressure. In coarctation the pressure is lower in the legs than in the arms. Automatic blood pressure monitors allow more accurate measurement.

If the pulses in all four limbs are easily felt and seem to be collapsing in quality the diagnosis of patent ductus arteriosus is suggested, there may be a continuous systolic murmur in the second left interspace below the clavicle.

Soft basal murmurs may come and go in the normal newborn infant, but harsh systolic murmurs are likely to be due to aortic or pulmonary stenosis. The most common form of congenital heart disease, ventricular septal defect (VSD), does not usually produce symptoms in the immediate neonatal period. It may take four weeks for the pulmonary vascular resistance to fall sufficiently to allow a significant pressure gradient between the ventricles to develop, and there may not be an appreciable left to right shunt until this happens.

Cyanotic heart lesions have been mentioned on page 297.

Laryngeal stridor

This may accompany inspiration in some newborn babies. It is worse with crying and quietens when the baby is asleep. There is often indrawing of the lower ribs. The cause is debatable, but it is usually attributed to congenital softening of the cartilage of the larynx, with infolding of the epiglottis during inspiration. The condition usually resolves by the time the infant is 1 year of age. Rarely, more severe stridor is caused by congenital anomalies such as a laryngeal web or cyst or a vascular ring.

Oesophageal atresia and tracheal fistula

See page 327.

Intestinal obstruction

See pages 305 and 327.

Imperforate anus

This abnormality must be looked for carefully at the first examination. The gap between the anal dimple and the blind rectal pouch may be only membrane thick or several centimetres wide. The rectal pouch may communicate with the vagina, urethra or bladder. The infant must be referred for surgical treatment at once.

Umbilical variations

The skin of the abdominal wall normally invests the base of the umbilical cord for a short distance and, when the cord separates the skin, dimples to form the naval. If the skin extends onto the cord further than usual, separation of the cord leaves a protruding cylinder of skin. Such a *cutis navel* needs no treatment and will be taken into the abdominal wall with growth. When the skin does not reach the base of the cord a wide raw area is left which heals by granulation and fibrosis – the *amnion navel.*

Meckel's diverticulum may form an intestinal fistula at the umbilicus. A persistent urachus may form a urinary fistula or a cystic swelling deep to the navel.

A single umbilical artery is found in a small number of infants and may occasionally be associated with other congenital abnormalities of the genitourinary tract or the cardiovascular system.

Umbilical hernia

The gap in the rectus sheath through which the components of the cord enter the abdominal cavity can be felt as a ring after separation of the cord. Normally this closes down, but sometimes an umbilical hernia forms. Most cases resolve spontaneously although a few will require surgical treatment later in childhood. The application of external pressure is never indicated.

Exomphalos

The infant is born with an extensive defect of the anterior abdominal wall and the intestines are extruded, usually covered by peritoneum. The condition looks very grave, but if no other gross congenital defect exists the viscera should be covered with sterile dressings and surgical advice immediately obtained. It is usually possible to repair the defect if the operation is performed in a neonatal surgical centre.

Cleft lip and cleft palate

These lesions cause surprisingly little difficulty in feeding. Breast feeding can be successfully achieved but bottle feeding may be more difficult, and it may be necessary to resort to cup and spoon. A cleft palate may permit milk to enter the nose and cause choking. Early reference to a plastic surgeon is advisable so that treatment can be planned. Some centres are now performing immediate closure of the cleft lip in the neonatal period.

Congenital dislocation of the hip

In the newborn infant this is a potential rather than an actual dislocation. The hips of the newborn are examined for excessive mobility or for a characteristic clunk felt on full abduction of the flexed thighs, which is suggestive of dislocation. Because congential dislocation of the hip is almost entirely preventable, it is important that all doctors who are involved with routine examination of the newborn should learn the technique of examination of the hips from a senior colleague who is experienced in the method. Orthopaedic advice must be sought in any doubtful case, and early follow-up and treatment may prevent trouble in later infancy.

Talipes equinovarus

The intrauterine position of the fetus tends to produce this deformity. When true adduction is present treatment by manipulation and splinting must be started at once.

Spina bifida and meningocele

Failure of fusion of the vertebral arches permits herniation of the meninges at any level in the spinal column, usually in the lumbar area. The herniation may be covered with skin or only by a bluish membranous roof, and the sac may include nerve roots or spinal cord (myelomeningocele), which can be recognized as a flat or raised neural plaque in the midline. The absence of the various coverings which protect the cord allows meningeal infection to occur early, but this can be prevented by immediate surgery to cover the defect. However, the overall prognosis is poor with the more severe lesions, with complete paralysis of legs, incontinence of urine and faeces, and the probable association with hydrocephalus. It is important that babies with a relatively good prognosis should be sent to a special centre where appropriate surgery can be performed without delay. Only experience can decide whether it is justifiable to operate on very severe cases.

Neural tube defects can be diagnosed *in utero* by amniocentesis and testing the amniotic fluid for α-fetoprotein (*see* p. 274). Testing the maternal serum for fetoprotein may serve as a preliminary screening test, but the diagnosis must be confirmed by amniocentesis before termination of pregnancy is considered. The defect may also be demonstrated by ultrasound examination.

The incidence of neural tube defects, including both spina bifida and anencephaly, varies from about 1 to about 7 per 1000 births, being highest in Ireland, South Wales, Northwest England and Southern Scotland, and in social classes IV and V. In addition, if a woman has had a child with a neural tube defect the risk is increased by about nine times over these figures. Claims that the incidence can be reduced by vitamin supplements in early pregnancy are being investigated.

Hydrocephalus

Hydrocephalus is caused by impaired circulation of the cerebrospinal fluid. The most common cause nowadays is obstruction to the flow of cerebrospinal fluid following intraventricular haemorrhage in the preterm infant. The head enlarges and the sutures and fontanelles are wide and bulging. There is sometimes an associated myelomeningocele. The condition may be present before birth due to congenital malformation and obstructs labour, or the baby may show slight enlargement of the head after birth. If hydrocephalus is suspected frequent cerebral ultrasound is performed and the head circumference is measured

every two to three days, if the rate of growth is much faster than normal a neurosurgical opinion is sought, as it is possible to prevent progression of the hydrocephalus by repeated lumbar puncture, intraventricular tap or by insertion of a valve.

Down's syndrome

This is caused by a chromosomal abnormality. In about 95 per cent of cases there are 47 chromosomes instead of 46. The extra chromosome is present because of non-disjunction of chromosome 21 (trisomy 21). In a small proportion of affected infants there are 46 chromosomes but one is abnormally large, probably number 15 which incorporates part of number 21 from a translocation.

The syndrome can often be diagnosed soon after birth. The infant has a flat face with slanting eyes, epicanthic folds, a snub nose, a mouth like an inverted bow, and often a protruding tongue. The head is round with a poorly developed occiput and unusual ears. The posterior and third fontanelle are often easily palpable. The infant is hypotonic with over-extensible joints. The hands show a single transverse palmar crease and incurving (clinodactyly) of the little finger and there is a simian cleft between the great and the next toe. Congenital heart disease may be detected.

The incidence of the syndrome is about 1.5 per 1000 births. The incidence rises sharply with maternal age and reaches 1 in 50 when the mother's age is over 40. Increased paternal age may also increase the risk. Chromosomal studies should be undertaken when a young mother gives birth to an affected infant. If the baby is found to have a translocation of chromosome 21, the discovery of translocation in either parent indicates a greatly increased risk of another affected child in any subsequent pregnancy. If it is found in the mother approximately 20 per cent of her later children may be affected; and if in the father the risk is about 6 per cent.

Down's syndrome may be diagnosed *in utero* by using chorionic villous sampling or amniocentesis to obtain fetal amniotic cells for tissue culture and chromosomal study. If the abnormality is found to be present termination of pregnancy should be considered. Such a test should be offered to women aged 38 and over (in some centres it is offered at 35), to those who already have an affected child and if either parent is known to have an abnormal chromosomal pattern, provided that they understand that the test carries some risk to the fetus. Maternal serum α-fetoprotein levels are generally lower if the mother has a fetus with Down's syndrome, probably due to reduced fetal production of that and other proteins. Hence Down's syndrome may be suspected among those with AFP levels below 0.4 multiples of the median for gestational age. If this is combined with hCG and oestrogen levels in the maternal blood a powerful prediction of Down's syndrome is produced. This puts more younger women in to the higher risk category and make amniocentesis and chromosomal testing for trisomy 21 worthwhile. Older women with high AFP values in their blood are less at risk of having a fetus with Down's syndrome.

Renal agenesis (Potter's syndrome)

This condition is often associated with oligo-hydramnios. Both kidneys fail to develop. The infant has wide set eyes, a flattened nose, a receding chin and low-set ears with poorly formed cartilage. The infant dies within a few hours.

Abnormalities of the male genitourinary system

All degrees of hypospadias and epispadias may be met. In the milder degrees of hypospadias it may be thought that the meatal orifice is not patent, but careful search will reveal a minute orifice on the ventral surface of the corona or shaft of the penis. The meatus is sometimes stenosed and so it is important to see the urinary stream, as meatotomy is sometimes required. Coronal hypospadias is also sometimes associated with curvature of the penis (chordee). In such cases it is important to avoid circumcision, as the surgeon may wish to use preputial skin during corrective operation at a later date.

Hydrocele may occur in the neonatal period, but requires no treatment as it usually resolves spontaneously within a few weeks.

Circumcision

There are no medical grounds for circumcision in infancy. Retraction of the foreskin may suggest the presence of phimosis, but if the prepuce is drawn gently forwards (as happens during micturition) it will be seen that it opens up to reveal an adequate channel. Indeed the foreskin should never be retracted in the baby, because this may lead to tearing and scarring and genuine phimosis as a result. The parents should be advised to leave the foreskin alone and allow it to retract normally as the boy grows. The presence of the preputial covering prevents meatal ulceration which could otherwise occur from the contact of wet napkins.

Ritual circumcision is practised on Jewish and Muslim infants and is usually performed on the eighth day. It is sometimes necessary to advise that the operation should be postponed if the infant is ill, jaundiced or shows undue loss of weight. It is wise to maintain a close watch for haemorrhage for the 12 hours following the circumcision, which is not always performed by the usual surgical technique.

Abnormalities of the female genitalia

Pseudohermaphroditism is usually due to the ad-renogenital syndrome. (*See Gynaecology by Ten Teachers.*) Hypertrophy of the clitoris may occur if the mother has been given large doses of prog-estogens for habitual abortion.

Labial adhesions

The female external genitalia may appear abnormal because adhesions between the labia minora obscure the urethral and vaginal orifices. The adhesions separate easily if the labia are drawn apart.

RESPIRATORY PROBLEMS

The establishment of breathing after birth is the most important function which the newborn infant must perform in order to adapt to extrauterine life. A number of respiratory problems which interfere with the normal adaptive processes at this stage are seen in the neonatal period.

Transient tachypnoea of the newborn

The absorption of fluid (mainly into the lymph-atics) and the progressive expansion of the alveoli by respiratory movements is usually rapid, occurring within a few minutes after birth, but total expansion may not be attained for some hours, especially in a preterm infant.

The tissues round the lung roots and the posterior parts of the lower lobes are the last to expand. When the process is particularly slow the infant may develop worrying symptoms. Some babies born by caesarean section, for example, may take some time to clear their lungs of fluid, and auscultation of the lung bases posteriorly may reveal fine crepitations. Such babies have rapid shallow respirations, often associated with an expiratory grunt, and cyanosis may be present. This condition is known as *transient tachypnoea of the newborn*. A radiograph of the chest will usually reveal the excess fluid by the presence of an 'air bronchogram' in some part of the lung fields and perhaps some hazy or streaky shadowing.

As a rule the only treatment necessary is to keep the baby warm, to increase the ambient oxygen until cyanosis is relieved and then to diminish the oxygen concentration as the condition improves. These babies should be nursed in an incubator where heart rate, temperature and respiration can be closely monitored. Blood gases should be measured at regular intervals of three to four hours. Continuous oxygen monitoring should be instituted by transcutaneous probe or by a saturation monitor. A chest radiograph should be performed to exclude other causes of respiratory distress. Rarely the condition deteriorates to such an extent that intubation and assisted ventilation is required. In most cases differentiation from neonatal pneumonia is not possible and antibiotics are given. In view of the possibility of infection by the Group B haemolytic streptococcus high doses of penicillin, preferably combined with gentamicin, are recommended pending the result of bacteriological reports (*see* p. 317).

Respiratory distress syndrome (hyaline membrane disease)

This condition is most commonly found in small preterm babies, but it also occurs in the infants of diabetic or prediabetic mothers; it is rare in term infants. Perinatal hypoxia is a predisposing factor. Caesarean section should not be associated with an increased incidence if care is taken to avoid hypoxia. With increasing skill in the management of preterm deliveries and early and effective resuscitation, the incidence of this disorder has fallen in recent years.

The syndrome occurs when there is deficiency of surfactant, either because of immaturity of the lungs or because the function of the Type II pneumocytes which produce it is temporarily depressed by hypoxia. After about 34 weeks gestation surfactant is normally produced in adequate quantities. When a decision to effect delivery before term is being considered the level of surfactant production can be checked by amniocentesis and measurement of the lecithin content of the amniotic fluid. Since absolute measurements will be dependent on the degree of dilution by amniotic fluid this is commonly expressed as a ratio of lecithin to sphingomyelin. When the L/S ratio is 2:1 or greater all should be well, but a ratio of under 1.5:1 means that there is a high risk of hyaline membrane disease, of the order of 75 per cent. There is some evidence that when the fetus has been subjected to stress, including that of labour, the L/S ratio is increased. There is also evidence that administration of corticosteroids to the mother will facilitate the production of surfactant if the steroids are given for at least 24 hours immediately preceding delivery. Betamethasone or dexamethasone are usually used. Difficulty in predicting the time of delivery, and possible risk of infection to the mother limit the use of this treatment. It is not usually effective at less than 28 weeks gestation.

The diagnosis is suspected when respiratory distress develops within two or three hours of birth with an expiratory grunt, increased respiratory rate to more than 60 per minute, indrawing of the lower chest and intercostal recession. In room air there is cyanosis, and on auscultation there are usually diminished breath sounds and fine crepitations throughout the chest; generalized oedema is often present. A radiograph of the chest has a ground-glass appearance or a reticular pattern, with an 'air bronchogram' where the air in the bronchi contrasts with the surrounding opaque lung fields. In fatal cases autopsy reveals almost airless lungs and a hyaline membrane lining the terminal air passages which takes up eosinophilic stains. Intraventricular haemorrhage is not uncommon.

As a result of the pulmonary disorder the Pa_{O_2} falls and the Pa_{CO_2} rises. The pH falls from respiratory acidosis, which leads on to metabolic acidosis.

Mildly affected infants recover with no more than good nursing care, warmth, graduated oxygen therapy and minimal handling, but the mortality overall may reach 20 per cent. With modern intensive care even severely ill infants can be saved, and since it is difficult to predict the course of the disease from the outset all affected babies should be transferred at an early stage to a centre with facilities for expert care, including umbilical arterial catherization, monitoring of arterial oxygen tension, administration of oxygen in high concentration, positive pressure ventilation and nasogastric feeding.

Infants with established disease require full support including provision of an adequate environment at the right temperature and humidity to minimize oxygen consumption. Added oxygen should be given to maintain the blood gases in the normal range and any serious acid–base disturbance should be corrected. An adequate fluid, electrolyte and glucose intake should be maintained. A significant proportion however, will develop increasing respiratory failure and require mechanical ventilation which may need to be continued for several days. Modern infant ventilators are highly flexible and the infant can be ventilated in a number of different ways until the most suitable rate and pressure has been found for the individual needs at any time. It is important to apply a positive end expiratory pressure (PEEP) on the ventilator as this maintains airway patency and prevents further alveolar collapse. Other measures which may be required include vasodilating drugs such as Tolazaline to open up the pulmonary vascular bed. Paralysis with pancuronium is required in selected cases if an infant cannot synchronize with the ventilator. All neonates with respiratory distress require antibiotics such as penicillin and gentamicin or a third generation cephalosporin, because of the risk of Group B streptococcal pneumonia mimicking respiratory distress syndrome.

Most neonates respond satisfactorily to this treatment and can be weaned from the ventilator. However, a significant proportion develop complications such as pneumothorax, pulmonary infection or chronic lung disease such as bronchopulmonary dysplasia. These infants require intensive treatment for a considerably longer period.

Although it is difficult to administer, attempts have been made to treat the disease with surfactant. Recent studies have reported a reduced mortality and morbidity with the use of various synthetic or animal surfactant preparations; however, the effects only last for a few hours. There is a theoretical risk that animal surfactant may cause immunological problems. Human surfactant is not easily available, although it could be harvested from amniotic fluid.

Pneumothorax

Pneumothorax is also a common complication for babies who require ventilation and it occurs in 15 to 40 per cent of cases. Because the air is being introduced under positive pressure it can also leak into the tissues leading to pulmonary interstitial emphysema and pneumomediastinum. Most of this air will absorb with time but air in the pleural cavity requires direct drainage, often with suction, in order to allow the lung to re-expand. Acute pneumothorax is associated with a rapid rise in carbon dioxide level and a reduction in oxygen, both of which result in increased cerebral perfusion accompanied by hypoxia. These effects can be damaging to the brain. There is a direct link between pneumothorax and intraventricular haemorrhage.

Infection with Group B streptococcus

Thsis organism requires special mention because in recent years it has become an important pathogen for the newborn baby. The infection is acquired from the maternal genital tract and the present rate of carriage in the UK is about 15 per cent. Colonization of the throat or the body surface occurs in 20–60 per cent of infants but only 1–2 per cent of those who are colonized develop systemic disease. The presenting features are identical to respiratory distress syndrome, and there is an increased risk of systemic infection in those who are of low birth weight, who have had prolonged rupture of the membranes and who have suffered from birth asphyxia. The respiratory rate is raised, with indrawing of the intercostal muscles, grunting and cyanosis. Chest X-ray shows extensive bilateral shadowing identical to that seen in hyaline membrane disease. Treatment consists of high dose penicillin and gentamicin and full respiratory support. Despite these measures the mortality rate is of the order of 50 per cent.

A late onset type of infection also occurs most commonly at the age of three to four weeks, although it is sometimes seen earlier than this, even during the first week. This results in meningitis, which also has a high morbidity and mortality. This is discussed on page 325.

Meconium aspiration syndrome

The passage of meconium before birth is seen in 8–15 per cent of deliveries. Infants who are asphyxiated commence gasping movements either *in utero* or immediately after birth and inhale meconium into the large and small airways. Meconium has a low pH and is irritant to the lungs so, apart from mechanical obstruction, aspiration results in a chemical pneumonitis. Any bacteria which may be present can also cause infection.

The clinical problems which are seen include respiratory distress but in this case the lungs are overinflated with patchy areas of a collapse-consolidation elsewhere. There is a high incidence of air leak leading to pneumothroax and pneumomediastinum in as many as 40–50 per cent of significantly affected infants. Treatment is preventive whenever possible, as most cases are associated with birth asphyxia. Suction of meconium from the upper airway and trachea after birth and before breathing is established is the next most important preventive measure that can be taken. For those who do develop symptoms ventilatory support is often required. There is a small but significant mortality but in those who survive complete recovery is usual.

Pulmonary haemorrhage

This condition occurs most frequently between the second and fourth days of life and is seen in infants who have had preceding birth asphyxia, infection, rhesus disease, meconium aspiration syndrome or acute left heart failure.

Treatment consists of correction of any clotting abnormalities which may be present, including the administration of fresh frozen plasma and vitamin K, and mechanical ventilation with a moderately raised end expiratory pressure which helps to prevent the development of associated pulmonary oedema.

Pulmonary haemorrhage is much less common than it used to be due to better perinatal management of the preterm infant.

Bronchopulmonary dysplasia

A proportion of infants who are ventilated develop longer term pulmonary problems secondary to the underlying disease and need treatment with high concentrations of oxygen and ventilation, particu-larly if high pressures are required. The most common complication of this type is bronchopulmonary dysplasia, which occurs in up to 20 per cent of ventilated infants. Such children require continuing respiratory support until they are more than one month of age. They also have chronic changes on the chest X-ray. These include generalized hazy shadowing with areas of chronic collapse consolidation alternating with areas of significant over-inflation and emphysema. More recently the emphysematous changes have been seen less frequently, particularly in extremely low birthweight infants (<1000 g at birth). Prolonged treatment with oxygen, and ventilation, is often required and may be necessary for a period of weeks, months or even years in some cases. Bronchoconstriction requiring the use of bronchodilators such as beta-agonists and theophylline is common. Some infants develop cor pulmonale, which requires treatment with diuretic therapy.

The long-term problems for these infants include failure to thrive and poor growth, recurrent respiratory infections, particularly during the first two years of life, and recurrent episodes of wheezing due to bronchial hyper-reactivity. As many as one-third die during the first year of life but those who survive show gradually improving lung function and most are able to lead a normal life, although they do have persistent abnormalities on respiratory function testing. The long-term effects of these chronic changes on the aetiology of adult lung disease is not yet known.

Apnoeic spells with cyanosis

Preterm infants are especially liable to periods of apnoea which may be life threatening, although if the baby is stimulated to breath within 15 seconds from the onset of apnoea normal respiration is usually re-established without much difficulty. Longer periods of apnoea may not respond to simple methods of stimulation and the baby requires resuscitation by bag and mask or intubation. This condition is usually due to immaturity of the respiratory centres in the very preterm infant. However, careful check should be made for other causes, particularly hypoglycaemia, infection such as septicaemia or meningitis and intraventricular haemorrhage. In some cases the apnoeic attacks are a form of seizure. If no other cause is found then the baby should be given parenteral or oral theophylline in carefully adjusted doses according to blood levels. This has been shown to reduce the frequency and severity of apnoeic attacks. Those who fail to respond to this treatment will require intubation and ventilation, which may have to be continued until the respiratory centres are sufficiently mature for such severe episodes to cease.

HAEMOLYTIC DISEASE

It is not yet understood why the maternal immune system does not reject the fetus, whose tissues must contain many factors inherited from the father which could excite the immune mechanisms. The placental barrier is far from perfect, as fetal trophoblast can be found in the maternal lungs and fetal red cells may enter the maternal blood, particularly during labour, and this may cause development of maternal antibodies. Although maternal HLA antibodies do not cause evident damage to the fetus, antibodies against red cells, granulocytes and platelets can be produced, causing haemolytic disease, neonatal neutropenia or neonatal thrombocytopenia. Of these haemolytic disease is the most common, with an incidence of at least 1 in 150 pregnancies.

In haemolytic disease the life span of the red cells of the fetus or newborn infant is shortened by the action of specific antibodies present on the infant's red cells but not present on the mother's red cells. These IgG antibodies come from the maternal plasma and, being small molecules, cross the placenta. Transfer is minimal before the 12th week of gestation, rises slowly to the 24th week, and then increases exponentially until term. Antibodies causing haemolytic disease may be produced by the mother against all known red cell antigens, but most commonly against A or B antigens, rhesus or Kell antigens. Because effective prophylaxis against haemolytic disease caused by rhesus antigen is available, disease caused by other antigens is now more frequently encountered, but it is still necessary to describe the rhesus antigens.

The rhesus antigens

In 1940 Landsteiner and Weiner showed that the red cells of 85 per cent of Caucasians contained a substance that they called the rhesus factor because of its similarity to an antigen found in the red cells of the rhesus monkey. Individuals possessing this factor were called Rh-positive and the others Rh-

negative. Five other antigens related to the rhesus system were subsequently found. Each of the six rhesus antigens (designated C, D, E, c, d, e) is carried on a single gene, and these genes are transmitted in groups of three on a single chromosome (chromosome 1). As the chromosomes are linked in pairs, any person will carry six genes linked in three pairs. Some common examples are CDe/cde, CDe/CDe, cde/cde, cDE/cde, cDE/cDE.

The gene that makes a person Rh-positive is D. This is inherited as a mendelian dominant, and if it is present in either of a pair of chromosomes the individual is Rh-positive; if it is present in neither the individual is Rh-negative. A homozygous Rh-positive father (DD) will pass the D gene to all his offspring, whereas a heterozygous Rh-positive father (Dd) will have an equal chance of having a Rh-positive or a Rh-negative baby by a Rh-negative woman. In European communities 15 per cent of individuals are Rh-negative, 38 per cent are homozygous Rh-positive and 47 per cent are heterozygous Rh-positive.

Rare cases of maternal immunization to one of the other antigens of the rhesus group have been described, but these are weak antigens.

Feto-maternal transfusion

Fetal red cells contain haemoglobin which is more resistant to denaturation with acid than adult haemoglobin. If a film of maternal blood is treated with acid and then stained, any fetal red cells which have entered the maternal circulation can be recognized and counted (Kleihauer and Betke test). By this test it can be shown that it is uncommon for significant feto-maternal transfusion to occur during pregnancy, but that it is a common event during labour, especially during the third stage. Manual removal of the placenta and caesarean section will increase the risk. Immunization is uncommon after spontaneous abortion, but the risk is increased after surgical procedures for termination of pregnancy. If the placenta is punctured during amniocentesis fetal blood may enter the maternal circulation, and external version may have the same effect.

It is probable that less than 0.1 ml of fetal blood is sufficient to cause the initial sensitization to rhesus D antigen, but the maternal response varies greatly. Because feto-maternal transfusion does not usually occur until labour, antibodies to this antigen are not commonly produced during a first pregnancy, but if the mother is sensitized she will show a rapid increase in antibody titre during any subsequent pregnancy in which the fetus is Rh-positive, presumably because of passage of minute amounts of fetal blood into her circulation.

It might be expected that immunization of a mother of blood group O to an A or B factor inherited by the fetus from the father would be common. Naturally occurring antibodies to A or B antigens have IgM molecular size and cannot cross the placenta, but smaller IgG antibodies to these antigens are acquired in significant amounts in many group O mothers. These can cross the placenta to destroy fetal cells of group A or B. Thus, haemolytic disease from ABO incompatibility may occur in a first pregnancy. Fortunately the disease is not usually so severe as that due to rhesus incompatibility, and less than 5 per cent of cases will need treatment.

Because there is now an effective method of preventing sensitization against D antigen (*see* p. 322) haemolytic disease from this cause ought to disappear. The incidence has been greatly reduced, but in rare instances fetal red cells enter the maternal circulation before preventive treatment is given, prophylactic treatment is overlooked, or sensitization occurs from mismatched blood transfusion, so that cases continue to occur, and it is still necessary to describe the condition and its management.

Clinical and pathological features of haemolytic disease

The basic pathological process is haemolysis of fetal red cells by the antibody passed across the placenta from the maternal plasma. The antibody coats the fetal red cells and leads to their destruction by the reticuloendothelial system. This blood destruction evokes hyperplasia or erythropoietic tissues in the fetus, and the outcome depends on whether new formation of cells keeps pace with their destruction.

In the most severe cases the fetus dies *in utero*, usually at some time after the 28th week. There is generalized oedema of the fetus (hydrops fetalis) with pleural, pericardial and peritoneal effusions. The primitive areas of red cell formation in the liver, spleen and lymphatic structures show activity. The placenta is enlarged and oedematous, and

histological examination shows abnormal persistence of the cytotrophoblast.

If the child is born alive the chief clinical features of haemolytic disease are jaundice, pallor and enlargement of the liver and spleen. The infant's blood shows reticulocytosis with many nucleated cells. At birth the haemoglobin level in the cord blood is the best guide to the severity of the disease, but the blood sample must be taken carefully to make sure that there is no clot in it. The disease is said to be severe if the haemoglobin level is 10 g/dl or below, of moderate severity with levels between 11 and 13 g/dl and mild with levels of 14 g/dl or above. There may be rapid increase in the jaundice after birth. Before birth the excess of bilirubin from the haemolysis is excreted into the mother's circulation by the placenta; hence the cord bilirubin level at birth is unreliable as an index of severity. After birth levels of unconjugated bilirubin rise very quickly because the liver of the newborn child has poor conjugating ability.

Unconjugated bilirubin is highly toxic to nerve cells if sufficient amounts of it cross the blood–brain barrier. Resultant brain damage particularly involves the basal ganglia, which may become bile-stained, hence the term *kernicterus*. The infant is irritable, has increased muscular tone, is reluctant to feed and in the worst cases shows hyperextension before death. In infants who survive there are varying degrees of spasticity, paralysis, deafness, visual defect and mental retardation.

Antenatal management

Every pregnant woman must have her blood group determined at her initial antenatal visit, and at the same time her serum is tested for antibodies. The direct antibody (Coombs') test is a non-specific test to show whether the red cells are coated with antibody. Ideally any woman whose serum contains antibodies should have the specificity of the antibody identified and the amount present determined. In practice, tests for rhesus, A and B, Kell, Kidd and Duffy antigens may be performed.

With rhesus antigens there is a correlation between the concentration of maternal serum antibody and the severity of the disease in the fetus. A direct quantitative measurement is made and if this is more than 4 IU an estimation needs to be done on the bilirubin in liquor amnii, or fetal blood samples should be examined.

Amniocentesis

Bilirubin is found in the liquor amnii as well as in the fetal tissues, and the amount of bilirubin in the liquor is a useful index of the severity of the disease in the fetus. Amniocentesis carries a small risk of damaging the placenta and causing the entry of fetal blood into the maternal circulation, but the risk can be reduced by ultrasound localization of the placenta and careful technique. For details *see* page 273. The liquor is centrifuged and then examined with a recording spectroscope. Estimations of the optical density of the fluid are made with light of varying wavelength. Bilirubin causes absorption of light of wavelength 450 nm, and the degree of change of optical density at that point is a measure of the bilirubin content. The results are recorded on a chart on which a line has been drawn representing standard levels of optical density for amniotic fluid. These levels vary with the age of the fetus, becoming lower as term approaches, and the chart is designed to allow for this. The height of the hump on the chart representing absorption of light at 450 nm indicates the bilirubin content. Standard charts are available that correlate the changes in optical density with the severity of the disease.

Fetal blood sampling

Fetal blood can be aspirated from the umbilical vein by cordocentesis from 18 weeks. The severity of haemolytic disease is shown by haemoglobin concentration and haematocrit readings (*see* p. 273).

Mode of delivery

Fetuses who are judged to be only mildly affected by haemolytic disease are left to proceed to term; those who are moderately affected may be delivered before term; a few who are severely affected and at great risk of early intrauterine death are treated by intrauterine blood transfusion (*see* below). The purpose of induction of labour before term is to deliver the fetus before intrauterine death can occur, and to enable the fetus to be treated by exchange transfusion immediately after birth. The timing of induction depends on the history of the outcome in previous pregnancies, and on repeated estimations of the bilirubin content of the liquor and of maternal antibody titres.

Labour is induced with prostaglandin pessaries, sometimes combined with amniotomy. Caesarean section may be considered for a fetus delivered before the 34th week.

Exchange transfusion after delivery (*see* p. 322) has lowered the mortality in haemolytic disease but has not eliminated it. In a few cases in which the fetus is severely affected but is judged to be too immature for safe delivery intrauterine transfusion is indicated. After accurate determination of the fetal position by ultrasound, a long needle is passed through the maternal abdominal and uterine walls into the fetal peritoneal cavity. Fresh Rh-negative blood, with partly packed cells, is injected slowly in volumes related to the estimated weight of the fetus and the degree of anaemia; 10 ml of blood for each week after the 20th week of pregnancy are given. Thus at 25 weeks 50 ml are injected. The red cells are taken up from the peritoneal cavity by the lymphatics. Among the severely affected fetuses treated by this method there is a mortality of up to 50 per cent, and the technique should only be carried out by those with special experience of it. With modern techniques it is possible to undertake antenatal blood sampling and to transfuse blood directly into the umbilical vein *in utero*. This may be combined with intraperitoneal transfusion giving both an immediate and a more long-lasting effect.

Postnatal management

The diagnosis has usually been made from the routine investigations during the antenatal period, but any infant becoming jaundiced within 24 hours of birth must be considered to be suffering from haemolytic disease until proved otherwise.

In haemolytic disease there will be a reticulocytosis of more than 5 per cent. The direct antiglobulin test (Coombs' test) will demonstrate antibody on the red cells in all cases except those due to anti-A or anti-B. In the latter cases the mother's group will be O, with haemolytic anti-A or anti-B IgG in her serum.

A very small group of infants with haemolytic anaemia and a negative direct antiglobulin test will be found to have an inherited defect of the red cells, such as glucose-6-phosphate dehydrogenase deficiency (*see* p. 311).

Treatment of the affected infant after birth

The objects of treatment are:

> to correct anaemia, thereby reducing the risk of death from heart failure
> to prevent kernicterus.

These objectives are achieved by exchange transfusion. By this procedure about 90 per cent of the infant's red cells, which are coated with antibody and destined for destruction, with consequent increase in serum bilirubin, are removed and replaced with red cells lacking the antigen to which the mother is immunized. One gram of haemoglobin produces 40 mg of bilirubin.

If the rhesus (D) blood group is involved the mother is Rh-negative and the fetus is Rh-positive, and Rh-negative blood would be transfused. For infants suffering from haemolytic disease due to anti-A or anti-B the blood used should be group O with the O plasma replaced by AB plasma, and of the same Rh type as the infant.

The exchange is carried out by passing a plastic catheter through the umbilical vein into the inferior vena cava. Twenty ml of blood is withdrawn and replaced by 20 ml of donor blood. In infants with raised venous pressure, who are usually the most anaemic infants, the initial withdrawal is increased to 40 ml. The procedure is repeated until 160 ml per kg has been exchanged; this amount usually gives the maximum exchange. Both withdrawal and replacement are carried out slowly, and the infant's heart rate is monitored with a ratemeter throughout the procedure.

The indications for exchange transfusion are:

> severely affected infants with umbilical cord haemoglobin concentration of less than 10 g/dl
> infants whose serum bilirubin concentration exceeds 120 μmol/L within 12 hours of birth
> infants in whom serial six-hourly estimations of serum bilirubin concentration indicate that the level is likely to exceed 340 μmol/L in the next few hours, even if they have already had an exchange transfusion. Lower levels of bilirubin are used to assess the need for exchange transfusion in preterm infants. The purpose is to prevent kernicterus.

Phototherapy, in which the infant is exposed to blue light, will assist in converting the bilirubin in the skin to a compound which is harmless to the brain. The conjunctivae must be protected from the light.

PREVENTION OF IMMUNIZATION AGAINST RHESUS ANTIGEN

It has been known for many years that if Rh-(D)-positive fetal cells are introduced into the circulation of an Rh-negative mother when there is ABO incompatibility between the mother and fetus, the fetal cells quickly disappear from her circulation, and rhesus immunization occurs infrequently. It was subsequently found that if 100 μg of anti-D γ-globulin is injected intramuscularly into an Rh-negative mother within 60 hours of the birth of an Rh-positive child, it will almost always prevent her forming anti-D antibodies. This dose of anti-D γ-globulin should be given to every Rh-negative woman who has no anti-D antibody in her circulation if she has:

> just given birth to an Rh-positive child, whether alive or stillborn
> had an abortion, therapeutic or otherwise
> had an external version
> had an amniocentesis and the aspirate was blood-stained
> had chorionic villus sampling.

This dose is sufficient to prevent immunization if less than 4 ml of fetal blood has entered the maternal circulation. Larger amounts occasionally enter. If the Kleihauer test shows that the proportion of fetal cells is greater than 1:1000 more than 4 ml of blood has come from the fetus, and if this has happened to be known the dose of anti-D γ-globulin should be increased.

INFECTION IN THE NEWBORN INFANT

The newborn infant has a low natural resistance to infection and may succumb to infections which are of low pathogenicity to adults, the organisms being carried by attendants who themselves have no symptoms. For this reason, carriers of streptococci in the throat, or individuals suffering from low grade staphylococcal infections or head colds, represent a great potential danger to infants in their care.

The newborn infant is at increased risk of infection because the natural barrier of the skin is easily broken, thus allowing access of organisms to the circulation. This may occur with scalp electrodes, tubes or drains inserted for various purposes or by direct skin trauma. The umbilical tissues which are undergoing spontaneous degeneration are another potential source and route of entry for infection. The cellular immune system is present and functional from an early stage of fetal life but phagocytosis is not so active as in the adult and is further suppressed by hypoxia. The antibody levels of IgA and IgM are also very low (*see* p. 241) although there are high levels of IgG from the mother in term infants. The preterm baby misses out on this important protection, especially before 34 weeks gestation.

The response to infection shown by newborn infants is very different from that shown by older children. Symptoms which denote neonatal infection are seldom local, but are systemic and merely indicate a general deterioration in health. The onset of serious infection in the newborn infant is often insidious, and it may be well established before it is realized that the infant is gravely ill. Vomiting and diarrhoea are commonly seen in infants suffering from infection which appears to be remote from the gastrointestinal tract. Refusal to feed, lethargy and sleepiness are common early signs in generalized infection.

The temperature response is seldom marked, and quite a severe infection may cause fever of only 0.5°C. With very severe infections there is often a subnormal temperature, slow or rapid pulse rate, reduced respiration rate, sleepiness and collapse without localizing signs. Apnoeic attacks are also common. The symptoms do not always point to the source of the infection and a careful clinical search for the source may be necessary. Frequently the help of the laboratory is required to localize the infective process. Examination of the urine, swabs from throat, ears and umbilicus, blood culture and sometimes lumbar puncture may be necessary to determine the nature of the infection.

General treatment

There are four main principles of treatment:

  the general condition of the infant must be maintained. Alterations may have to be made in the feeding routine. If the infant tires easily feeds may be given in smaller amounts at shorter intervals. The total daily intake must be sufficient for the infant's needs and must compensate for any unusual losses from diarrhoea. If the infant cannot take adequate fluid by mouth intravenous infusion or tube feeding may be necessary

  if the lungs are involved or there is cardiovascular failure oxygenation must be maintained. If anaemia occurs great benefit may be derived from a small transfusion of 15 ml/kg body weight of packed red blood cells

  the temperature must be kept within reasonable limits by the application of warmth, or by cooling if pyrexia is present

  the infection must be controlled by an appropriate antibiotic. The range of bactericidal drugs is very wide, and if the organism causing the infection is known and its sensitivities have been determined the correct drug for the case can be employed. The newborn infant may show reactions to antibiotics which do not occur in older patients, and care to give the correct dose is very important. Certain drugs have special disadvantages for neonatal use:

  chloramphenicol is cleared from the body after conjugation as glucuronide. Since glucuronide conjugation is at a low level in the early days of life the drug may accumulate in the body. Newborn or premature babies may show collapse and hypothermia after treatment with this drug – the 'grey-baby syndrome'. It must be used with great discretion, and the blood levels should always be monitored

  tetracycline should never be given to newborn infants as it may cause yellow staining of the deciduous teeth.

In the newborn infant it is not desirable to await the result of the laboratory investigations, which may take 48 hours, before starting treatment. Empirical treatment is begun as soon as the signs of infection have been detected, using the antibiotics which are thought most likely to overcome the infection. Most commonly used are a combination of a penicillin with an aminoglycoside or a third generation cephalosporin. Metronidazole is used for suspected anaerobic infection and antifungals for systemic mycotic infection.

RESPIRATORY TRACT

Head cold and nasal cattarh

When a young infant contracts a cold in the head the nasal secretions may cause embarrassment during feeding and the infant may be fretful at this time. The real danger to the infant is in the supine position, when infected secretions drain down the back of the throat and with the poor cough reflex, may pass the barrier of the larynx and be aspirated into the lungs where infection can cause collapse and consolidation by blocking a bronchus, especially the right middle lobe bronchus. These infants are best nursed on a firm mattress which is raised at the head end to an angle of about 20°. Another possible hazard for a snuffly baby is apnoea during sleep when both nostrils are blocked, and this is one of the possible causes of sudden infant death. Nasal drops can perpetuate local irritation, but they may be beneficial for one or two days.

Otitis media

The relatively straight and wide eustachian tube forms an easy channel for ascending infection, or for the passage of infected secretions. The symptoms are those of low grade fever, irritability and general malaise and the site of infection is only discovered on full routine examination, which must always include examination of the tympanic membranes. Spread of infection to the meninges is a possible danger. Early diagnosis and antibiotic therapy are essential.

Pneumonia

The infection is usually a descending infection from the upper respiratory tract to the lung, especially if there is already another lesion such as atelectasis or there has been inhalation of mucus, food or vomitus. Cough is an uncommon symptom in infancy, and attention is usually drawn to the disease by a rising respiration rate, cyanosis, pallor or a slight rise in temperature, with anorexia and general malaise. Examinations of the chest may show little that is abnormal. The presence of fine râles may be all that is found. A chest radiograph is essential.

The essentials of treatment are to maintain oxygenation, which may require an oxygen tent, to ensure an adequate fluid intake and to give an appropriate antibiotic. Nose and throat swabs are taken to discover the offending organism and its sensitivities. Early onset pneumonia with Group B streptococcus is considered on page 317.

MOUTH

Infection of the buccal mucosa and tongue by *Candida albicans* is not infrequent in bottle-fed or debilitated infants. It may also occur during delivery if the mother has vaginal thrush. There are greyish-white plaques which resemble milk curds but which cannot be wiped off. The constitutional upset is slight, but the soreness of the mouth may cause the baby to refuse feeds. Rarely, thrush spreads down the gastrointestinal tract and cause oesophagitis. Sore buttocks may be caused by thrush. During antibiotic therapy the lungs may be invaded by the fungus which multiplies under cover of the antibiotic which inhibits the normal bacterial flora.

Treatment is by local application of nystatin 100 000 units in 1 ml of fluid which is swabbed around the mouth four times daily for one week. Perineal infection is treated with nystatin ointment.

GASTROENTERITIS

See page 306.

INFECTION OF THE URINARY TRACT

This is as common in the male newborn infant as in the female. Symptoms suggestive of infection with or without physical signs should always call for investigation of the renal tract. Renal tenderness is seldom found, and the predominant symptoms may be vomiting, diarrhoea and reluctance to feed, some babies develop jaundice. The temperature may be only slightly raised. Culture of a clean specimen of urine often shows coliforms, *Streptococcus faecalis* and infrequently *Bacillus pyocyaneus* or *B. proteus*. This finding should not be taken as evidence of renal infection unless pus cells are also found in the urine. The discovery of five to ten leucocytes in each high power field and of 10^5 organisms per ml is highly suggestive of renal infection. In doubtful cases it may be necessary to culture a specimen obtained by suprapubic aspiration.

Many infants with pyelonephritis suffer from a congenital malformation of the renal tract causing some degree of obstruction or ureteric reflux, such infections are often resistant to treatment which demands a full course of the appropriate antibiotic. All infants with proven urinary tract infection require renal ultrasound and a micturating cystogram.

SEPTICAEMIA

Neonatal septicaemia is one of the most serious and potentially fatal conditions of the newborn period. The infant presents in a variety of ways but mainly with systemic signs such as lethargy, anorexia, pallor, mottling of the skin and sometimes jaundice. Variations in temperature control are common and apnoeic attacks may be a feature. As the infection worsens more ominous signs such as vomiting, abdominal distension and respiratory grunting on expiration may appear. If the platelet count is low from toxic bone marrow suppression or from disseminated intravascular coagulation there may be bleeding from puncture sites or petechial haemorrhages into the skin.

The most common organisms at present causing neonatal septicaemia are *Staphylococcus epidermis*, Group B streptococci, *Staphylococcus aureus*, *Escherichia coli*, *Streptococcus faecalis* and *Pseudomonas aeruginosa*. Other organisms which are increasingly seen are *Listeria monocytogenes*, *Candida albicans* and certain anaerobes.

Treatment is supportive and includes the correction of acid–base disturbance and of any clotting deficiency and the reversal of shock with appropriate fluids and blood products. The choice of antibiotics will depend on the likely organism, but they are started as soon as the appropriate cultures have been taken from the baby. The usual agents are penicillin or flucloxacillin in combination with an aminoglycoside such as gentamicin or tobramycin. Aminoglycosides should never be used without monitoring the blood levels. The new third generation cephalosporins such as cefotaxime or ceftazidime are increasingly being used as they have a wide spectrum of activity and are relatively non-toxic. Metronidazole is given when anaerobes may also be involved as, for example, in necrotizing enterocolitis. If systemic candidiasis is found amphotericin and 5 flucytosine are used. The length of treatment is determined by the culture results and the response. Despite all these measures there is still a significant mortality from this condition.

OSTEOMYELITIS

Infection of a long bone or the maxilla may be a complication of staphylococcal infection, usually of the skin or umbilicus. Three to six weeks after the initial infection there is general malaise with low grade fever, followed by reluctance to use a limb. Redness and swelling, and occasionally the development of septic arthritis in a contiguous joint may follow. Full antibiotic treatment and orthopaedic advice about the drainage of pus are essential.

MENINGITIS

Neonatal meningitis is another serious condition which, although relatively uncommon, still carries a high mortality, and there is significant morbidity among survivors. A lumbar puncture should always be performed if there is the slightest suspicion of this problem or if there are signs of infection without localizing features. The most common causative organism in the UK is now the Group B streptococcus. Other organisms include *E. coli*, staphylococci and pneumococci; *L. monocytogenes* and *C. albicans* are becoming more common. The disease rarely presents in a classical form and there may only be general signs of deterioration in the baby's condition.

Treatment is with systemic antibiotics including chloramphenicol. Blood levels should always be monitored. The third generation cephalosporins also show good CSF penetration and are useful in this disease. Intraventricular antibiotics may be indicated if there is ventriculitis. A number of patients are left with permanent neurological sequelae.

SKIN INFECTION

The most common skin infection is an eruption of small pustules caused by staphylococci. The soft skin of the infant is easily traumatized by clothing or rubbing with the towel after the bath. The infecting organism may be present in the nose or on the skin of nurses or doctors, or may be transferred from other infected babies. The umbilicus is often colonized, and the infection spreads from there.

Pemphigus neonatorum is a bullous or vesicular eruption caused by streptococcal or staphylococcal infection. It is now rarely seen. Large fluid-containing blisters raise the outer skin layers, which are easily rubbed off to leave raw areas which become secondarily infected. If the lesions are widespread there is a high mortality. (Another unrelated variety of pemphigus occurs in cases of congenital syphilis, in which bullae appear on the palms and soles.)

Any infant with a skin infection should be isolated. An appropriate antibiotic is given systematically; local antibiotics not used as they may cause sensitivity reactions.

CONJUNCTIVITIS

Conjunctivitis in the newborn gives rise to anxiety because in the past gonococcal infections sometimes caused serious damage. In every significant case of conjunctivitis smears should be taken and swabs plated directly onto selective medium for gonococci. If facilities are available for tissue culture of chlamydia a swab from the lower conjunctival fornix is sent to the laboratory in special chlamydial transport medium, but a rapid diagnosis can be made by looking for chlamydial inclusion bodies in conjunctival scrapings.

For treatment topical antibiotics such as aureomycin alone are used. Systemic antibiotics are given in severe cases. Chloramphenicol suppresses chlamydial infection, obscuring the diagnosis without eradicating it. If gonococci are found, intravenous injections of benzyl penicillin 30 mg/kg every 24 hours are given eight- or 12-hourly for seven days. Penicillin eye drops are instilled at hourly intervals initially. For strains producing β-lactamase similar injections of cefotaxime 100 mg/kg every 24 hours are given.

If chlamydia are found, or if there is a poor response to treatment, erythromycin succinate 50 mg/kg per 24 hours is given orally in divided doses. Topical treatment with tetracycline eye drops (1 per cent) may be added.

It is important to establish the diagnosis of chlamydial conjunctivitis, first because it implies the presence of chlamydia in the mother's genital tract and the possibility of urethritis in the father which should be diagnosed and treated; and second because chlamydial pneumonia is an occasional complication in the baby, the cause of which would otherwise be obscure, and which requires erythromycin for effective treatment.

Dacryocystitis

The nasolacrimal duct may be blocked by infection and pus can be expressed by pressure in the angle between the inner canthus and the nose. Most cases resolve spontaneously over a period of time, but if not, the help of an ophthalmic surgeon must be sought, with a view to probing the duct.

UMBILICAL INFECTION

The stump of the umbilical cord desiccates and separates, usually by the seventh day, leaving a raw area which heals by granulation. Until healing is complete this is a warm moist region that provides an excellent site for colonization by bacteria. Not only may these organisms cause mild local infection, but they can be carried to other infants in whom they may cause serious infections. Chlorhexidine in spirit should be applied to the area, followed by hexochlorophane dusting powder.

Infection with a virulent organism may be followed by spread of infection along the umbilical vein to the bloodstream and liver, with septicaemia, jaundice and haemolytic anaemia. The infant becomes ill with general signs of infection, and often enlargement of the liver. A swab from the navel and a blood culture to establish the nature and sensitivities of the infecting organism is followed at once by full antibiotic treatment. Unless early aggressive treatment is given the prognosis may be poor.

HIV INFECTION

Infants born to HIV-positive mothers (women infected with human immunodeficiency virus) are antibody positive at birth and have a risk of approximately one-third of remaining antibody positive after 15 months. They are not clinically unwell during the neonatal period but half will develop signs of disease between six months and two years. Because of the risk of transmission of the virus they should not be breast fed, although in developing countries, where adequate milk substitutes are not available, breast feeding may be preferable. The initial immunization schedule, except for BCG, should be followed if the child is clinically well, as this will provide some protection later when immunity begins to wane.

SURGERY IN THE NEWBORN

A variety of conditions which affect the newborn require surgical intervention either immediately or electively some time later. Most of these are due to congenital malformations and an increasing number are now being diagnosed antenatally on ultrasound. The science of intrauterine surgery is also developing in relation, for example, to hydrocephalus and hydronephrosis with the promise of new techniques for other conditions in the future. Careful follow-up of infants who have undergone surgery for congenital abnormalities is required to assess long-term function, since such early problems are often associated with significant damage and a poor prognosis.

Infants requiring surgery should be transferred to a specialized unit where there is a high level of expertise in dealing with the particular problems that can arise pre- and postoperatively.

Some conditions have already been considered elsewhere. These include cleft lip (*see* p. 313), necrotizing enterocolitis (*see* p. 307), hypospadias (*see* p. 315), circumcision (*see* p. 315), exomphalos (*see* p. 313), umbilical hernia (*see* p. 313), spina bifida (*see* p. 313), imperforate anus (*see* p. 313) and hydrocephalus (*see* p. 314).

OESOPHAGEAL ATRESIA AND TRACHEO-OESOPHAGEAL FISTULA (TOF)

Oesophageal atresia, with or without tracheo-oesophageal fistula, occurs in approximately 1:3500 births. The possibility must be borne in mind in every infant who demonstrates persistent salivation and drooling after birth or who has difficulty with the first feed. There is a high incidence of hydramnios during pregnancy and oesophageal atresia should be considered in all patients with this complication. Oesophageal atresia usually occurs just above the level of the bifurcation of the trachea (in 85 per cent of cases) and is most commonly associated with a tracheo-oesophageal fistula in which the lower oesophagus joins the trachea just above the carina. Less than 10 per cent of cases have oesophageal atresia without a fistula. A tracheo-oesophageal fistula on its own also occurs but is very rare. In the classic form of oesophageal atresia the upper oesophageal pouch fills with saliva or milk which then spills over into the trachea and down into the lungs. Gastric acid can regurgitate in the lower segment through the fistula and into the bronchi, again causing irritation and pneumonitis. Half of these babies have other congenital malformations particularly of the bones, heart or genitourinary systems. The infant should be given a thorough examination to exclude these before surgery is undertaken.

Any suspicion that swallowing is not normal should lead to prompt investigation by attempting to pass a moderately stiff catheter through the oesophagus into the stomach. A soft catheter may coil up in the segment above the atresia and delude the observer into believing that it has passed into the stomach. The aspiration of acid secretion and the emptying of the stomach of air provide proof that the oesophagus is patent. Failure to pass the catheter more than half way down the oesophagus proves the presence of atresia. The catheter should be radio-opaque so that its position can be confirmed with X-rays. Directly the diagnosis is established the infant is transferred to a paediatric surgical unit with frequent suction during the journey. Surgery in specialized units offers an excellent chance of survival and good function in the longer term.

CONGENITAL ATRESIA OF THE GUT

Duodenal atresia or stenosis

This condition occurs in about 1:6000 babies. It may be detected on ultrasound prenatally when a double bubble shadow is seen in the stomach and duodenum with empty gut beyond. In the immediate neonatal period it presents with vomiting, which is bile-stained, and failure to pass meconium. A radiograph of the abdomen in the erect position shows a double bubble of air in the stomach and proximal duodenum but no gas beyond this level. The lesion is associated with Down's syndrome in up to one-third of cases and as many as half of the children with this condition also have other congenital malformations. Treatment is surgical and shows good results providing there are no other significant abnormalities.

Jejunal and ileal atresia

This occurs in about 1:5000 infants. Single or multiple atretic segments of the small bowel result in vomiting, abdominal distension and failure to pass meconium after birth. An erect or lateral decubitus abdominal film will show gaseous distension of the bowel with fluid levels present above the site of the lesion. Treatment is surgical. There is also an association with cystic fibrosis and these infants should have a sweat test to exclude this disease.

Meconium ileus

Almost all infants with meconium ileus suffer from cystic fibrosis, in which there is an abnormal pancreatic secretion into the bowel. During intrauterine life the meconium is abnormally digested and becomes packed into the lower ileum, forming a mass of putty-like consistency and appearance. This may be seen as abnormal bowel shadowing on ultrasound as early as 18–20 weeks gestation. Immediately after birth the infant develops vomiting and abdominal distension and fails to pass meconium. X-ray examination shows gaseous distension and fluid levels in the small bowel with lack of gas and a mottled opacity in the areas of the inspissated meconium. Treatment is surgical, often involving resection of small bowel which is non-viable followed by end to end anastomosis to enable the remaining bowel to function normally. All such infants require a sweat test which usually confirms a diagnosis of cystic fibrosis following which the infant will need life-long treatment for this condition and its complications.

CONGENITAL HYPERTROPHIC PYLORIC STENOSIS

Symptoms arising from the obstruction caused by hypertrophy of the circular muscle of the pylorus are uncommon before the second week of life. The condition occurs five times more often in male than in female infants. The symptoms are projectile vomiting, failure to gain weight and constipation. The infant usually feeds eagerly despite the vomiting which occurs at the end of feeds, and will accept re-feeding immediately after having vomited. As a rule the vomit does not contain bile.

With continued vomiting the infant's condition deteriorates, becoming dehydrated with loss of skin turgor, depression of the fontanelle and dryness of the mouth. The loss of chloride in the vomit causes a low plasma chloride level and compensatory alkalosis. Careful examination, with the baby relaxed during a feed, reveals gastric peristaltic waves and a pyloric tumour is felt. The condition is treated surgically by Ramstedt's pyloromyotomy, which gives excellent results provided that dehydration and chloride deficiency are first corrected.

HIRSCHSPRUNG'S DISEASE

This is caused by absence of ganglion cells in the myenteric plexus of the bowel. In the majority of cases this is found in the lower portion of the large bowel and rectum. Occasionally much more extensive disease is found involving the small bowel but this is unusual. There is an association with Down's syndrome. The overall incidence is about 1:5000 births. Infants presenting soon after birth fail to pass meconium and develop abdominal distension. This may be difficult to distinguish from meconium ileus. Examination shows the rectum to be empty but the anal tone is good. Meconium is usually passed rapidly after the examination is complete. The diagnosis is made by suction rectal biopsy. Treatment is surgical. A colostomy is usually performed in the first instance and at a later stage definitive surgery is undertaken to resect the aganglionic bowel and reconstruct the normal anatomical passage.

IMPERFORATE ANUS

See page 313.

ABNORMALITIES OF THE DIAPHRAGM

Diaphragmatic hernia

The incidence of this condition is 1:4000 births. Congenital failure of development of one side of the diaphragm presents a difficult diagnostic problem. Persistence of the posteriorly situated pleuroperitoneal sinus on either side allows the abdominal contents to herniate into the pleural cavity. This occurs more commonly on the left side, and at an early stage of fetal life when there is still a universal mesentery, so that almost all the intestine can enter the thorax. Such herniae cause cyanosis from birth. The diagnosis may be suspected if heart sounds are heard on the right and bowel sounds in the chest, and is proved by X-ray examination. During transfer to surgical care assisted respiration may be necessary with an endotracheal tube, and the stomach and gut should be kept deflated with another tube.

Infants with diaphragmatic hernia have hypoplasia of the lung on the affected side. This can lead to major respiratory problems postoperatively and in the longer term if the lung is significantly reduced in size. There is also a reduced alveolar count on the other side indicating that the intrauterine events have a major effect on lung growth generally.

Eventration of the diaphragm

Occasionally the diaphragm fails to develop the normal musculature and is a non-contractile fibrous septum which is pushed up high into the chest. Bowel sounds are heard in the chest, the lungs are poorly expanded, and the infant is cyanosed. X-ray examination shows the abnormal position of the diaphragm. Some infants succumb, and survivors may have frequent chest infections. An operation to plicate the diaphragm is often necessary.

Hiatus hernia

Herniation of the cardiac end of the stomach through the oesophageal hiatus may cause vomiting. The infant regurgitates small amounts between feeds and fails to thrive. The condition is demonstrated by a barium swallow. Sometimes no hiatus hernia can be found, and the diagnosis of gastro-oesophageal reflux or lax cardia is made. When regurgitation of gastric acid occurs there is likely to be oesophagitis, with blood or altered blood in the vomit. This can be investigated using continuous pH monitoring of the lower oesophagus.

Thickening the feeds and posturing the infant are usually sufficient to relieve the symptoms. The infant is placed in the prone position on a firm mattress which is elevated to an angle of 30°. Thickening of the feeds can be achieved without the addition of salt or increasing the calorie content by adding small amounts of powdered carob bean (Nestargel, Carobal), starting with one scoop to 150 ml of feed. For a breast fed baby the powder is mixed with a little water and given before the feed. In severe cases a Nissen's fundoplication of the gastro-oesophageal junction is necessary.

ECTOPIA VESICA

This is a very rare condition occurring more often in boys than girls in approximately 1:30 000 births. There is epispadias and the bladder mucosa is exposed directly onto the anterior abdominal wall with an associated dysgenesis of the symphysis pubis. The anus is anteriorly situated and there may also be associated exomphalos. There is a high incidence of associated upper renal tract abnormalities as well. Treatment is surgical but it is complicated and must be carefully planned by an expert in order to achieve the best long-term results.

URETHRAL VALVES

This is a condition in male infants which often presents after birth although there may have already been significant damage to the urinary tract *in utero*. Prenatal ultrasound diagnosis is possible although many present after birth with signs such as bladder enlargement, a poor urinary stream, recurrent urinary tract infections or abdominal swelling due to hydronephrosis. Full investigation of the urinary tract and renal function should be undertaken and treatment is by endoscopic surgery. The long-term prognosis depends on how much damage there has been to renal function by the time the diagnosis is made.

UNDESCENDED TESTES

This occurs in 3 per cent of term infants and is usually unilateral. Bilateral undescended testes are associated with a significant incidence of other abnormalities particularly of the genitourinary tract. Many descend spontaneously, particularly during the first year of life. In those which do not, surgery is indicated before school age.

INGUINAL HERNIA

This is relatively uncommon in term infants but there is a high incidence in preterm babies, particularly those who are very small. The treatment is surgical although this can be delayed if the infant is very small provided close observation is being maintained. Urgent surgery is required if the hernia becomes acutely tense and cannot be reduced.

10

MEDICO-LEGAL PROBLEMS IN OBSTETRICS

The rapid increase in litigation against British doctors at the present time is a matter for concern. The combined specialities of Obstetrics and Gynaecology are among the foremost targets of such claims. Not only does this mean that large sums of money have to be paid in compensation but it also means there may have to be changes in the style of practice. Defensive medicine, which results from these changes, implies unnecessary and expensive investigations and a hasty recourse to caesarean section.

So far as the financial aspects are concerned obstetric claims and awards now lead the way in the sheer magnitude of the sums of money involved. Settlements for the brain damaged infant, for example, are at present approaching £1 million. Until the 1st of January 1990 these sums of money had to be paid by the medical profession itself through its defence societies. They explained the high level of subscriptions to these societies. In the USA the individual doctor has personal insurance and any large claim can be recovered from the fees charged to patients. This is not possible in the UK in the context of a National Health Service but from the beginning of 1990 NHS claims are to be paid from Government funds thus removing the threat of a huge decrease in the number of young doctors entering the speciality of obstetrics and gynaecology. Doctors in private practice will need to subscribe to a defence system as in the past. Many doctors support the no-fault system used in New Zealand. By this method compensation is decided by a committee, and is appropriate to the disability or discomfiture incurred; doctors are not named.

LITIGATION IN OBSTETRICS

Obstetrics is unusual in that the obstetrician is dealing with two patients – the mother and the developing baby. This makes the task doubly demanding particularly in the present climate of what is rapidly becoming a consumer orientated service. Parents have, quite rightly, a high expectation for the best outcome of pregnancy – a healthy, normal baby and a mother unscathed physically by pregnancy and delivery and fulfilled emotionally by the experience.

Advances in obstetrics have been considerable over the past ten or fifteen years and, as a result perinatal, and particularly maternal, mortalities and morbidities have diminished. These results have been associated with techniques such as ultrasound scanning, cardiotocography and fetal blood sampling. Many mothers find these techniques unacceptably 'invasive' in the sense that they feel that they interfere with the normal process of labour, the privilege of the mother and father to enjoy the experience of childbirth and their freedom of choice in planning the method of delivery. If obstetricians are not aware of these attitudes then hostility can arise and from this it is a short step to complaint and, of course, litigation.

We can therefore define the most important broad principles to avoid litigation and to maintain a good relationship between parents and obstetrician. Some of these principles apply equally to gynaecology, and indeed to all specialties. They are of equal importance.

Communication

Time and again failure of communication between doctor and patient is the root cause of litigation. If more time had been spent with the patient, not only giving explanations but ensuring that they were understood, and in answering questions, many a claim would never arise.

Time is often short in obstetrics, not only because of the demands which the specialty makes on frequently inadequate numbers of staff, but also because action – on behalf of a distressed baby for example – must be taken swiftly. But as doctors and midwives develop their skills in talking to patients, speed need not be sacrificed in achieving understanding and co-operation.

Recording

Closely allied to communication is the need to make clear and concise notes written and signed at the time of, or just after, an event and containing not only the course of action decided upon but also exactly what was said to the mother and her partner.

Irritating and time consuming though these records may be they can ultimately avoid or modify potentially serious litigation.

The consent form should be signed whenever possible in obstetrics, as in any other specialty, although it may not be regarded by a Court of Law as evidence of *informed* consent. Unless action has to be taken so urgently that consent cannot be obtained, explanation should be given to the patient over and above the standard words used in hospital consent forms and that this has been done should be recorded in the patient's case notes.

Again adequate records and full explanation made after the event will go a long way in avoiding legal action. It goes without saying, however, that a doctor who takes urgent action to save life without proper consent is most likely to be supported in a Court of Law. But the court will not necessarily be supportive in a less than life and death situation where no evidence exists that information was given to the patient or a relative.

Observation

In many ways the part which the obstetrician plays throughout pregnancy, and even during labour, is that of observer. Pregnancy and delivery are essentially physiological processes and the midwife, who assists in a practical sense during labour, also has to play a part in the avoidance of unhappy litigation. The obstetrician, however, bears the greater responsibility. Antenatal care is concerned with observing the mother and the fetus closely for early warning signs such as hypertension, poor intrauterine growth and abnormal lie. Forearmed is forewarned and at the booking visit the doctor must take into account any points in the medical, obstetric or family history which may be of importance to the forthcoming pregnancy, recording the facts in the notes for future observers.

Most hospitals now run special high risk antenatal clinics for women with actual or potential problems, so that they may be seen by the more senior and experienced members of the obstetric team who are able to provide a high degree of vigilant observation and thus reduce the risk of litigation.

Referral

Junior obstetric staff should not take decisions without discussing the case with their seniors. Midwives too should share responsibility with medical personnel when their experience tells them that it is advisable.

Litigation is most liable to arise during:

PREPREGNANCY AND GENETIC COUNSELLING

Before pregnancy a couple may wish to seek advice. This may be because of their age, because of a family problem such as a Down's syndrome child, because of the medical condition of the mother (diabetes for example) or because of a previous difficult delivery. Many hospitals have been fortunate enough to be able to establish prepregnancy counselling clinics to which enquiring patients can be sent by their family doctors. The clinics should be conducted by experienced doctors giving sound, correct advice because if the wrong advice is given and problems result litigation may well follow. For many straightforward conditions the non-specialized doctor can give advice but in more complex circumstances specialized advice must be obtained.

Hospitals may not have geneticists available but there is almost always a district centre to which patients may be sent or where information may be obtained from an expert. The non-specialist should never be tempted to give advice on such matters unless absolutely sure of the facts.

Possible legal action may also arise following prenatal diagnostic tests themselves. Amniocentesis carries a 0.5–1 per cent risk of abortion; chorion villus biopsy carries a higher risk. Ultrasound is safe but fetoscopy may be followed by miscarriage.

These procedures must be carried out by an expert, following comprehensive counselling on the risks involved. It should be explained that amniotic fluid may not be obtained, chromosome analysis may not be accurate or cell culture may fail.

Written consent must be obtained for all the invasive procedures with the implication that such consent is informed.

PREGNANCY

Antenatal care is, as we have seen, an exercise in diligent monitoring. There is a risk that repetition creates boredom which in turn may lead to carelessness.

There are a few simple rules:

Frequent appointments

The mother should be seen at frequent intervals. Shared care with the general practitioner is a good method of decreasing the burden on antenatal clinics but the ultimate responsibility lies with the hospital under whose care the mother has booked. She should be seen by the obstetrician at important stages such as at 28 and 36 weeks.

Identify at risk cases

Special at risk cases must be identified and preferably seen in a special antenatal clinic by the more senior doctors available there.

Discussion of problems

Junior doctors must be encouraged to discuss all problems, however minor they may seem, with their seniors.

Check records

At every visit the patient and her records should be scrutinized, dates should be checked, histories confirmed and notes made on the symptoms, if any, the findings on obstetric examination and the advice given.

If a problem arises later and a move is made towards litigation the patient's records will be scrutinized in detail by doctors, lawyers and the defendant's and plaintiff's experts alike. Inadequate antenatal care and poor records then become difficult to defend.

SPECIFIC PROBLEMS IN PREGNANCY

There are, of course, innumerable possible areas in antenatal care which could become subjects for litigation. Some of the common ones are:

The small-for-dates baby

In this situation intrauterine prenatal anoxia may occur, with the risk of a brain-damaged baby after delivery. These babies can be identified using a variety of techniques from the simple clinical ones such as regular weighing of the mother and measurement of the fundal height to the more sophisticated techniques of serial ultrasound measurements and the latest biophysical tests. Once detected the mother ought to be admitted to hospital for intensive monitoring of her fetus, including cardiotocography and placental function tests. The management requires experience and scrupulous records should be kept.

Medical conditions in association with pregnancy

Diabetes

This is perhaps the most commonly encountered medical condition and carries grave risks to the fetus and to the mother unless adequately managed. The best results are obtained in units where the expertise of a senior obstetrician and a diabetic physician are combined, preferably at a joint clinic. Once again, careful record keeping is essential

Pre-existing hypertension

This is not common in obstetric patients since they represent a young population. Mutual sharing of the responsibility between obstetrician and physician is again desirable; in pregnancy-induced hypertension the responsibility is usually entirely that of the obstetrician. It is useful in such cases to have a unit protocol for management which guides junior staff on action to be taken and is of value if litigation arises. However, it should not replace records of events and decisions written at the time.

Underlying good antenatal care are high levels of awareness, early and adequate treatment, appropriate referral for senior opinions, full explanations to patients and accurate, signed, note keeping. These steps will not avoid complaints but they will go a long way to protect doctors and midwives from litigation.

Postmaturity

See page 132.

LABOUR AND DELIVERY

Women have a high expectation of a safe delivery but also want a fulfilling and satisfying experience. Some may make special demands, that they should, for example, be allowed to adopt unusual positions for delivery, such as squatting, or sitting upright. Some insist on no mechanical monitoring by the cardiotocogram during labour; that the baby should be delivered in the dark; that the cord be left uncut while the baby is handed directly to the mother to be put immediately on the breast.

These and similar requests put the midwife and obstetrician in somewhat of a dilemma. If the requests of the mother are refused then complaints may arise. If they are agreed to and something goes wrong, for example, failure to resuscitate the baby adequately, litigation may follow.

In many maternity units now a compromise has been reached. A so-called birth plan is given to the mother during the antenatal period in which she can mark off her particular requests and discuss them with the midwives and the doctors in advance of labour. Full and frank discussion takes place with tact and understanding on the part of the advisers. Any difficulties or disagreements which arise should be noted. Once more the recurrent theme is communication and recording.

In the conduct of labour itself the most scrupulous vigilance is required on the part of the attendants. Traditionally, when problems arise the midwife will call the doctor on duty, who is often of quite junior status. It is imperative that a junior doctor seeks help from a senior colleague (usually a Registrar) where there is the slightest doubt over management and that the Registrar, in turn, must never hesitate to discuss the situation with the consultant. It is advisable that the time when a senior is called is recorded in the notes and the outcome of discussions noted. Too often a defence will fail because of lack of adequate recording.

Improvements in the organization of medical cover for the labour ward are being made in some hospitals. Sessions are frequently given to consultants purely for labour ward work and supervision. A junior staff team is assigned to labour ward duties, free from outpatient clinics or theatre sessions so that their availability to the labour ward is immediate and the midwifery staff know at once who to turn to when a problem arises.

Health Authorities with increasing awareness of the potential for litigation in obstetrics are appointing extra medical staff and ensuring that facilities are adequate.

Occasionally problems may arise which are not particularly associated with the process of labour. Retention of swabs and breakdown of the episiotomy or caesarean section wounds are examples. Frank discussion and good records are important again.

INSTRUMENTAL DELIVERY

The indications for forceps delivery are given on page 279 and the criteria which must be observed before the forceps are applied are given on page

280. There is no place in modern obstetrics for a difficult forceps delivery and certainly there is no place for a junior doctor applying forceps without the closest supervision. Damage to the fetus may range from tentorial tears and intracerebral haemorrhage to superficial trauma to the face. Any of these may lead to litigation. A baby who is brain damaged during delivery carries huge awards against the obstetrician, amounting in some cases to £1 million. Rotation and delivery with Kielland's forceps demands particular expertise and should only be undertaken by a fully trained and experienced operator.

BREECH DELIVERY

Many obstetricians feel that because of the potential risk to the fetus born as a breech and in the present climate of litigation, delivery should always be by caesarean section. But caesarean section carries its own intrinsic risk to mother and baby and with careful antenatal assessment of the mother's pelvic size, the size of the fetus and any other complicating features there would seem to be no reason why a vaginal delivery should not be allowed. The most careful watch must be kept over the progress of the labour by a team consisting of a senior midwife and assistant, an experienced obstetrician (usually of Registrar or Senior Registrar status) and the junior doctor. The most experienced obstetrician should be in charge of the delivery, at which there should also be an anaesthetist and a paediatrician.

One useful feature of modern labour ward practice is the protocol in which is written out the policy of a department largely for the benefit of new doctors and midwives. It should not supercede adequate record keeping but does at least provide some evidence of what is normal practice in that department.

CAESAREAN SECTION

There are many potential sources of litigation connected with this procedure. Failure to carry out the operation soon enough; carrying it out against the wishes of the patient; trauma (especially to the bladder) during the operation and postoperative complications, to name but a few. Full explanation of the reasons for caesarean section should be made to the patient so that her signed consent can be said to be informed. Careful surgery by an experienced operator will avoid complaint but complete documentation of the details of the surgery is also important.

ANAESTHETIC PROBLEMS IN OBSTETRICS

Inadequate pain relief from an epidural may be a source of complaint. Provided the procedure is explained to the patient, rash promises are not made and consent is obtained, then problems should be avoided.

Awareness during anaesthesia is well publicized and particularly refers to awareness during caesarean section. It is, of course, an anaesthetic problem but it is worth observing once more that an experienced anaesthetist should always be available for the labour ward and full details of anaesthetic agents used should be recorded.

FETAL HYPOXIA

At the present time fetal hypoxia and its relation to brain damage is giving rise to much discussion.

The huge awards that fetal hypoxia carries against the medical profession is a source of difference of opinion. Until such time as a clear causal link between fetal hypoxia and other factors, such as prolonged fetal distress in labour or instrumental delivery and subsequent handicap, can be established it is difficult for a court not to link these factors to handicap on the basis of *res ipse loquitur*.

Congenital abnormality, intrauterine growth retardation, prematurity, maternal health and particularly smoking and alcohol habits are all possible causal background factors for subsequent handicap in the baby. But the final insult of labour and delivery may seem to be the precipitating factors and doctors, lawyers and the public tend to pin the entire blame on what is seen as mismanagement. A baby handicapped by cerebral palsy is indeed a tragedy for the infant and parents alike and compensation often seems right. Whether this should be made virtually on the automatic assumption of obstetric blame is another matter.

Fetal hypoxia may be avoided by detecting and paying special attention to high risk cases in the antenatal clinic, including the small-for-dates baby, women who have had a previous premature delivery and those with associated medical problems such as hypertension or diabetes.

The following steps are also helpful:

judicious induction of labour in conditions such as pre-eclampsia

careful monitoring of the fetus during labour and where any doubt on a fetal heart tracing exists referral to a senior, more experienced doctor

the greater use of fetal blood pH measurements

skilled instrumental delivery

earlier recourse to caesarean section when fetal distress arises

good anaesthesia

experienced paediatric attendance at delivery so that adequate and immediate resuscitation can take place.

Such measures will ensure a minimum risk of cerebral handicap to the baby and if they are carefully recorded and communicated adequately to the parents litigation may be avoided.

THE POSTNATAL PERIOD

Once a baby has been safely delivered and proves to be sound and healthy many a criticism of the conduct of labour and delivery will disappear. Usually discomforts and disappointments quickly recede, but not always, and it may be some time after the mother and baby have been discharged from hospital that murmurs of discontent reach the hospital authorities.

These frequently relate to what the parents consider to be unkind or inconsiderate handling by the staff, inadequate explanations and neglect of what the public feel are minimal standards of care. They almost always reflect a poor level of communication, a recurring word in all medico-legal considerations. This kind of complaint can usually be dealt with by a swift response, giving explanations and offering a face-to-face meeting between the complainant and the obstetrician involved. At such meetings, whatever may be the approach of the parents, the medical and nursing staff should always remain polite, understanding and sympathetic, not aggressively on the defensive. Careful records of such meetings should be kept.

But many complaints in the postnatal period may reach litigation level. Examples are the broken down or poorly healed episiotomy with resultant dyspareunia or even apareunia, always (understandably) a source of discontent; a secondary postpartum haemorrhage or uterine infection necessitating a further admission to hospital; failure to detect problems in the new born baby which may become worse after discharge from hospital (jaundice for example). These complications are more likely to arise where early discharge has been inappropriately permitted.

Vigilance in the postnatal period must be scrupulous if such problems are to be avoided. Discussions with the mother, taking time to give proper explanations; careful note keeping and sharing of responsibility are important if medico-legal difficulties are to be avoided, however difficult they are to maintain in the midst of a busy programme.

HOME CONFINEMENT

It is necessary to consider this topic under litigation since requests are often made by mothers nowadays to be allowed to deliver at home. There seems no doubt that hospital is safer for delivery, as there is immediate access to medical staff, anaesthetics, blood transfusion and operating theatres. But it does not necessarily provide the ideal psychological environment and to some women this is of overriding concern.

But who bears legal responsibility if something goes wrong at a home confinement? Health Authorities have an obligation to ensure that midwifery services are available for home delivery. General practitioners can opt out of attendance during labour but in an emergency the doctor on call must attend. In most districts the midwives have direct access to a hospital emergency service (flying squad) which will respond immediately to a request for help. So on the face of it legal responsibility may devolve on the midwife on the spot, which in effect means the Health Authority; on any general practitioner called to attend the case; on the flying squad team and on the obstetric doctor who is usually of registrar status.

Most authorities have looked at the question of home confinements bearing in mind their possible medico-legal consequences. Domino schemes for early discharge after delivery and the provision of general practitioner delivery suites attached to the hospital labour ward are offered as an alternative. In the latter a mother can be delivered by her midwife and attended by her own doctor and return home a few hours after delivery. The advantage is that all the facilities of the labour ward and specialist obstetric expertise are at hand. But the obstetric team is of course dependent on being notified of problems by the general practitioner or district midwife and it is upon them that initial responsibility rests.

As far as home confinements are concerned two points must be made. Adequate and proper advice must be given to the woman requesting a home confinement and in the case of the patient pursuing her demands against advice, clear notes to this effect must be made. In some parts of the country general practitioners may have direct access to consultant obstetricians to approve of an arrangement or to advise otherwise. In a few District Health Authorities a nominated consultant is available for reference during such a home labour if any problems arise. The responsibility then becomes the obstetrician's.

Where does the parents' responsibility lie when harm results to a baby when it can be shown that they were acting contrary to medical advice? The following statement from the Congenital Disabilities (Civil Liability) Act 1976 summarizes the position:

'If it is shown that the parent affected shared the responsibility for the child being born disabled, the damages are to be reduced to such an extent as the Court thinks just and equitable, having regard to the extent of the parents' responsibility'.

The obstetrician's duty is to the mother and the unborn child with the aim of improving care both in the antenatal period and during delivery. It would be a tragedy if increasing litigation deflected from the proper application of skills and experience, or worse still caused young doctors to turn away from entering the specialty. Viewed in its proper context the knowledge of potential litigation should raise the standard of the obstetrician's care of patients. Meticulous recording, close observation, ready recourse to other opinions, maintenance of a high standard of postgraduate education, communication and counselling skills are the basis for good practice and certainly the basis for avoiding litigation.

11

VITAL STATISTICS

Vital statistics are essential for the planning of health services, and are used by hospitals, regions and countries for this purpose. They allow obstetricians to compare their work with that of others, so as to show where progress might be made or where failures have occurred. Because childbirth is usually normal and any one person has limited experience of abnormal cases, pooling of results is necessary if false impressions are to be avoided.

THE COLLECTION OF OBSTETRICAL STATISTICS

The following account relates to England and Wales, but many other countries collect vital statistics to a similar degree.

In England and Wales a national census is taken every 10 years. All births, marriages and deaths are notified to the Registrars, and from these notifications statistics are computed and regularly published. Many maternity hospitals compile their own statistics and prepare an annual summary, and even when this information is not published it is of interest to those concerned and may help them to improve their practice.

Birth rates

In the UK the average number of children per family is less than 2.1; this no longer replaces the population. From the Registrars' returns the birth rate is calculated. The *crude birth rate* is the number of live births per 1000 total population. Since this population includes men, children and women beyond childbearing age it is more imformative to relate the number of live births to the number of women aged between 15 and 44. This gives the *general fertility rate*, which is expressed as the number of live births per 1000 women of these ages (*see* Figs 11.1 and 11.2).

There was a fall in the total annual number of births from 1885 to 1940, then there was an increase each year until 1964, after which the annual number fell. There has been a slight rise since 1976. There were 693 100 total births (live and still) in England and Wales in 1986, and the fertility rate was 66/1000.

In unsophisticated areas of the world, where little contraception is practised, the crude birth rate is of the order of 50, against which the rate of 13.8 for England and Wales is small. Yet in the developing countries the total population may not rise much, because with lack of development go high stillbirth and infant mortality rates. When these fall because of better medical services and greater wealth, the community reaction is often a wider use of contraception, in the knowledge that then most children born alive will survive.

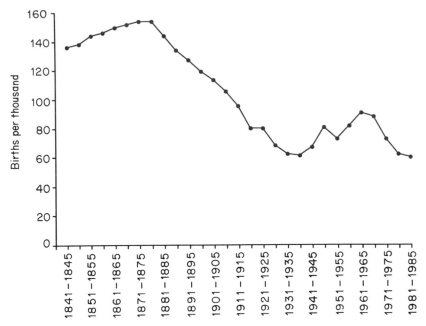

Fig. 11.1 The general fertility rate for England and Wales from 1841–1985. Showing numbers of births per thousand women aged 15–44

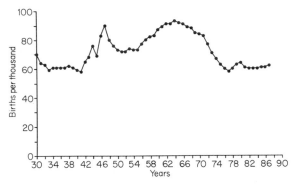

Fig. 11.2 The general fertility rate for England and Wales from 1930–1987. Showing the numbers of births per thousand women aged 15–44

Obstetrical statistics

From the obstetrician's point of view the Maternal Mortality and Perinatal Mortality Rates are of obvious importance, as they give some indication of the standard of practice and of the health of women. The number of deaths during infancy is an index of the work of paediatricians and also of public health measures directed against infectious diseases but, as will be shown later, the death of an infant in the first week after delivery often has an obstetric cause.

MATERNAL MORTALITY

In the nineteenth century the number of deaths of women from childbearing was appalling. Deaths were chiefly from sepsis but also from eclampsia, disproportion and other complications of labour, and haemorrhage. Even in 1928, long after the introduction of aseptic surgery, for every 1000 births 4.28 women died; that is to say that any woman embarking on pregnancy had a 1 in 250 chance of dying. With such results it is not surprising that the first task of obstetricians was to make childbearing safer for the mother, and the fate of the fetus was, at that time, of lesser consideration. In recent years the maternal mortality has fallen to such low levels that it is no longer so useful as an index of obstetric failure or success, and now more attention is given to fetal and neonatal mortality. Nevertheless, every maternal death is still a major tragedy, and maternal mortality studies are of great importance for everyone who practises obstetrics (Fig. 11.3).

In the 62 years since 1928 the maternal mortality

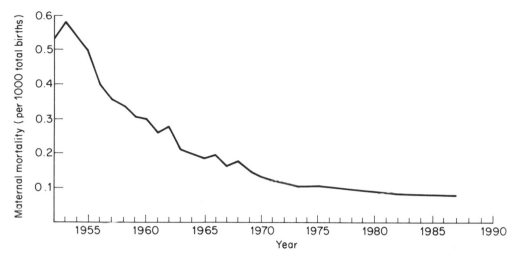

Fig. 11.3 Maternal mortality for England and Wales per 1000 total births (excluding abortion) for the years 1952–1987

has fallen from over 4 to 0.08 per 1000 total births. This has been due to several groups of factors:

the control of infection
blood transfusion
a readier recourse to operative treatment which has been made safer by advances in anaesthesia and resuscitation
the improvement in the health and nutrition of women, who are therefore in better health when they become pregnant.

Nevertheless there is still room for improvement, as a closer look at the causes of death will show.

Statistical data about maternal mortality based on death certification is published annually by the Registrar General in England and Wales and, from 1985, in the rest of the UK. Much additional information about maternal deaths is derived from the *Reports on Confidential Enquiries into Maternal Deaths*. When a woman who is or has recently been pregnant dies, the District Medical Officer sends a detailed form to be filled in by the doctor who was in charge of the patient. Any midwives or nurses who have knowledge of the case may also write reports. At no time is the identity of the person connected with the medical or nursing care of the patient disclosed, and because of this each person giving evidence may be completely frank and unbiased, and nobody filling in the form need fear recriminations of any kind from anybody.

After the form is filled in it is sent to a regional assessor, a senior obstetrician of standing in the region, who gives his or her opinion about the cause of death. A senior pathologist assess the autopsy findings and if the patient had an anaesthetic the opinion of an anaesthetist will also be sought. In their report the assessor tries to judge whether the death was avoidable or unavoidable. These terms are not meant to imply criticism of those concerned with the case, but to ask whether the patient, her family, the doctor and the midwife, and anyone else concerned, had made the fullest possible use of all available services and help. If there had been shortcomings in the use of services

Table 11.1 Direct causes of maternal death elicited by The Confidential Enquiries 1982–1984 (England and Wales)

	Rate per 10^6 maternities
Hypertensive diseases of pregnancy	10.0
Pulmonary embolism	10.0
Amniotic fluid embolism	5.6
Anaesthesia	7.2
Abortion (including sepsis)	4.4
Haemorrhage	3.6
Ectopic pregnancy	4.0
Sepsis (including abortion)	0.8
Ruptured uterus	1.2
Other direct causes of death	8.4
	48.2

and administration, or if the standard of professional care had been lower than should be expected, then the death would be classified as avoidable. This is not to say that it could have been avoided, but only that some factor was present which, if foreseen, might have made the outcome different. The results of these enquiries are published at three-yearly intervals.

Table 11.1 summarizes some of the conclusions of the last Report.

Hypertensive diseases of pregnancy

The incidence of these conditions has been falling slowly during the last thirty years in Britain, but they are still one of the greatest single causes of maternal death. The slow improvement may have resulted from improved antenatal care, and also from better living standards and better general health. One of the major aims of antenatal care from the earliest days has been the prevention of eclampsia by early recognition and treatment of pre-eclamptic hypertension and proteinuria.

Deaths from eclampsia and hypertension were associated with an avoidable factor in three-quarters of the cases, when the factor was calculated. The most common group were patients who refused antenatal care or who would not cooperate by accepting advice about admission to hospital. Doctors were sometimes at fault by delay in acting on signs of severe hypertension and instituting efficient treatment. These women must be under the care of a consultant obstetrician and not in general practitioner units. Smaller units should be prepared to transfer those patients most affected by the condition to larger, regional centres for better care of the mother and the baby.

Pulmonary embolism

This is a sudden and dramatic cause of maternal death. In the Reports from 1964 onwards a third of the deaths occurred during pregnancy, while two-thirds followed delivery. Of the postpartum deaths, one-third followed caesarean section, although only one-twentieth of all the women were delivered by this method, so that the risk of pulmonary embolism is much greater after section than after vaginal delivery. The risk of pulmonary embolism is higher in women aged over 34 years, in those who are overweight, and in those who have an operative delivery of any kind. Most of the deaths during pregnancy occurred suddenly and unexpectedly, and it is difficult at present to see how they could be prevented. After delivery warning signs of deep venous thrombosis were seldom present. Possibly more women in high risk categories should be given prophylactic anticoagulant treatment.

The use of oestrogens to inhibit lactation is one cause of deep venous thrombosis and pulmonary embolism; their use for this purpose has largely been abandoned (see p. 238).

Abortion

In 1968 a major change in practice occurred when the Abortion Act of 1967 came into operation. Since then there has been a steady fall in the number of deaths following abortion, without any great rise in the number of deaths following therapeutic termination of pregnancy, despite over 165 000 terminations being notified each year among women resident in England and Wales.

In the three years covered by the latest Report on Confidential Enquiries into Maternal Deaths (1982–84) abortion accounted for 4.4 per cent of all deaths. There were 77 deaths reported in the 1970 report just after the Abortion Act came in, but only 11 deaths in the 1982 report. Of these seven were after legal abortion and four after spontaneous abortion. No woman died from illegal abortion in the three years under review. This is the first time that no deaths from illegal abortion have been reported by any country in which accurate statistics are kept.

Haemorrhage

Maternal deaths associated with both antepartum and postpartum haemorrhage have fallen steadily since 1950. Placental abruption remains one of the most serious complications of pregnancy. For these cases monitoring of the central venous pressure is essential, and large amounts of blood are required to treat hypovolaemia. A third of the deaths from haemorrhage occur in cases of placenta praevia, but these have been greatly reduced since the introduction of conservative management and better diagnosis by ultrasound methods of examination.

The number of deaths from postpartum haemorrhage was sharply reduced in the 1950s by the prophylactic use of ergometrine in the third stage of labour. A woman who has had a postpartum haemorrhage is at risk of having another in a subsequent pregnancy; she must always be booked for delivery at a hospital with a blood bank and facilities for immediate transfusion. The existence of a flying squad must not be an excuse for delivering such a patient outside a consultant unit.

Ectopic pregnancy

Deaths from this cause have been reduced, but not at the same rate as deaths from other causes. The number of deaths in each triennial Report has fallen from 59 in 1952–54 to 10 in 1982–84. Almost half the patients died at home or in the ambulance before admission to hospital, showing that the flying squad should be used more often. Another quarter died in hospital before operation. It is essential to operate immediately the diagnosis of ectopic pregnancy has been made. The operation should not wait for resuscitative measures; these should proceed while the operation is being performed, because once the bleeding vessels are secured improvement usually follows quickly.

Infection

Before 1936 puerperal sepsis was the largest single cause of maternal mortality. Since the introduction of sulphonamides and then antibiotics, and with better understanding of the mode of spread of infection, infection is a much less common cause of death, but it is often an associated factor in fatal cases. In the 1982–84 Report there were only two deaths from sepsis; vigilance must be maintained if sepsis is not again to become an important cause of maternal death.

Amniotic fluid embolism

In the three years covered by the 1982–84 Report there were 14 deaths from this cause, and about half of these patients had an associated coagulation disorder. The common symptoms were sudden collapse soon after rupture of the membranes, particularly when the uterine contractions were strong. The collapse was often accompanied by a fit, and the patient was usually dyspnoeic and cyanosed, with frothy blood-stained sputum. Confirmation of the diagnosis is possible if amniotic cells are recognized in the sputum. This condition should be kept in mind in cases of sudden collapse, for it is a difficult diagnosis to make. Treatment with oxygen and steroids can save some patients, whilst the ensuing coagulation disorder needs correction.

Uterine rupture

In the last Report there were only three deaths from this cause. With persisting haemorrhage and shock the uterine cavity should always be examined if there is any possibility of uterine rupture, and laparotomy should not be delayed.

Apart from the causes of maternal death which have been mentioned above, two other factors (not direct causes of death) require special mention: anaesthesia and caesarean section.

Anaesthesia

In the Report on Confidential Enquiries into Maternal Deaths the deaths associated with anaesthesia are classified under the headings of the conditions for which treatment was required. However, in the Report for 1982–84 it is stated that 18 deaths were directly due to anaesthesia, with avoidable factors in most; the death rate from this cause does not seem to be falling. Several women died from inhalation of gastric contents during general anaesthesia. In other cases there was difficulty in intubation, injudicious use of drugs, or incorrect administration of epidural anaesthesia by inexpert doctors. Cardiac arrest occurred in some cases, but there was usually some other discernible cause.

For general anaesthesia during labour a skilled and experienced anaesthetist is required. Patients may be dehydrated after a long labour, and although they may not have been given food for some hours the stomach may still contain food taken before that, and gastric juice will still have been produced. Such women should be intubated in the head-up position, with controlled pressure over the cricoid. A wider use of epidural block will help to reduce mortality.

Caesarean section

In the Report for 1982–84 there were 44 deaths within 42 days of caesarean section. These cases were classified under the headings of the conditions for which the operations were performed, but from information obtained separately from the Hospital Inpatient Enquiry the number of caesarean sections can be calculated. In this triennium there was a mortality rate of 0.24 per 1000 operations. This shows that the mortality following section is about four times greater than that of vaginal delivery but, of course, the conditions calling for treatment by caesarean section may themselves be dangerous.

Further analysis shows that in the same triennium the mortality rate for emergency caesarean section was 0.37 per thousand compared with 0.09 for elective operations (a ratio of 4:1). The conditions under which emergency surgery is performed carry greater risks and a shift from emergency to elective operations could reduce some of the maternal mortality from caesarean sections.

Deaths from associated and intercurrent conditions

There has been a fall in the number of deaths from cardiac disease in each triennial Report. That for 1952–4 included 121 deaths, whereas the Report for 1982–84 included only 17, 11 acquired and 6 from congenital heart disease.

A wide variety of medical and surgical disorders and accidents caused the remaining deaths, but in most of them there was no avoidable obstetric factor.

STILLBIRTHS AND NEONATAL DEATHS: PERINATAL MORTALITY

Stillbirths and neonatal deaths are notifiable in Britain, and for statistical accuracy it is essential to use correct definitions.

Stillbirth

The term *stillbirth* refers to any child delivered after the 28th week of pregnancy that does not afterwards breathe or show any sign of life. If the heart is beating after delivery, although there is no sign of respiration, the death should not be recorded as a stillbirth but as a neonatal death. A child born dead before 28 weeks gestation should not be recorded as a stillbirth, in spite of the fact that many other babies born before this time have survived. Many other countries of the Western world use different definitions involving 24 or even 22 weeks of gestation or, more precisely, a birth weight above 500 g. It is probable that in the United Kingdom a change will come soon, probably using 24 weeks as the new cut-off point.

The stillbirth rate is defined as the number of stillbirths per 1000 total births.

Neonatal death

The neonatal period is defined as the first 28 days of life, and the *neonatal death* rate as the number of infants dying in that period per 1000 *live* births. *Early neonate death* occurs in the first week of life.

Infant mortality rate

This is defined as the number of infants dying in the first year of life per 1000 *live* births. The neonatal period is included.

Perinatal mortality rate

As a measure of obstetric success or failure another rate is often preferred to any of the foregoing. The *perinatal mortality rate* is defined as the number of stillbirths (born dead after 28 weeks) together with the number of neonatal deaths in the first week of life per 1000 total births. This is a more useful index for obstetric purposes because deaths in the first week are often related to factors occurring during pregnancy or delivery, whereas deaths in the rest of the neonatal period are more often due to paediatric causes.

In the last thirty years the stillbirth rate has fallen from about 19 to about 5 per 1000 total births; the neonatal death rate from 20 to 4; the infant mortality rate from about 34 to about 10 per 1000 live births and the perinatal mortality rate from about 39 to about 9 per 1000 total births (Fig. 11.4).

CAUSES OF PERINATAL DEATH

In determining the cause of stillbirth or neonatal death the clinical events and the postmortem findings must both be considered. In about 25 per cent of stillbirths the fetus is macerated and, because of autolysis of the tissues, the autopsy gives incomplete information about the cause of death. In many cases the final cause of death is asphyxia, but post-mortem examination may not

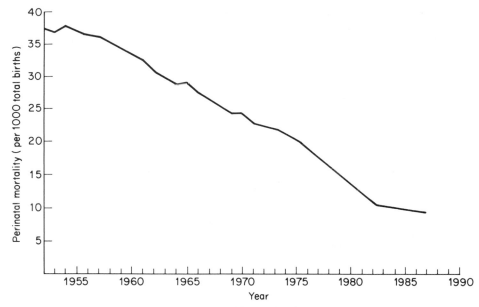

Fig. 11.4   Perinatal mortality per 1000 total births for the years 1952–1987 (England and Wales)

be able to distinguish between the various obstetric causes of this, such as placental insufficiency, antepartum haemorrhage, long labour or cord compression. Asphyxia is a mode of death rather than a cause of death, and the obstetric history may be the only clue to the basic cause. The post-mortem examination may reveal unsuspected congenital abnormalities and intracranial lesions.

The chief cause of death varies according to the times of death.

Antepartum fetal death

This is usually due to asphyxia from placental bed insufficiency or placental separation, a cord accident, haemolytic disease or maternal diabetes.

Intrapartum death

In intrapartum death asphyxia is again the usual final event, and may result from interference with placental bed blood flow during uterine contractions, but any preceding cause of placental bed insufficiency will increase the risk. In addition intracranial haemorrhage or other injuries may occur during labour. A few severe congenital abnormalities are incompatible with survival during delivery, but in many such cases recorded as

Table 11.2   Primary necropsy finding. Percentage indices in 395 perinatal deaths

Intrauterine asphyxia (stillborn)	26.3
Congenital abnormalities	21.5
Stillbirth with no anatomical lesion	14.9
Resorption atelectasis (with and without respiratory distress syndrome)	13.7
First week deaths with intrauterine asphyxia	7.6
Immaturity	6.8
Incompatible blood group	2.8
Intracranial birth trauma	1.8
Other	4.6
	100

stillbirths the fetal heart is beating at delivery, and they should be recorded as neonatal deaths.

Table 11.2 shows the necropsy findings in cases studied during the British Births survey of 1970.

Neonatal death

Neonatal death may occur as a sequel to complications of pregnancy or labour. Asphyxia or cerebral haemorrhage before or during birth may leave such metabolic or physical injury that the infant dies soon after delivery. In addition respiratory distress may occur after delivery from hyaline membrane formation, pulmonary haemorrhage, pneumonia or other intrathoracic lesions. Severe malformations may also cause early neonatal death.

Fetal maturity at delivery

Whatever the cause of fetal hazard, the maturity of the fetus has a great effect on the outcome. About 50 per cent of all infants who suffer perinatal death weigh less than 2500 g at birth, and about half of these babies are delivered before the 38th week.

The old fashioned definition of prematurity was a baby weighing less than 2500 g at birth. This definition had the great advantage of simplicity: the weight was usually accurate, but it included two groups of babies. First were those delivered after preterm labour but who were of appropriate birth weight for their gestation; for example, a baby born at the 34th week would be expected to weigh about 2000 g. Secondly there were those who were born underweight for their period of gestation; for example a baby born weighing 2000 g after a proven gestation of 39 weeks would be light-for-dates. The first group are born early because of premature myometrial action or early rupture of the membranes. The second group have suffered from intrauterine malnutrition, from placental bed insufficiency and have a higher risk of hypoxia during labour; they have a higher mortality and morbidity rate than the first group.

The aetiology of low birth weight is partly related to the mother's background, including her genetic disposition, nutrition in early childhood, past disease and social upbringing, but also to placental function. The chief causes of death in immature babies are hyaline membrane disease, atelectasis and intraventricular haemorrhage.

Another group of preterm babies must be considered. Induction of labour is not infrequently necessary to remove the fetus from a hostile intrauterine environment. In such conditions as hypertension and diabetes the obstetrician may judge that life outside the uterus may be safer than inside, and this is an iatrogenic cause of immaturity.

Environmental and social background of the mother

The perinatal death rate has been used as a measure of the quality of obstetric services, but it also

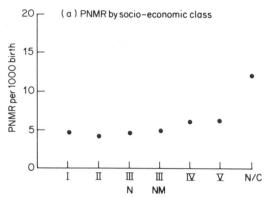

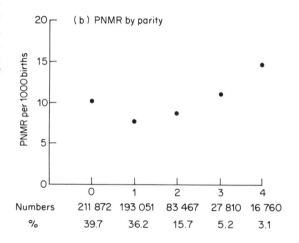

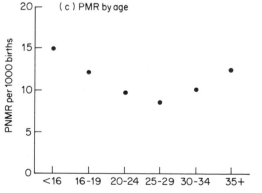

Fig. 11.5 Effects of age, parity and social class on perinatal mortality (England and Wales, 1985)

assays the total health of women in a country. Three major factors affect a woman's performance in pregnancy: her age, her parity and her social class (Fig. 11.5).

The first two factors often go together, but girls under 20 and women above the age of 35 have the highest risk at any parity. The first baby and those born fourth or later in the family have a higher perinatal mortality rate than do the second or third babies in any particular age group. The social class of a married woman is adjudged from her husband's occupation as classified in an index of occupations prepared by the Registrar General. The husband's occupation is considered because there is greater differentiation in male than in female occupations, some 80 per cent of women being either housewives or engaged in clerical work. This classification reflects the socio-economic background of married women, but leaves about 20 per cent of women unclassified because they are unmarried, and these women cluster at the worst end of the spectrum of perinatal mortality. In consequence, in many studies, if a woman is unmarried but living in stable union her partner's occupation is taken as an index of the couple's socio-economic class. The classification reflects the mother's past nutrition and health, and her education and attitudes. Perinatal mortality is lowest in Social Class I (the professional group) and highest in Social Class V (unskilled) and the unmarried.

Social class is related to other factors; for example maternal height derived from genetic inheritance and nutrition during childhood. The composition of the population varies from the South East to the North West of Britain, the proportion of Social Classes IV and V rising towards the north. The perinatal mortality in different regions of Britain is affected by this, but multifactorial analysis shows that geographical differences are not just the result of social class, but also reflect such factors as the use the women make of the obstetric facilities available.

To summarize, the perinatal mortality will usually be lowest in mothers aged between 20 and 30, of Social Class I or II, whose height is over 165 cm, having their second or third babies. The results will be worst in small women over 35, of Social Class IV or V, having a fourth or subsequent baby.

It follows, therefore, that the following groups of women should be booked for antenatal care and delivery in well-equipped consultant obstetric units:

women with obstetric abnormalities, or a history of past abnormalities which are likely to recur
mothers under 20 or over 30 years of age
women having their first, or their fourth or subsequent babies
women under 160 cm (63 inches) in height
women of social Class IV or V and women who are unsupported.

International differences

Politicians and administrators often make much of the differences in international levels of perinatal mortality rates. Ignoring the different definitions used, the obstetrician will recognize the great variation in the populations of various countries, the variety of reproductive patterns and the socio-economic differences. Figure 11.6 shows the perinatal death rates for a group of countries since 1945. All the reported rates are decreasing at much the same rate with some narrowing of the differences in forty years. However, those countries that start with a higher rate (e.g. Scotland) still rank high in 1980 while the lower groups in 1945 (e.g. Norway and Sweden) are still low. All have good services but the populations of some are more deprived than others.

It is probable that the international differences in perinatal mortality can be explained in part by differences in birthweight distribution. In Sweden, which has a low perinatal mortality rate, only 4 per cent of babies born weigh less than 2500 g; in

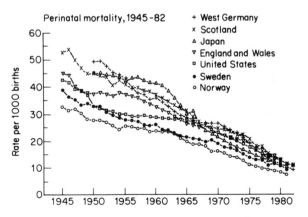

Fig. 11.6   The comparison of perinatal mortality rates in certain countries per 1000 total births since 1945

England and Wales the proportion is 7 per cent. Japan is a country where the proportion of babies of low birthweight has fallen in the last 20 years, and with this fall there has been a sharp improvement in perinatal mortality.

THE REDUCTION OF PERINATAL MORTALITY

The three major causes of perinatal mortality are congenital abnormality, low birthweight and hypoxia, and these account for about 75 per cent of all perinatal deaths. The remaining causes include birth injuries, haemolytic disease and infection. Deaths from all these causes are being reduced as obstetric care and skill improve, but to an uneven degree.

Congenital abnormalities

The incidence of congenital abnormalities varies from one population to another, implying that there are genetic or environmental causative factors which need to be identified, and may need to be treated by measures wider than those of conventional therapy. For example, in a recent year in England and Wales 1.88 babies per 1000 live births died from congenital malformations, while during the same year in Sweden the figure was only 1.47 per 1000. The difference may seem small, but the higher rate represents 200 more deaths in England and Wales each year.

At present the management of congenital abnormalities involves their detection early enough in pregnancy to allow termination of the pregnancy. The abnormal fetus is removed from the perinatal mortality figures, but of course this does not treat the basic problem. The two abnormalities most easily detected are Down's syndrome and defects of the neural tube.

Some reduction in perinatal mortality from congenital defects may be achieved by providing protection against known teratogens, for example by rubella vaccination before pregnancy and the avoidance of harmful radiation and certain drugs during pregnancy.

Perinatal mortality may also be reduced by dealing promptly with those lesions which can be relieved by neonatal surgery, such as occlusion of the intestinal tract or certain cardiovascular abnormalities (*see* p. 327).

Low birthweight

As stated above, this heading includes two groups of babies; those expelled from the uterus too early but of correct size for gestational age, and those light-for-dates babies below the 10th centile for their maturity.

In the first group mortality might be reduced by identifying those who are at higher risk for preterm labour, for example women who have had vaginal termination or preterm labour in a previous pregnancy. Cervical incompetence may be treated by an encircling stitch. If uterine contractions occur they may be checked with a β-mimetic drug. If labour is imminent or actually proceeding the woman should be taken to a hospital with a special care unit for the newborn. This may mean moving her by ambulance in early labour. The fetal lung surfactant system may be made more mature by giving the mother steroids.

The second group of babies are protected by careful monitoring of fetal growth. This is done by clinical examination, but more precisely by repeated ultrasound estimations of the fetal abdominal circumference and other fetal dimensions. Rest in bed may improve uterine blood flow, but if fetal growth is not progressing adequately the fetus is best removed from the adverse uterine environment by induction of labour or caesarean section.

Both groups of infants benefit enormously if they are delivered in a fully equipped hospital, with expert obstetric and paediatric staff. The fetus is then monitored carefully during labour, resuscitation is immediate and skilful, and the newborn infant is looked after in a special care unit with experienced paediatric staff.

Hypoxia

This is still one of the major causes of perinatal mortality. Death can occur before labour from placental failure, or during labour if the uterine contractions are so prolonged or frequent that they progressively overcome the natural resistance of the fetus to stress. The fetus that has already suffered from relative placental insufficiency during pregnancy is at special risk if hypoxia is added during labour. Reduction of perinatal mortality will result from identification of fetuses at high risk by recognizing impaired fetal growth during pregnancy, with the aid of placental bed function tests. Any fetus thought to be at high risk requires special care during labour, with continuous monitoring of the fetal heart rate and intermittent checks of the pH of scalp blood. Again, proper care can only be given in adequately equipped hospitals with experienced obstetric staff, and also facilities for neonatal resuscitation.

Such care will not only reduce perinatal mortality but also diminish perinatal morbidity. It is hard to measure morbidity in economic terms, but the cost to the family and to the community of caring for a handicapped child is enormous, and the emotional distress to the parents is beyond computation.

Index

NOTE

Page numbers in *italics* refer to pages on which figs/tables appear.

Abbreviations used in subentries:

DIC Disseminated intravascular coagulation
LOA Left occipitoanterior position
LOT Left occipitotransverse position
PPH Postpartum haemorrhage
ROP Right occipitoposterior position

Bronchiectasis during
    pregnancy   110
Bronchitis during pregnancy   110
Bronchoconstriction   318
Bronchopulmonary dysplasia   318
Brown adipose tissue   241, 299
Brow presentation   23, 157, 188–
    190, *189*
    caesarean section indication   289
    management   190

Caesarean hysterectomy   292–293
Caesarean section   287–293, 335
    abnormal uterine action   289
    in abruptio placentae   79, 289
    anaesthesia for   175, 290–292
    breech delivery   195, 289, 335
    in cephalopelvic disproportion,
        indications   207, 288–289
    in cord presentation and
        prolapse   215, 290
    dangers to fetus and
        mother   293, 343–344
    emergency   215, 290
    fetal malpresentations
        indicating   289
    history of   288
    indications   207, 224, 288–290
    low birthweight babies   213
    lower segment   *291*, 292
        anaesthesia   175, 290–292
        scars   221, 222
    maternal mortality   293, 343–
        344
    medico-legal considerations   335
    in placenta praevia   82, 83
    postoperative care   293
    in prolonged labour   *180*, 181–
        182
    repeated   290
    respiratory distress syndrome
        and   316
    scars, rupture of   221, 222, 224,
        290, 293
    shoulder impaction   200
    sterilization with   292
    technique   290, 292
    twin delivery   141, 289
    upper segment ('classical'),
        in placenta praevia   83
        scar rupture   221, 222, 290
        technique   290, 292
Calcium   10
    maternal and fetal
        requirements   30, 43
Calcium gluconate   308
Calorie requirements

in anuria   80
of newborn infants   245
in pregnancy   29, 43
Candida albicans infections   46,
    324
Caput succedaneum   156, *183*, 184,
    301–*302*
    causes, oedema   156, 301–*302*
    in obstructed labour   *210*, 211
Carbohydrates in pregnancy   43,
    110–113
    see also Diabetes mellitus
Carbon dioxide, partial pressure in
    pregnancy   31
Cardiac abnormalities, fetal,
    ultrasound detection   58
Cardiac arrhythmias, in
    pregnancy   107
Cardiac failure, in pregnancy   107,
    109
Cardiac massage, newborn
    infant   297
Cardiac output
    fetal   16
    in pregnancy   30, 106
Cardiac surgery, in
    pregnancy   108–109
Cardiomyopathy of
    pregnancy   107
Cardiotocograph   90, 131
Cardiovascular causes of
    cyanosis   297–298
Cardiovascular changes during
    pregnancy   30, 106–107
Cardiovascular drugs, effect on
    fetus   47
Carneous mole   143, 144, 146
Carob bean   329
Carpal tunnel, oedema in   46, 87
Casein   252
Catheterization of bladder   164,
    236, 280
    infections   259
Caudal block   174
Cellulitis
    breast   261
    pelvic   257, 258, 259
Central nervous system,
    abnormalities,
    ultrasound   *58*
Cephalhaematoma   *302*
Cephalic presentation   49, 157
    preterm labour
        management   213
    see also Delivery
Cephalopelvic disproportion   205–
    209

caesarean section
    indication   207, 288–289
    diagnosis   205–206
        during labour   206
        radiological   206–*207*
    exclusion by palpation   52
    management   207–209
    prolonged labour due to   180–
        181, 277
Cephalosporins   325
Cephradine   145
Cerebral haemorrhage   303
    maternal   93
Cerebral lesions, pregnancy-
        induced hypertension/
        eclampsia   93
Cerebral palsy   301, 303, 335
Cerebral thrombophlebitis   120
Cervical ectropion   27
Cervical pregnancy   149
Cervical smear   41, 67, 238
Cervicogram (cervimetric
        graph)   179, *180*
Cervix
    adenomatous polypi   149
    amputated   64
    assessment, Bishop score   *53*,
        276
    carcinoma   67, 122
        caesarean hysterectomy   293
    changes during pregnancy   27,
        34
    dilatation   152, *154*, 155, 179
        active and latent phases   164,
            179, *180*
        assessment   *53*
        failure to progress in
            obstructed labour   210
        for forceps delivery   280
        in prolonged labour   *180*
    erosion   149, 238
    fibromyomata   65
    incompetence   27, 146, 152, 213
    intraepithelial neoplasia
        (CIN)   67
    lacerations   221, *225*, 225, 232
        abortions due to   143
        extensive, rupture of
            uterus   223
        forceps delivery   286
        repair of   *225*
    retroverted uterus   63
    ripening, prostaglandins in   276
    shortening (taking up)   27, *154*
    softening and blue
        discoloration   27, 34
    stenosis   289